ACUTE CORONARY SYNDROMES

Edited by **Mariano E. Brizzio**

Acute Coronary Syndromes
Edited by Mariano E. Brizzio

Published by InTech
Janeza Trdine 9, 51000 Rijeka, Croatia

Publishing Process Manager Molly Kaliman

Technical Editor Teodora Smiljanic

Cover Designer InTech Design Team

Additional hard copies can be obtained from orders@intechopen.com

Acute Coronary Syndromes, Edited by Mariano E. Brizzio
p. cm.
978-953-307-827-4

For EU product safety concerns:
IN TECH d.o.o., Prolaz Marije Krucifikse Kozulić 3, 51000 Rijeka, Croatia,
info@intechopen.com or visit our website at intechopen.com.

Meet the editor

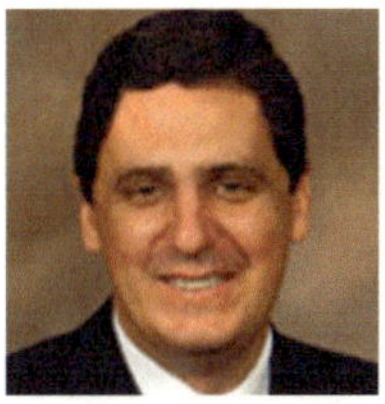

Mariano E. Brizzio, MD PhD is a Faculty member at Columbia University's College of Physicians & Surgeons. Born in Buenos Aires, Argentina, Dr Brizzio received his medical degree from the University Of Buenos Aires School Of Medicine in 1989. He completed extensive training in general and cardiovascular surgery in various medical institutions in Buenos Aires, including residencies in general surgery at the Hospital Churruca-Visca and in cardiovascular surgery at the Instituto Sacre Coeur in 1993 and 1995 respectively, followed by a research fellowship in cardiovascular surgery and the subsequent completion of his PhD degree in 1996. In 2003 he moved to the United States where he completed his fellowship in advance cardiothoracic surgery at the renowned Cleveland Clinic. This was followed three years later whenhe joined Columbia University in New York to continue his clinical and research career in cardiovascular surgery. Dr Brizzio has participated in clinical research in the developing of an artificial heart, minimally invasive cardiothoracic surgery, coronary artery disease and blood conservation techniques.

Contents

Preface

This book has been written with the intention of providing an up-to-the minute review of acute coronary syndromes. Atherosclerotic coronary disease is still a leading cause of death within developed countries and not surprisingly, is significantly rising in others. Over the past decade the treatment of these syndromes has changed dramatically. The introduction of novel therapies has impacted the outcomes and surviving rates in such a way that the medical community need to be up to date almost on a "daily bases".

It is hoped that this book will provide a timely update on acute coronary syndromes and prove to be an invaluable resource for practitioners seeking new and innovative ways to deliver the best possible care to their patients.

Mariano E. Brizzio, MD
Editor in Chief
The Valley Heart and Vascular Institute, Ridgewood, New Jersey
USA

1

Antiplatelet Therapy in Cardiovascular Disease – Past, Present and Future

Mariano E. Brizzio
The Valley Heart and Vascular Institute, Ridgewood, New Jersey
USA

1. Introduction

Platelet activity has a very important role in the pathogenesis of atherosclerosis disease. In addition to being part of the coagulation system, they contribute to all phases of the atherosclerosis process (1) The "intervention" in the platelet activity has been played a central role in the treatment of coronary artery disease (CAD) (2).
Aspirin is considered the foundation antiplatelet therapy for patients at risk of cardiovascular events. However, in the last few decades many different agents were introduced to have a more effective antiplatelet action and improve treatment outcomes in coronary syndromes.
In this chapter you will find a systematic review of all the antiplatelet agents available: mechanism of action, pharmacokinetics, side effects, evidence of effectiveness and their use in clinical settings. A special emphasizes will point out agents that are in investigational stage and what are the future perspectives.

1.1 Platelet mechanisms of action

Platelets play a critical role in the normal coagulation system by "preventing" bleeding after blood vessels are damaged. In addition they contribute to different phases of the atherosclerotic process (1). Rupture of a previously formed atherosclerotic plaque exposes collagen, smooth-muscle cells and von Willebrand factor (vWF) all of which trigger platelet activation and massive aggregation (3). The result of this accumulation of platelets is thrombosis. Acute coronary syndrome (ACS) is a consequence of the occlusion of an atherosclerotic vessel by the thrombotic process. As described before, collagen and vWF in addition to thromboxane A2 (TXa2), thrombin and adenosine diphosphate (ADP) are the most powerful platelet activators (4). When a platelet is activated a conformational change occurs in a receptor located in the platelet membrane called glycoprotein IIb/IIIa which promotes platelet aggregation (5).
Antiplatelet agents that target critical steps of the thrombotic mechanism described above have been developed in the last three decades. However, treatment with these agents can sometimes increase the risk of "undesirable" bleeding complications (6).

2. The traditional anti-platelet agents

Many anti-platelet agents have been tested and used as an effective treatment in arterial thrombosis. Acetyl salicylic acid, commonly known as **aspirin** was the first anti-platelet agent used and proven to be effective to reduce the incidence of myocardial infarction and stroke in many high risk vascular patients (2).The recurrence of vascular events in patients treated with aspirin alone ranges between 10 – 20% within five years of the initial event (2-7).

Aspirin is effective by blocking the synthesis of TXa2, a powerful platelet activator.

In the last decade, the thienopyridines such as **clopidogrel** have been used to improve outcomes in the treatment of ACS. This anti-platelet agent irreversibly blocks the P2Y12 receptor, precluding the platelet activation by ADP (2). Its anti-platelet mechanism of action clearly differs from aspirin. In the majority of cardiovascular patients the combination of clopidogrel and aspirin has additive beneficial effects when compared with clopidogrel or aspirin alone (8). Clopidogrel also has some limitations, which have prompted the development of newer anti-platelet agents which interact at different sites of the coagulation cascade.

The following figure reflects the site of action of the common antiplatelet agents (figure 1)

3. The thromboxane A2 antagonist

Dipyridamole (Persantine) acts as a thromboxane synthase inhibitor, therefore lowering the levels of TXA2 and thus stops the effects of TXA2 as a platelet activator (9).

Also can causes systemic vasodilation when given at high doses over a short period of time. The latter, due to the inhibition of the cellular reuptake of adenosine into platelets, red blood cells and endothelial cells leading to increased extracellular concentrations of adenosine (9). It also inhibits the enzyme adenosine deaminase, which normally breaks down adenosine into inosine. This inhibition leads to further increased levels of extracellular adenosine, producing a strong vasodilatation (9).

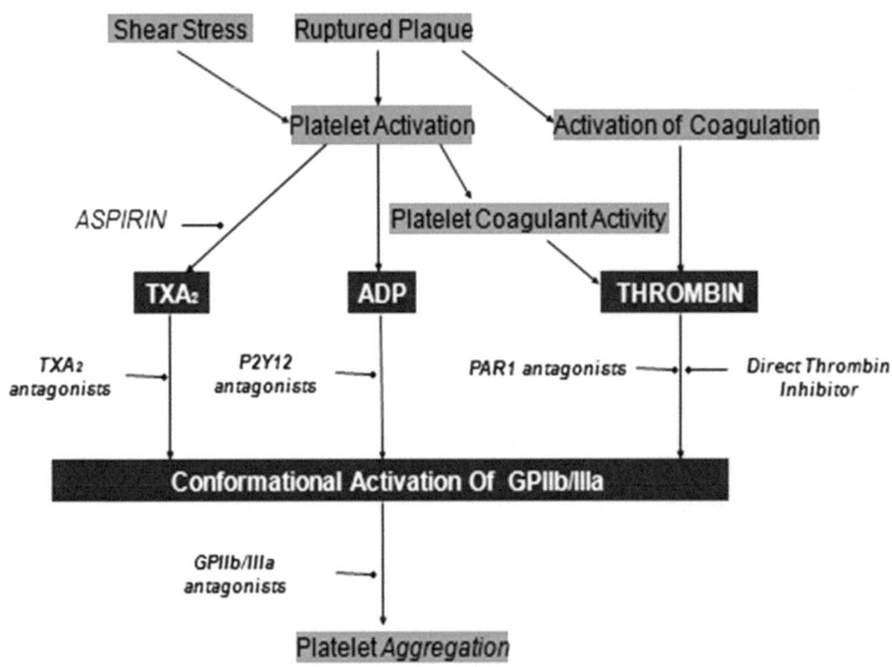

Antiplatelet agents nowadays
Inhibits the synthesis of TXa2
Aspirin
TXa2 antagonist
Dipyridamole Terutroban
P2Y 12 antagonist
Ticlopidine Clopidogrel Prasugrel Ticagrelor Cangrelor
Glycoprotein IIb/IIIa antagonist
Abciximab Tirobiban Eptifibatide
Protease-activated receptor 1 antagonist
Vorapaxar
Direct thrombin Inhibitor
Bivalirudin

Modified release dipyridamole is used in conjunction with aspirin (under the trade names Aggrenox in the USA or Asasantin Retard in the UK) in the secondary prevention of stroke and transient ischemic attack. This practice has been confirmed by the ESPRIT trial (9). A triple therapy of aspirin, clopidogrel and dipyridamole has been investigated, but this combination led to an increase in adverse bleeding events (10).

Via the mechanisms mentioned above, when given as 3 to 5 min infusion it rapidly increases the local concentration of adenosine in the coronary circulation which causes vasodilation. Vasodilation occurs in healthy arteries, whereas stenosed arteries remain narrowed. This creates a "steal" phenomenon where the coronary blood supply will increase to the dilated healthy vessels compared to the stenosed arteries which can then be detected by clinical symptoms of chest pain, electrocardiogram and echocardiography when it causes ischemia. Flow heterogeneity (a necessary precursor to ischemia) can be detected with gamma cameras and SPECT using nuclear imaging agents such as Thallium-201 and Tc99m-Sestamibi (9).

Terutroban is a selective antagonist of the thromboxane receptor. It blocks thromboxane induced platelet aggregation and vasoconstriction (11). As of 2010, it is being tested for the secondary prevention of acute thrombotic complications in the Phase III clinical trial. However, the recent publication of the finalized trial PERFORMS shown no clinical advantage in comparison with patients with aspirin monotherapy in preventing strokes (12). At the time of this publication its use in clinical practice is not approved in the USA.

4. Other P2Y 12 antagonist

Ticlopidine an anti-platelet drug in the thienopyridine family inhibits platelet aggregation by altering the function of platelet membranes by irreversibly blocking ADP receptors. This prevents the conformational change of glycoprotein IIb/IIIa which allows platelet binding to fibrinogen (13). It is used in patients in whom aspirin is not tolerated, or in whom dual anti-platelet therapy is desirable (in combination with Aspirin). Because it has been reported to increase the risk of thrombotic thrombocytopenic purpura (TTP) and neutropenia, its use has largely been supplanted by the newer drug, clopidogrel, which is felt to have a much lower hematologic risk (14).

Prasugrel, a novel thienopyryridine was approved for clinical use in the USA by the Food and Drug Administration (FDA) in 2010. Unlike clopidogrel, which undergoes a two-step, CYP450-dependent conversion to its active metabolite, prasugrel only requires single-step activation. Prasugrel is a more potent platelet inhibitor with faster action and inhibition. Also, it has been estimated that due to its "easy metabolism" its genetic resistance is less likely (15). In other words, prasugrel has a significantly lower incidence of hypo-responsiveness in comparison with clopidogrel (15). However, the risks of bleeding in these patients are greater than clopidogrel (16).

Ticagrelor is the most novel class of anti-platelet drugs, the cyclopentytriazolopyrimides, which also inhibit the P2Y12 receptor as the thienopyryridines. However, it has a simpler and faster metabolism (rapid onset of action) high potency and most importantly reversibility (17). The latter, makes this drug safer in regards of bleeding complications.

Cangrelor, an ATP analog, is an investigational intravenous anti-platelet drug. This agent has biphasic elimination and possesses the advantages of high potency, very fast onset of action and very fast reversibility after the discontinuation (16).This gives a considerable advantage over other ADP antagonist in patients who might need immediate surgery. However, after initial treatment, patients who received intravenous infusion of Cangrelor often require continued treatment with one of the oral P2Y12 antagonists, something that one must take into consideration (16).

5. Glycoproteins IIb/IIa antagonist

Abciximab, more known as the ReoPro is an antibody against glycoprotein IIb/IIIa receptor. It had a lot of popularity within interventional cardiologist 10 years ago. It is barely used today. It was replaced by newer IV agents. Abciximab has a plasma half-life of about ten minutes, with a second phase half-life of about 30 minutes. However, its effects on platelet function can be seen for up to 48 hours after the infusion has been terminated, and low levels of glycoprotein IIb/IIIa receptor blockade are present for up to 15 days after the infusion is terminated (18).

Tirobiban (Aggrastat) is a synthetic, non-peptide inhibitor acting at glycoprotein (GP) IIb/IIIa receptors. It has a rapid onset and short duration of action after proper intravenous administration. Platelet activity returns to normal 4 to 8 hours after the drug is withdrawn (19).

Eptifibatide (Integrilin) is the newer anti-platelet drug which inhibits the glycoprotein IIb/IIIa inhibitor. It belongs to the class of the so-called arginin-glycin-aspartat-mimetics and reversibly binds to platelets. Eptifibatide has a short half-life, 3 to 5 hours after the discontinuation platelet activity recovers to normal levels (20).The drug is the third inhibitor of GPIIb/IIIa that has found broad acceptance within interventional cardiologists nowadays.

6. Proteasa-activated receptors antagonist

Vorapaxar (formerly SCH 530348) is a thrombin receptor (PAR-1) antagonist based on the natural product himbacine. It is an experimental pharmaceutical treatment for acute coronary syndrome as a very powerful platelet inhibitor (21).In January 2011, the clinical trial was halted for patients with stroke and mild heart conditions due to safety reasons. It is unknown if it will continue.

7. Direct thrombin inhibitors

Bivalirudin (Angiomax) is a specific and reversible intravenous direct thrombin inhibitor. Clinical studies demonstrated consistent positive outcomes in patients with stable angina, unstable angina (UA), non-ST segment elevation myocardial infarction (NSTEMI), and ST-segment elevation myocardial infarction (STEMI) undergoing PCI in 7 major randomized trials (22). Coagulation times and platelet activity return to baseline approximately 1-6 hour following cessation of bivalirudin administration (23).

8. Conclusions

Antiplatelet therapy plays a crucial role in the treatment of coronary patients. The continuous introduction of new agents is geared to improve results in patient ongoing percutaneous coronary interventions. However, the side effects of theses should be monitored closely. In the end, the ideal management of patients with acute coronary syndrome should be to be a collaborative effort between cardiologist and surgeons to assure the best outcomes possible.

9. References

[1] Hoffman M et al.Activated factor VII activates Factor IX on the surfaces of activated platelets. Blood Coag Fibrinolyis. 1998:9; 61-65.

[2] Antithrombotic triallist's collaboration. Collaborative meta-analysis of randomized trials of antiplatelet therapy for prevention of death, myocardial infartion, and stroke in high risk patients. BMJ 2002;324:71-86

[3] Heemskerk JW. Funtion of glycoprotein VI and intgrelin in the procoagulant response of single, collagen-adherent platelets. Throm Hemost 1999;81:782-792

[4] Jin, J, Kunapuli, SP. Coactivation of two different G protein-coupled receptors is essential for ADP-induced platelet aggregation. Proc Natl Acad Sci USA 1998;95:8070-74

[5] Heechler B, et al. The P2Y1 receptor in necessary for adenosine 5'-diphodphate-induced platelet aggregation. Blood 1998;92:152-159

[6] Brizzio, ME, Shaw, RE, Bosticco B, et al. Use of an Objective Tool to Assess Platelet Inhibition Prior to Off-Pump Coronary Surgery to Reduce Blood Usage and Cost. Journ Interv Cardiol. 2011 In press

[7] de Werf F et al. Dual antiplatelet therapy in high-risk patients. Euro Heart J . 2007:9:D3-D9 MC,

[8] Metha SR, Peters RJG, Bertrand ME, et al., for the Clopidrogel in Unstable angina to prevent Recurrent events (CURE) Trial Investigators. Effects of pretreatment with clopidogrel and aspirin followed by long-term therapy in patients undergoing percutaneous coronary intervention: the PCI-Cure study. Lancet 2001;358:527-33.

[9] Halkes PH, van Gijn J, Kappelle LJ, Koudstaal PJ, Algra A (May 2006). "Aspirin plus dipyridamole versus aspirin alone after cerebral ischaemia of arterial origin (ESPRIT): randomised controlled trial". Lancet.2006; 367: 1665–73.

[10] Sprigg N, Gray LJ, England T, et al. (2008). Berger, Jeffrey S.. ed. "A randomised controlled trial of triple antiplatelet therapy (aspirin, clopidogrel and

dipyridamole) in the secondary prevention of stroke: safety, tolerability and feasibility". PLoS One. 2008 Aug 6;3(8):e2852

[11] Sorbera LA, Serradel N, Bolos J, Bayes M. Terutroban sodium.Drugs of the Future 2006;31 (10):867-873.

[12] Hennerici, M. G.; Bots, M. L.; Ford, I.; Laurent, S.; Touboul, P. J. "Rationale, design and population baseline characteristics of the PERFORM Vascular Project: an ancillary study of the Prevention of cerebrovascular and cardiovascular Events of ischemic origin with teRutroban in patients with a history oF ischemic strOke or tRansient ischeMic attack (PERFORM) trial". Cardiovascular Drugs and Therapy 2010; 24 (2): 175.

[13] Berger PB. Results of the Ticlid or Plavix Post-Stents (TOPPS) trial: do they justify the switch from ticlopidine to clopidogrel after coronary stent placement? Curr Control Trials Cardiovasc Med. 2000; 1(2): 83–87.

[14] Bennet CL, Davidson CJ, Raisch DW, et al. Thrombotic Thombocytopenic purpura with ticlopidine in the setting of coronary artery stents and stroke prevention. Arch Intern Med. 1999;159:2524-2528.

[15] Wiviott S et al. Prasugrel versus clopidogrel in patient with acute coronary syndromes. N Engl J Med 2008;357:2001-2015

[16] Raju NC, Eikelboom, Hirsh J. Platelet ADP-receptor antagonist for cardiovascular disease:past, present and future. Nature Cini Pract 2008;5(12):766-779

[17] Wallentin, Lars; Becker, RC; Budaj, A; Cannon, CP; Emanuelsson, H; Held, C; Horrow, J; Husted, S et al. Ticagrelor versus Clopidogrel in Patients with Acute Coronary Syndromes". N Engl J Med 2009;361 (11): 1045–57.

[18] Tcheng, JE; Kandzari, DE; Grines, CL; Cox, DA; Effron, MB; Garcia, E; Griffin, JJ; Guagliumi, G et al. "Benefits and risks of abciximab use in primary angioplasty for acute myocardial infarction: the Controlled Abciximab and Device Investigation to Lower Late Angioplasty Complications (CADILLAC) trial." Circulation 2003;108 (11): 1316–23

[19] Shanmugam G. Tirofiban and emergency coronary surgery. Eur J Cardiothorac Surg 2005;28:546-550

[20] Mann H, London AJ, MannJ. Equipoise in the Enhanced Supression of the Platelet IIb/IIIa Receptor with Integrilin Trial (ESPRIT): a critical appraisal. Clin Trials June 2005 vol. 2 no. 3 233-243

[21] Chackalamannil S . "Discovery of a Novel, Orally Active Himbacine-Based Thrombin Receptor Antagonist (SCH 530348) with Potent Antiplatelet Activity". J of Medic Chemis 2008 51 (11):3061-04

[22] Kushner FG, Hand M, Smith SC Jr, et al. 2009 Focused Updates: ACC/AHA Guidelines for the Management of Patients With ST-Elevation Myocardial Infarction (Updating the 2004 Guideline and 2007 Focused Update) and ACC/AHA/SCAI Guidelines on Percutaneous Coronary Intervention (Updating the 2005 Guideline and 2007 Focused Update): a Report of the American College of Cardiology Foundation/American Heart Association Task Force on Practice Guidelines. J Am Coll Cardiol. 2009 Nov 18.

[23] Stone GW, McLaurin BT, Cox DA, et al.; for the ACUITY Investigators. Bivalirudin for patients with acute coronary syndromes. N Engl J Med. 2006;355:2203-2216.

2

Thrombotic Inception at Nano-Scale

Suryyani Deb and Anjan Kumar Dasgupta
Department of Biochemistry, University of Calcutta
India

1. Introduction

Seeing is believing, but the reverse, namely, disbelieving the unseen may often go against the spirit of scientific exploration. This is particularly true for nano-scale objects interacting almost invisibly with biological cells, tissues or organs. Interestingly many of the biological sub-cellular components (e.g. proteins, DNA)have nano-scale dimension. The apparently innocent (chemically inactive) and tiny particulate matter originating from various natural or artificial sources (e.g., pollutant) have been shown to be toxic at different physiological levels. The famous saying by Jeevaka, the legendary physician of the Jataka tales, that there is no herb in the world that is not a drug, however follows. What is toxic in some context have important therapeutic value elsewhere. Nanoparticles do interfere with the thrombo-static equilibrium. While this shift on one hand is a matter of concern, it may provide us a tool to handle or diagnose diseases in which such equilibrium is shifted. One of the finest models to test this dual aspect of the nano-scale objects is Acute Coronary Syndrome (ACS), a leading cause of death in the global scenario. What is known today regarding the effect of nanoscale objects may really be a tip of iceberg and with the advent of smarter nanoparticles one may think of more versatile use of nanotechnology in the management of ACS.

2. Role of platelets in Acute Coronary Syndrome (ACS)

ACS is a complex and multi-factorial disease (Badran et al., 2009). ACS is an umbrella like term which includes mainly three diseases i). **ST elevated myocardial infarction (STEMI)**, ii). **Non ST elevated myocardial infarction (NON STEMI),** and iii) **unstable angina**. The patho-physiological event of ACS can be divided into four phases:

a. Atherosclerotic plaque formation.
b. Rupture of an unstable plaque.
c. The acute ischemic event.
d. Long term risk of recurrent coronary event.

2.1 Platelet basic physiology

Platelets play a pivotal in manifestation of ACS. Platelets are discoid in shape, with approximate number density 150,000-300,000/µl, and dimension of the order of 2000-4000 nm. Derived from megakaryocyte (figure 1) (Thompson, 1986) they contain mitochondria, peroxisomes, endoplasmic reticulum. They also contain granules and glycogen bodies.

Granules occur as i) **dense granules (δ)**, ii) **alpha granules (α)**. Dense granules mainly contains ATP, ADP, serotonin etc., whereas alpha granules contain fibronectin, fibrinogen, platelet activation factor (PAF) etc. (Marcus et al, 1966; Flaumenhaft et al, 2005). Ca^{++}, one of the most important factors for platelet action, is stored in endoplasmic reticulum and released into the cytoplasm, during platelet activation (Nesbitt et al, 2003). Open canalicular system (OCS) is a channel like protrusion inside the platelet where granules release their contents (Escolar & White, 1991). Recently role of mRNA and mi-RNA has been shown to play important roles in platelet aggregation (Calverley et al, 2010; Rowley et al, 2011; Nagalla et al, 2011).

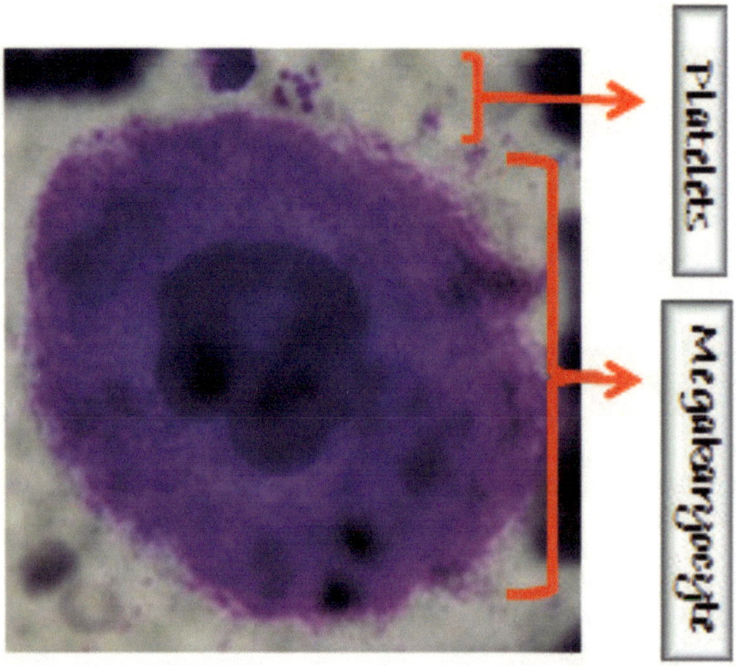

Fig. 1. Precursor megakaryocyte and progenitor platelets: Represents microscopic image (20X) of a megakaryocyte in the bone marrow. Platelets generated from the megakaryocyte can be seen in 12 o'clock position of the megakaryocyte.

When exposed to agonists, platelets become activated and this is followed by an aggregatory response (Patscheke, 1979). In systemic blood flow platelets remain in resting phase, without being activated (Marcus et al, 1991). Physiological agonists like collagen, thrombin, ADP, ATP etc. are not associated with the normal blood flow. Even if a trace amount of ADP and ATP are present, they are broken down by the phosphatase activity of CD39 (Marcus et al, 1997). At wound site, sub endothelial layers get ruptured. Hence Von Willebrand factor (vWf) and collagen get exposed causing activation of platelets (Nyman , 1980; Tschopp et al., 1980). After the primary phase of activation and aggregation, platelet granules are released, this leads to enhancement of local concentration of agonists (e.g. granule secreted ADP, ATP, serotonin etc.). This triggers irreversible secondary phase platelet aggregation with fibrinogen, which is further followed by cessation of bleeding (Decie and Lewis 2003) (figure 2).

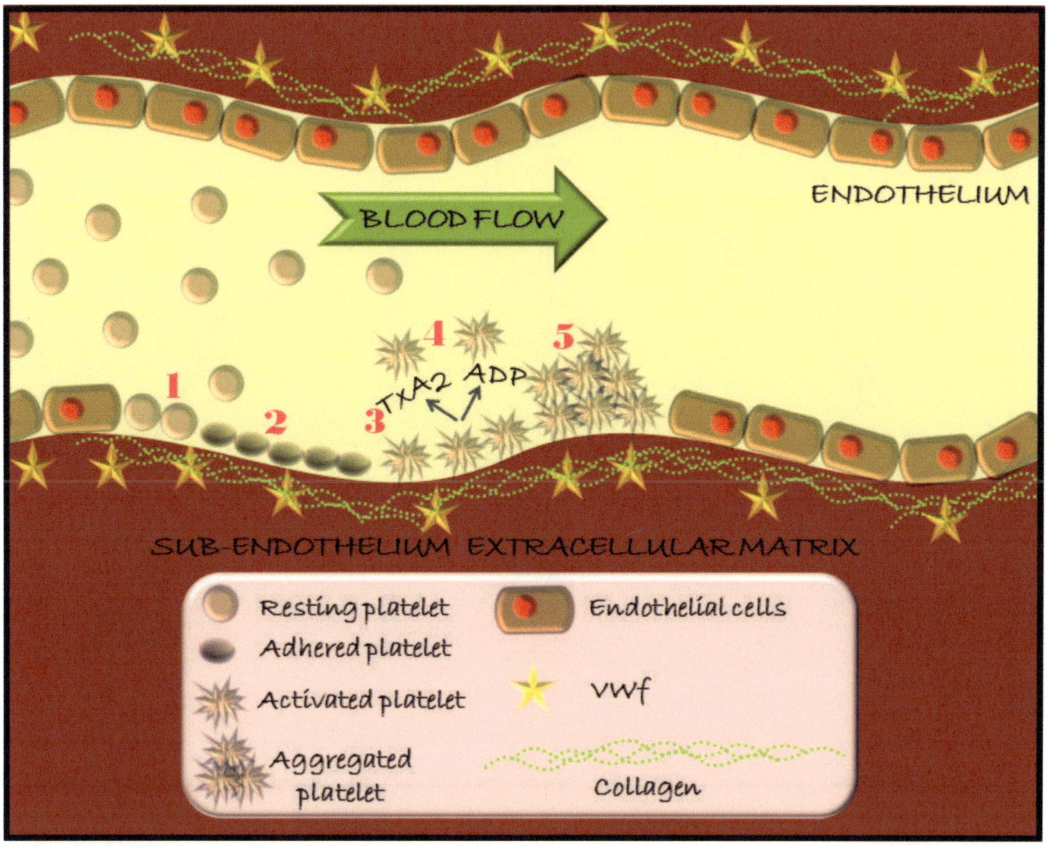

Fig. 2. Schematic diagram of platelet activation and aggregation. In the resting conditions platelets, maintain their discoid form and flow in circulation. Upon injury, platelets become exposed to sub-endothelial collagen and vWf (1) adhered on it (2). This is followed by activation and shape changes (3). The next phase is granules release and secondary phase aggregation (4) and lastly the stable platelet plaque forms(5).

The detailed mechanism of platelet function depends on the complex intracellular signalling pathways. This leads to platelet activation by simulating a series of physiological events. Briefly, after binding of agonists, the corresponding receptors trigger downstream signalling cascades and initiates Ca^{++} mobilisation from endoplasmic reticulum. Platelet granules release (α and δ), platelet shape change and the thromboxane A2 (TXA2) production then follows. The cumulative effects of these events initiate activation of fibrinogen receptor (GPIIbIIIa) and triggering of primary phase aggregation. The released granules-content (ADP, ATP etc.) along with TXA2 activate other resting platelets resulting the secondary phase aggregation (Kroll & Schafer, 1989; Ashby, 1990) (figure 3). The important signalling molecules that help the above process through a complex interplay among different G-protein coupled receptors, integrin receptors, second messengers, kinases, phosphatise and Ca^{++} mobilisation etc (Dorsam & Kunapuli, 2004; Wu e al., 2006,2010; Roberts et al.,2004; Karniguian et al., 1990; Farndale, 2006; Spalding et al., 1998; Patscheke , 1980; Clifford et al., 1998; Hoffman et. al. 2009).

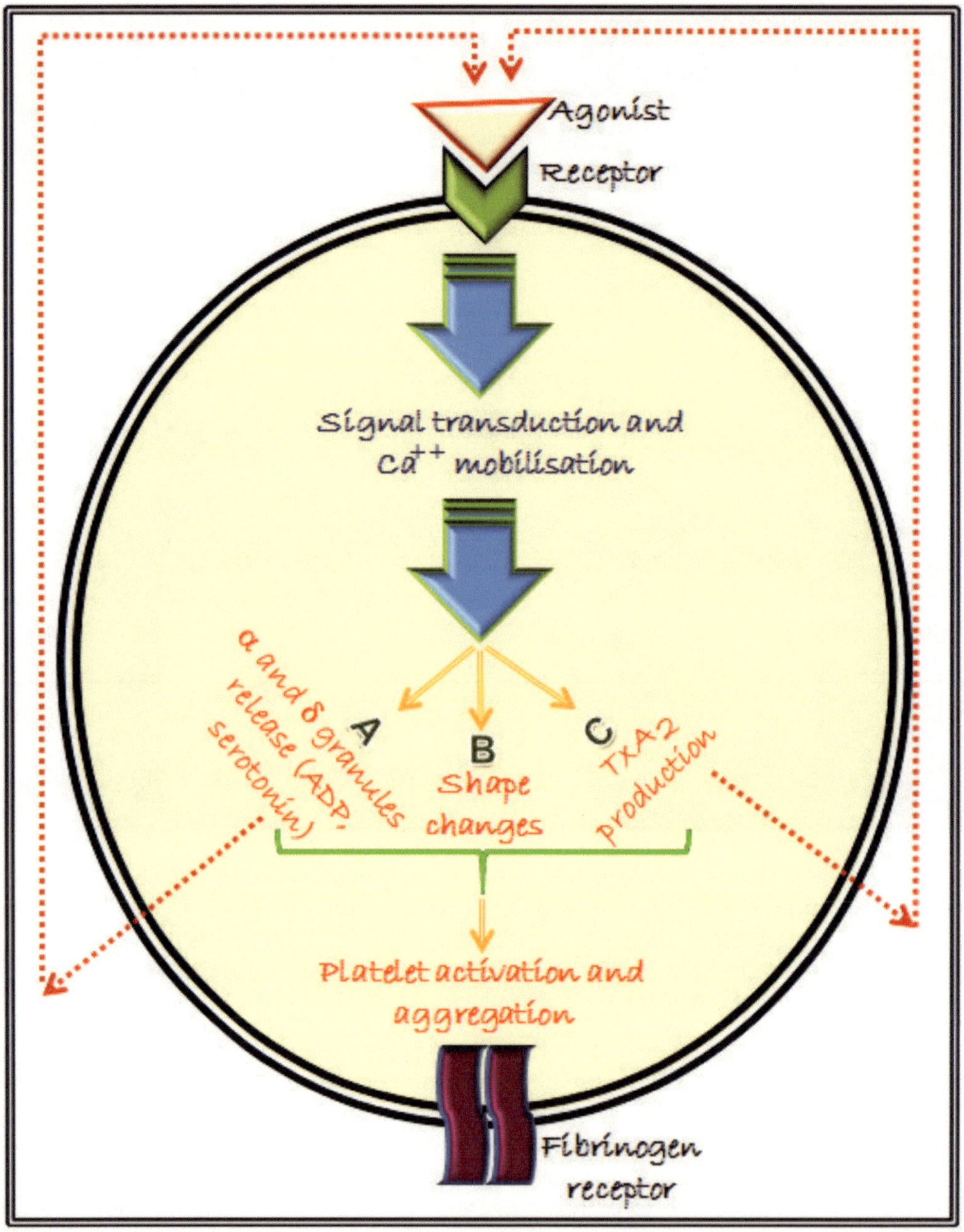

Fig. 3. Schematic diagram of agonists induced platelet activation. Binding of agonists with corresponding receptors, triggers downstream signalling cascade, and causes mobilisation of intracellular Ca^{++}. The initial Ca^{++} flux branches itself into three major signalling events: A (alpha and dense granules release), B (platelet shape change), C (TXA_2 production). The three signalling events cumulatively determine the activation and aggregation. The released chemicals (ADP,ATP etc) from granules and the TXA2, further activates other resting platelets and initiates the secondary phase of aggregation.

2.2 Platelet in ACS

It may be contextual to focus on the pathological role of platelets in ACS. Platelet thrombosis plays a central role in the pathogenesis of Acute Coronary Syndrome (ACS) by the formation of thrombi at the site of the ruptured atherosclerotic plaque (figure 4) (Massberg et al., 2003; Kottke-Marchant, 2009; Lakkis et al., 2004).

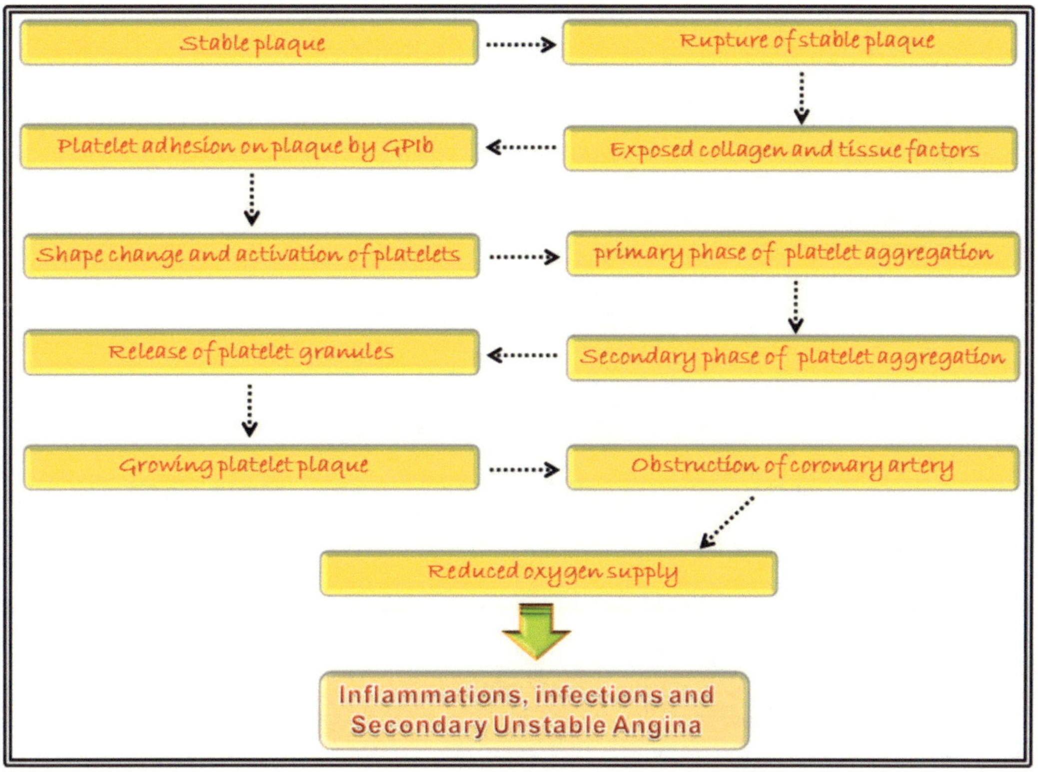

Fig. 4. Flow chart illustrating the role of platelets in thrombus formation.

Thus, the main therapeutic regime for the treatment of ACS is use of anti-platelet drug that inhibits platelet hyper aggregation (Faxon, 2011; Guha et al., 2009; Aragam & bhatt, 2011; Born & Patrono, 2006). Table 1 describes a list of such drugs, while their mode of action is illustrated in figure 5.

In the normal platelet aggregation process, downstream signalling induces fibrinogen receptor activation (GpIIbIIa). GpVI is the collagen receptor. P2X1 is the receptor of ATP and acts as Ca^{++} channel. P2Y1 is high affinity ADP repector and P2Y12 is low affinity ADP receptor, where the former one is G_q and the later one is Gi coupled. Gz coupled alpha 2a are adrenergic receptors for epinephrine, where G_s coupled PGI2R are the receptors of prostaglandin I_2 (PGI2) or prostaglandin E1 (PGE1), these being inhibitory receptors. Protease-activated receptor 1 (PAR1), protease-activated receptor 4 (PAR4), are coupled with Gq and G_{13} these being the receptors of thrombin. Thromboxane A_2 (TxA_2) receptor TP is also coupled with G_q and $G_{13.}$ Released TxA2 (b in figure 5) and ADP (a in figure5) further act on their corresponding receptors. The second messengers and other signalling mediators include, (DAG) diacylglycerol; (PLCβ) phospholipase C β; (PKC) protein kinase C; (PIP_2)

Mode of Action	Name of the drugs
Cyclo-oxygenase inhibitors (COX1), (1)	Aspirin
P2Y12 receptor inhibitors(2)	Clopidogrel, Prasugrel, Ticlopidine
Phosphodiestarase inhibitors(3)	Cilostazole
Glycoprotein GPIIbIIIa inhibitors(4)	Abciximab, Eptifibatide, Tirofiban
Adenosine uptake inhibitors(5)	Dipyridamole

Table 1. List of anti-platelet drugs – their mode of action and generic names. The most common drugs are described in the first two rows.

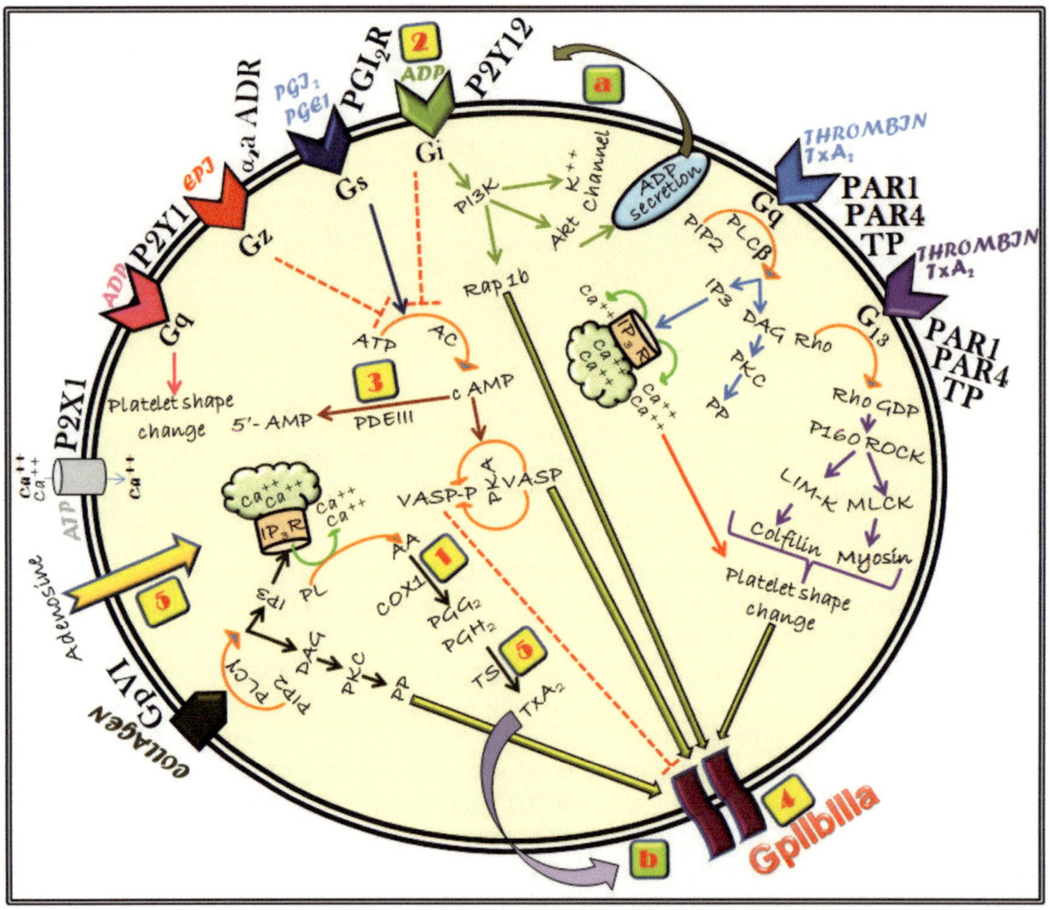

Fig. 5. Target sites for anti-platelet drugs in platelet signalling pathway- different downstream signalling pathways are shown. The drug targets described in Table 1 are represented by the corresponding numbers (see text for elaboration).

phosphotidylinositol-4,5-biphosphate; (PLC_{γ}) phospholipase C γ; (PLC_{β}) phospholipase C γ; (IP_3) inositol triphosphate; (IP_3R) inositol triphosphate receptor; (PP) protein phosphorylation; (PLA_2) Phospholipase A_2; (AA) arachidonic acid; AkT and Rap1B (which are serine /threonine kinase), (PI3K) phosphatidylinositol 3-kinase; (AC) adenylyl cyclase; (PKA) phosphokinase A; (cAMP) cyclic adenosine mono phosphate; (VASP) vasodialator stimulated phosphor protein; (P160 ROCK) a Rho activated kinase, (MLCK) myosine light chain kinase, (LIM-K) LIM kinase; (PGG2) prostaglandin G2; (PGH2) prostaglandin H2; (PL) membrane phospholipids; (COX1) cyclooxygenase 1; (TS) thromboxane synthetase and (PDEIII) phosphor di-esterase III. As platelets are the key player in ACS, any extra-physiological environmental materials that can alter platelet signalling circuit is of great challenge in combating the disease. This is the context where nanotechnology can come in picture.

3. Nano-interface

Nanotechnology has the potential to interfere with basic biological mechanisms because of their tunable electrical, magnetic and optical properties, and small size (Chen et al., 2005; Gobin et al., 2007; Fu et al., 2007). This tunability makes them potential tool in diagnostics (e.g. bio-imaging) therapy and a smart combination of both of these properties (Smith et al., 2008; Peng et al., 2000; Li et al., 2003; Murry et al., 2000).

Some of advancement of nanotechnology inspired application include improved imaging contrast agents by SPIONS (super-paramagnetic iron oxide nanoparticles), targeted delivery of drugs, molecular chaperons and agents to kill specific cancer cells (Yu et al., 2011; Petkar et al., 2011; Patra et al., 2007). Another exclusive application involve magnetic induction (radio frequency) heating or laser induced heating of designer particles, with desirable material and shape attributes (Peterman et al., 2003; Plech et al., 2004). The hyperthermic killing of tumor cells, is one of the most important examples (Rao et al., 2010; Huff et al., 2007). The recently reported chaperon properties of nanoparticles can also have important biomedical potential (Singha et al., 2010). Interestingly there are only few report on haematological (Elias & Tsourkas 2009; Baker, 2009; Walkey et al., 2009; Wickline et al., 2005) and cardiological applications (Lanza et al., 2006; Iverson et al., 2008) of nanotechnology.

4. Nanotechnology in ACS and platelet contexts

Nanotechnology is important in ACS because of several reasons. A simple application is imaging of plaques, conventional methods being grossly inadequate for such purpose (Nikolas, 2009; Wicklinea & Lanza, 2003). Secondly, the targeted delivery of therapeutic agents using nanoparticles to the areas of injured or dysfunctional vascular wall that inhibit the plaque progression is of significant importance in the ACS context (Nikolas, 2009).

Furthermore, nanoparticle based assay can be used for the detection of myocardial injury in patients with ACS (Wilson et al., 2009). In the therapeutic regime , an important use of nanotechnology is to increase the amount of HDL in circulation interning delivery of cholesterol to liver, thus minimizing the risk associated with ACS (Luthi et al., 2010).

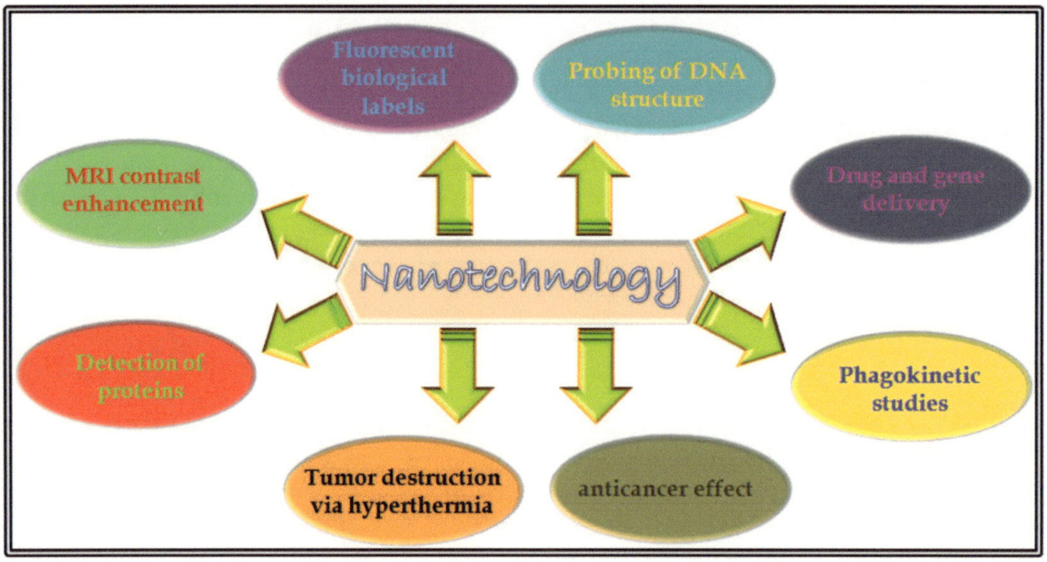

Fig. 6. Diverse applications in nanotechnology

In most of the above mentioned cases (diagnosis, drug delivery or treatment) the primary entry route of nanoparticle is through circulation where they interact directly with blood cells. Conversely exposure to unwanted nanoparticles (e.g. gas phase exhaust from car or industry) inhaled by human, that can penetrate the alveolar space and interfere with circulation may lead to cardiovascular diseases (Yamawaki & Iwai, 2006; Mohmmad et al., 2011; Chen et al., 2008). In both cases such interaction deserves a special attention.

In case of ACS patients, if nanoparticles activate platelets then they may induce life threatening alarm. Till now there are a number of papers (Geys et al., 2008; Oberdörster et al., 2007; Deb et al., 2007,2011; Wiwanitkit et al., 2009; Radomski et al., 2005; Shrivastava et al., 2009; Koziara et al., 2005; Mayer et al., 2009; Li et al., 2009; Ramtoola et al., 2010; McGuinnes et al., 2010; Nemmar et al., 2003; Gulati et al., 2010; Cejas et al., 2007; Wilson et al., 2010; Rückerl et al., 2007) about the effect of nanoparticles on platelets (Table. 2.) where most of the citations show that nanoparticles can induce platelet aggregation. What makes a nanoparticle pro-aggregarory (Geys et al., 2008; Oberdörster et al., 2007; Deb et al., 2007,2011; Wiwanitkit et al., 2009; Radomski et al., 2005; Mayer et al., 2009; McGuinnes et al., 2010; Nemmar et al., 2003; Cejas et al., 2007; Wilson et al., 2010; Rückerl et al., 2007; Miller et al., 2009), inert (Li et al., 2009; Ramtoola et al., 2010; Gulati et al., 2010) or even anti-platelet in nature (Shrivastava et al., 2009; Koziara et al., 2005; Miller et al., 2009) is of great importance in development of ACS based nano-drugs, risk assessment in ACS , and also in evaluating resistance to ACS related drugs (Guha et al., 2009; Jogns et al., 2006; Michelson et al., 2006).

TYPE OF NANOMATERIALS		EFFECT ON PLATELETS
Carbon NP	Carbon nanoparticle (C_{60})	Inert
	Standard urban particulate matter	Activation
	Multiwall carbon nanotube	Activation
	Single wall carbon nanotube	Activation
	Mixed carbon nanotube	Activation
Metallic NP	Gold nanoparticle	Activation
	Iron nanoparticle	Activation
	Cupper nanoparticle	Activation
	Cadmium sulphide nanoparticle	Activation
	Cadmium sulphide nanorod	Activation
	Quantum dots	Activation
	Silver nanoparticle	Anti-platelet effect
Polymer NP and Bio- derived NP	Short collagen related peptide	Activation
	Amidine White Polystyrine Latex NP(+ve)	Activation
	Aminated Polystyrine Latex NP (+ve)	Activation
	Carboxylated Polystyrine Latex NP (-ve)	Activation
	Unmodified Polystyrine Latex NP	Inert
	PNIPAAM	Inert
	PEG coated PNIPAAM	Inert
	poly(D,L-lactide-co-glycolide) (PLGA)	Inert
	Chitosan nanoparticles	Inert
	Human and Bovine derived NP	Anti-platelet effect
	Hydroxyapatite	Anti-platelet effect
	E78 NPs	Anti-platelet effect
	PEG coated E78 NPs	Anti-platelet effect
Aerosol	Ultra fine particles	Activation
	Ambient Particulate Matter	Activation

Table 2. Nanoparticle effects on platelets – the Table enlists how the platelet response varies with variation in nano-material as well as the corresponding nano-surface configuration. NP is nanoparticle.

5. Platelet nanoparticle interaction – A deeper insight

A different paradigm of nanotechnology application has recently got considerable interest. How thrombotic response is modulated by nanoparticles has recently become a new paradigm in nano-medicine. Till today, the exact mechanisms of how nano-surface exposure or uptake of nanoforms alter the platelet response are not known. Most of the metallic nanoparticles, carbon nanoparticles, aerosol and polymer nanoparticles induce platelet aggregation (Mayer et al., 2009; McGuinnes et al., 2011). A few nanoparticles remain inert for platelet or induce anti-platelet effect (Li et al., 2009; Ramtoola et al., 2010; Gulati et al., 2010). Interestingly in case of some polymer nanoparticles, surface conjugation induces varying response to platelets (McGuinnes et al 2010). One needs deeper insights in induced platelet signalling to explain such varying response to nanoparticles with a characteristic surface property.

As mentioned earlier, anti-platelet drug therapy is the most important therapeutic regime for ACS patients. A major fall-out of the conventional therapeutic approach is the sizable incidence of drug resistance among ACS patients (Guha et al., 2009; Jogns et al., 2006; Michelson et al., 2006). There are indications that nanotechnology can help diagnosis of drug resistance (Deb et. al. 2011).

Again, metallic nanoparticles can induce platelet aggregation depending on the physiological state of the platelets. For a given nano-drug such response can show inter individual variations, and there is evidently a scope of judging the safety of such drugs depending on the extent of induced alteration in platelet function. It may be important to note that under certain conditions nanoparticles can be hazardous to both normal individuals as well as ACS patients. Table 3 summarises the overall ACS risk associated with nanoparticles :

Phenomenon	Risk Factors
< 60 nm nanoparticle.	Safe in context to thrombotic risk.
Resting platelets + nanoparticle.	No thrombotic risk.
Anti-platelet drug like clopidogrel or reo-pro.	No thrombotic risk.
Rupture plaque (where vascular bed is open) + Nanoparticle of any size.	High thrombotic risk.
Some special surface modification	tunable

Table 3. Overview of thrombotic risk factors of nanoparticles.

5.1 Excitability of the nanoparticle mediated pro-aggregatory response

Metallic nanoparticle (made of gold, copper, iron, cadmium sulphide and quantum dots) induced platelet aggregation is intriguing as the profile change of such aggregation fully depends on the physiologic conditions of the platelets (e.g. pre-activation) (Deb et al., 2007, 2011; Geys et al., 2008). Non-metallic carbon nano-tube or polymer based nanoparticles on the other hand induce platelet aggregation without any pre-activation, their pro-aggregatory effect depends mainly on hydrophobic collapses (Radomski et al., 2005) or charge-charge interaction among platelets and nanoparticles (McGuinnes et al., 2010). At critical concentrations of ADP or in presence of a threshold shear force, which mildly activates the platelets, they become most sensitive to nano-particles (figure 7). In other words, the nanoparticles in such cases serve as agonists. On the other hand, when platelets are in resting condition most of the metallic nano-forms seems to be inert.

Unlike optimal size response (of nanoparticles) observed in case of cancer cells, the nano-response in platelets increases monotonically with decreasing size of nanoparticles (Deb et al., 2011). This phenomenon occurs also in case of polystyrene nanoparticles (Mayer et al., 2009). This size attribute is similar to entry of the nanoparticles through inhalation. Smaller the size of the nanoparticle, lesser in the efficiency of the clearance by alveolar macrophages, which in turn increases their (nanoparticle) deposition in alveolar cell leading to entry into circulation (Yamawaki & Iwai, 2006). Thus, smaller nanoparticles pose a higher risk in the ACS scenario.

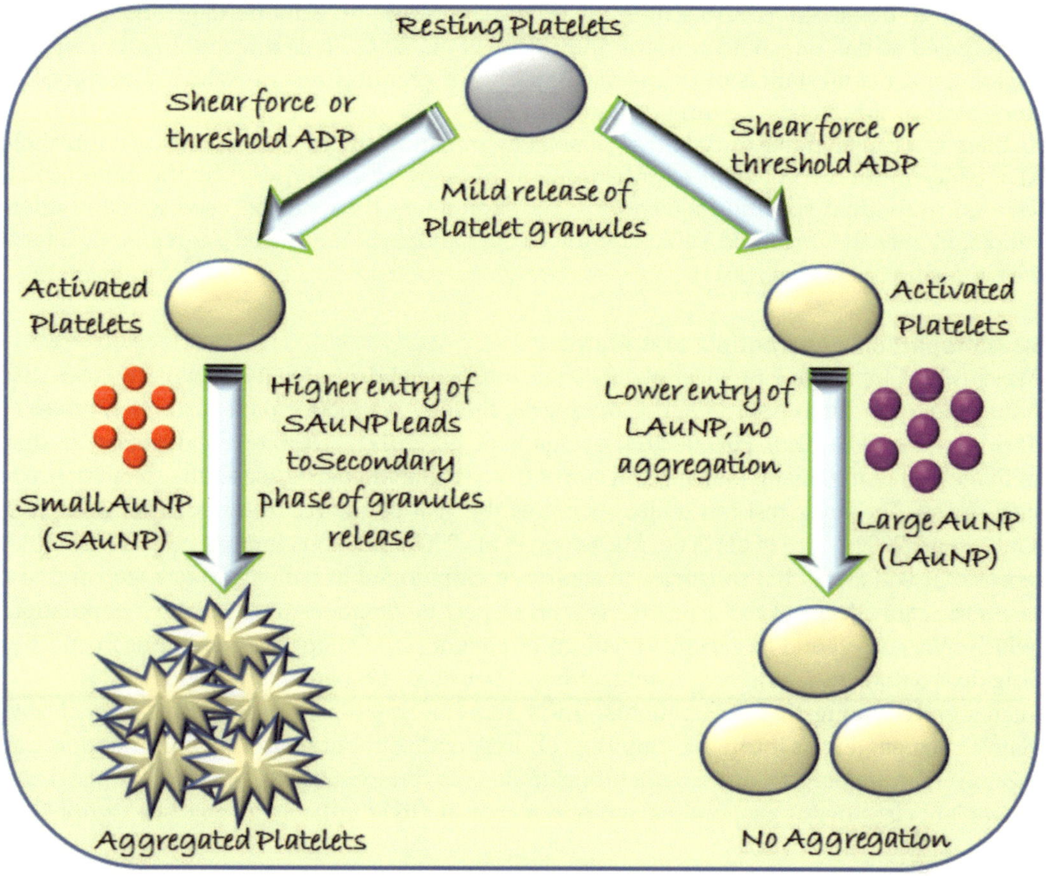

Fig. 7. Nanoparticle Size Response. Gold Nanoparticle induced platelet response [see Deb et. al. 2007,2011] is dependent on nanoparticle size, smaller particle showing aggregatory effects.

Though the exact molecular mechanism of metallic-nanoparticle platelet interaction is yet to be established, systemic response like release of platelet granules (both α and δ) have been observed in presence of nano-particles. In presence of apyrase (scavenge ADP released from δ granules), or anti-platelet drug clopidogrel (block P2Y12 purinergic receptors, thus inhibit secondary wave of aggregation, which is the signature of granules release) nano-particle induced aggregation inhibited. In presence of Arg-Gly-Asp-Ser (RGDS) (a tetra-peptide, which binds to fibrinogen receptor GpIIbIIIa, mimicking the anti-platelet drug Reo-Pro), nano induced platelet aggregation is again inhibited. This reflects that nanoparticles induced aggregation is not due to any physico-chemical agglomerate formation. Consequently, metallic nano-forms are unlikely to activate platelets from patients under anti-platelet drug therapy (Deb et al., 2011). Alternatively, conjugation of anti-platelet drugs (or combined administration of such drugs) can help to reduce the thrombotic risk of nanoparticle based drug formulation.

5.2 Platelet Response as a measure for nano-safety

In the suspended condition, metallic nanoparticle induced platelet aggregation is highly dependent on the local ADP concentration. A transition of deaggregation to aggregation occurs at a threshold concentration of ADP. Interestingly, nanoparticle effect is most pronounced at this threshold concentration (Deb et al., 2007). This threshold nano-response is perhaps a manifestation of primary triggering of granules release which undergoes an auto-catalysis, ultimately leading to aggregation.

As there is a considerable variation of platelet aggregation among individuals, the threshold ADP concentration and extent of enhancement of aggregation induced by the nanoparticle have an individual specific fingerprint. The parameters thus can be used as nano-safety indices. Higher the threshold value and lower the nanoparticle induced aggregation, safer is the nano-drug (Deb et al., 2011).

5.3 Nanoparticles and antiplatelet drugs

Aspirin and Clopidogrel are most widely used anti-platelet drugs for ACS .In many cases dual antiplatelet drug (both Aspirin and Clopidogrel) therapy is used for patient safety (Born et al, 2006, Guha et al., 2009, Faxon 2011, Aragam et al., 2011) Despite the benefits of dual antiplatelet therapy, many patients still suffer from cardiovascular disease due to resistance to such drugs. The drug resistance also increases the risk of the recurrent occurrence of ACS (Guha et al., 2009; Jogns et al., 2006; Michelson et al., 2006). It is thus important to have a quick sensor that will assess the resistance to aspirin or clopidogrel in patients in one step and also assess the equivalence of the drug effects with respect to variations in geographic populations (which may correspond to genetic variations of patient population) and variations in effective drug dose among different drug manufacturers (Deb et al., US patent application, 2011).

Interestingly among the ACS patients, one's showing resistance to the conventional anti-platelet drugs (e.g. aspirin or clopidogrel) respond differentially to gold nanoparticle (~20nm) as compared to one's responding to it. This differential response can be used as a convenient classifier of responders and non responder to antiplatelet drugs **(see figure 8).**

5.4 Nano-material nano-surface and nano-response

Though most of the nano induced response is pro-aggregatory in nature, a few reports Mention inert nature of some nanoparticles (Li et al., 2009; Ramtoola et al., 2010; Gulati et al., 2010). As most of the nano-particles induce platelet aggregation, so it can be said the aggregatory nature of nano surface depends on its diameter rather than its component material. But this conjecture is not applicable to all nano-forms. Charged surface (aminated - positively charged or carboxylated - negatively charged) polystyrene latex nano-forms are capable of inducing platelet aggregation, whereas unmodified latex beads are unable to do so. Interestingly, the modes of aggregation for positive and negatively charged nanoparticles are different. For carboxylated nanoparticle the aggregation is due to the upregulation of surface adhesion molecules, whereas aminated nanoparticles alter the platelet membrane and interact with the anionic phospholipid (Mayer et al., 2009; McGuinnes et al., 2010). Though both of the charged particles are capable of inducing platelet aggregation, the negatively charged larger particles (larger than 60nm) are shown to be less toxic in the platelet activation context (Mayer et al., 2009).The lesser toxicity of the such particle is probably due to less entry and charge repulsion between nano particles and platelets. Human cell derived nanoparticles that actually accentuate platelet granules release, inhibit platelet aggregation. This paradox is possibly due to the reduction of platelet-platelet interaction in presence of nanoparticle (Miller et al., 2009). Negatively charged Polyethylene glycol (PEG) coated nanoparticles from Microemulsion precursor (PEG-E78) induces platelet inhibition (Koziara et al., 2005). Importantly, in both pro-aggregatory or antiplatelet responses , the nanoparticles are effective inducer when added in the pre-incubation stage. Neither the inhibition nor the aggregatory response are observed once the aggregation is initiated by an agonist (Koziara et al., 2005; Deb et al. 2007, 2010). Similar argument holds good for anti-platelet effect of silver nanoparticles prepared with a certain surface attributes (Shrivastava et al., 2009). Silver nanoparticles with a different surface conjugations again show pro-aggregatory effects (Deb et al., 2011 (in press)).

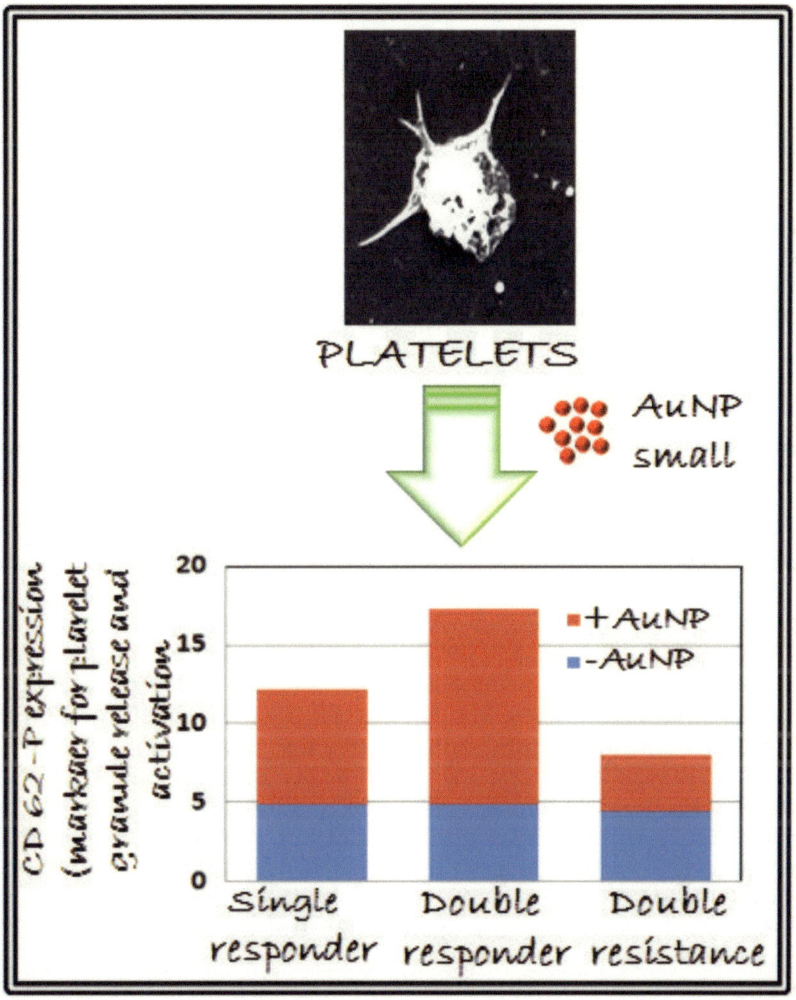

Fig. 8. Nanosensor for Drug Resistance in ACS [89]-Using Nanoparticle effect to discriminate between responder and non-responder of antiplatelet drugs (e.g. aspirin and clopidogrel).

The important question that crops up here is whether in the platelet context it is the nano-surface conjugation or the nano-material that play the lead role. It follows that by modulating the nano-surface, one can tune the thrombotic level, the desirable level depending on the patient status. For ACS, the desired state is a nanoform that attenuates the aggregatory response, and in case of hemorrhage the situation may be complimentary in nature.

6. References

Aragam KG, Bhatt DL. Antiplatelet therapy in acute coronary syndromes.J Cardiovasc Pharmacol Ther. 2011 Mar;16(1):24-42. Epub 2010 Oct 5.

Arnida, Malugin A, Ghandehari H. Cellular uptake and toxicity of gold nanoparticles in prostate cancer cells: a comparative study of rods and spheres.J Appl Toxicol. 2010 Apr;30(3):212-7.

Ashby B, Daniel JL, Smith JB. Mechanisms of platelet activation and inhibition.Hematol Oncol Clin North Am. 1990 Feb;4(1):1-26.

Badran HM, Elnoamany MF, Khalil TS, Eldin MM.Age-related alteration of risk profile, inflammatory response, and angiographic findings in patients with acute coronary syndrome.Clin Med Cardiol. 2009 Feb 18;3:15-28.

Baker JR Jr. Dendrimer-based nanoparticles for cancer therapy.Hematology Am Soc Hematol Educ Program. 2009:708-19.

Born G, Patrono C.Antiplatelet drugs.Br J Pharmacol. 2006 Jan;147 Suppl 1:S241-51.

Calverley DC, Phang TL, Choudhury QG, Gao B, Oton AB, Weyant MJ, Geraci MW. Significant downregulation of platelet gene expression in metastatic lung cancer.Clin Transl Sci. 2010 Oct;3(5):227-32.

Cejas MA, Chen C, Kinney WA, Maryanoff BE. Nanoparticles that display short collagen-related peptides. Potent stimulation of human platelet aggregation by triple helical motifs.Bioconjug Chem. 2007 Jul-Aug;18(4):1025-7. Epub 2007 Jun 21.

Chen J, Saeki F, Wiley BJ, Cang H, Cobb MJ, Li ZY, Au L, Zhang H, Kimmey MB, Li X, Xia Y. Gold nanocages: bioconjugation and their potential use as optical imaging contrast agents. Nano Lett. 2005 Mar;5(3):473-7.

Chen Z, Meng H, Xing G, Yuan H, Zhao F, Liu R, Chang X, Gao X, Wang T, Jia G, Ye C, Chai Z, Zhao Y. Age-related differences in pulmonary and cardiovascular responses to SiO2 nanoparticle inhalation: nanotoxicity has susceptible population. Environ Sci Technol. 2008 Dec 1;42(23):8985-92.

Chithrani BD, Ghazani AA, Chan WC. Determining the size and shape dependence of gold nanoparticle uptake into mammalian cells.Nano Lett. 2006 Apr;6(4):662-8.

Clifford EE, Parker K, Humphreys BD, Kertesy SB, Dubyak GR.The P2X1 receptor, an adenosine triphosphate-gated cation channel, is expressed in human platelets but not in human blood leukocytes.Blood. 1998 May 1;91(9):3172-81.

Deb S, Chatterjee M, Bhattacharya J, Lahiri P, Chaudhuri U, Pal Choudhuri S, Kar S, Siwache O P, Sen P, Dasgupta A K.Role of purinergic receptors in platelet-nanoparticle interactions.Nanotoxicology 2007. 1:93-103.

Deb S, Patra HK, Lahiri P, Dasgupta AK, Chakrabarti K, Chaudhuri U. Multistability in platelets and their response to gold nanoparticles. Nanomedicine. 2011 Feb 26. [Epub ahead of print]

Deb S, Dasgupta AK. One step nanosensor for single and multidrug resistance in acute coronary syndrome (acs).Pub No: US 2011/0053172 A1

Deb S, Raja SO, Dasgupta AK, Sarkar R, Chattopadhyay AP, Chaudhuri U, Guha P, Sardar P. Surface tunability of nanoparticles in modulating platelet functions. Blood Cells, Molecules, and Diseases. 2011 [in press].

Decie and Lewis. Practical Heamatology. 9th edition. Edited by S M Lewis, B J Bain, I Bates. Chapter 16 - Investigation of Haemostasis.

Dorsam RT, Kunapuli SP. Central role of the P2Y12 receptor in platelet activation.J Clin Invest. 2004 Feb;113(3):340-5.

Elias A, Tsourkas A. Imaging circulating cells and lymphoid tissues with iron oxide nanoparticles.Hematology Am Soc Hematol Educ Program. 2009:720-6.

Escolar G, White JG.The platelet open canalicular system: a final common pathway.Blood Cells. 1991;17(3):467-85; discussion 486-95.

Farndale RW. Collagen-induced platelet activation.Blood Cells Mol Dis. 2006 Mar-Apr;36(2):162-5. Epub 2006 Feb 7.

Faxon DP. Optimizing antiplatelet therapy in acute coronary syndrome and percutaneous coronary intervention.Catheter Cardiovasc Interv. 2011 May 26. doi: 10.1002/ccd.23163. [Epub ahead of print]

Flaumenhaft R, Dilks JR, Rozenvayn N, Monahan-Earley RA, Feng D, Dvorak AM. The actin cytoskeleton differentially regulates platelet alpha-granule and dense-granule secretion. Blood. 2005 May 15;105(10):3879-87. Epub 2005 Jan 25.

Fu A, Gu W, Boussert B, Koski K, Gerion D, Manna L, Le Gros M, Larabell CA, Alivisatos AP. Semiconductor quantum rods as single molecule fluorescent biological labels. Nano Lett. 2007 Jan;7(1):179-82.

Geys J, Nemmar A, Verbeken E, Smolders E, Ratoi M, Hoylaerts MF, Nemery B, Hoet PH. Acute toxicity and prothrombotic effects of quantum dots: impact of surface charge. Environ Health Perspect. 2008 Dec;116(12):1607-13. Epub 2008 Jul 18.

Gobin AM, Lee MH, Halas NJ, James WD, Drezek RA, West JL. Near-infrared resonant nanoshells for combined optical imaging and photothermal cancer therapy. Nano Lett. 2007 Jul;7(7):1929-34. Epub 2007 Jun 6.

Guha S, Mookerjee S, Guha P, Sardar P, Deb S, Roy PD, Karmakar R, Mani S, Hema MB, Pyne S, Chakraborti P, Deb PK, Lahiri P, Chaudhuri U.Antiplatelet drug resistance in patients with recurrent acute coronary syndrome undergoing conservative management.Indian Heart J. 2009 Jul-Aug;61(4):348-52.

Guha S, Sardar P, Guha P, Deb S, Karmakar R, Chakraborti P, Mookerjee S, Deb PK, De R, Dutta A, Chaudhuri U. Dual antiplatelet therapy in ACS: time-dependent variability in platelet aggregation during the first week.Indian Heart J. 2009 Mar-Apr;61(2):173-7.

Guha S, Sardar P, Guha P, Roy S, Mookerjee S, Chakrabarti P, Deb PK, Chaudhuri U, Deb S, Karmakar R, Dasgupta AK, Lahiri P.Dual antiplatelet drug resistance in patients with acute coronary syndrome.Indian Heart J. 2009 Jan-Feb;61(1):68-73.

Gulati N, Rastogi R, Dinda AK, Saxena R, Koul V. Characterization and cell material interactions of PEGylated PNIPAAM nanoparticles.Colloids Surf B Biointerfaces. 2010 Aug 1;79(1):164-73. Epub 2010 Apr 10.

Hoffman R, Edward J. Benz Jr et.al.Hematology Basic Principles and Practice. Edition 5. Chapter116 - The Molecular Basis of Platelet Activation 2009.

Huff TB, Tong L, Zhao Y, Hansen MN, Cheng JX, Wei A.Hyperthermic effects of gold nanorods on tumor cells.Nanomedicine (Lond). 2007 Feb;2(1):125-32.

Iverson N, Plourde N, Chnari E, Nackman GB, Moghe PV. Convergence of nanotechnology and cardiovascular medicine : progress and emerging prospects.BioDrugs. 2008;22(1):1-10.

Johns A, Fisher M, Knappertz V. Aspirin and clopidogrel resistance: an emerging clinical entity.Eur Heart J. 2006 Jul;27(14):1754; author reply 1754-5. Epub 2006 Jun 2.

Karniguian A, Grelac F, Levy-Toledano S, Legrand YJ, Rendu F. Collagen-induced platelet activation mainly involves the protein kinase C pathway. Biochem J. 1990 Jun 1;268(2):325-31.

Kottke-Marchant K. Importance of platelets and platelet response in acute coronary syndromes.Cleve Clin J Med. 2009 Apr;76 Suppl 1:S2-7.

Koziara JM, Oh JJ, Akers WS, Ferraris SP, Mumper RJ. Blood compatibility of cetyl alcohol/polysorbate-based nanoparticles. Pharm Res. 2005 Nov;22(11):1821-8. Epub 2005 A

Kroll MH, Schafer AI.Biochemical mechanisms of platelet activation.Blood. 1989 Sep;74(4):1181-95.

Lakkis N, Dokainish H, Abuzahra M, Tsyboulev V, Jorgensen J, De Leon AP, Saleem A. Reticulated platelets in acute coronary syndrome: a marker of platelet activity.J Am Coll Cardiol. 2004 Nov 16;44(10):2091-3.

Lanza G, Winter P, Cyrus T, Caruthers S, Marsh J, Hughes M, Wickline S.Nanomedicine opportunities in cardiology.Ann N Y Acad Sci. 2006 Oct;1080:451-65.

Li JJ, Wang YA, Guo W, Keay JC, Mishima TD, Johnson MB, Peng X. Large-scale synthesis of nearly monodisperse CdSe/CdS core/shell nanocrystals using air-stable reagents via successive ion layer adsorption and reaction. J Am Chem Soc. 2003 Oct 15;125(41):12567-75.

Li X, Radomski A, Corrigan OI, Tajber L, De Sousa Menezes F, Endter S, Medina C, Radomski MW.Platelet compatibility of PLGA, chitosan and PLGA-chitosan nanoparticles./ Nanomedicine (Lond). 2009 Oct;4(7):735-46.

Luthi AJ, Patel PC, Ko CH, Mutharasan RK, Mirkin CA, Thaxton CS.Nanotechnology for synthetic high-density lipoproteins.Trends Mol Med. 2010 Dec;16(12):553-60. Epub 2010 Nov 17.

Marcus AJ, Broekman MJ, Drosopoulos JH, Islam N, Alyonycheva TN, Safier LB, Hajjar KA, Posnett DN, Schoenborn MA, Schooley KA, Gayle RB, Maliszewski CR. The endothelial cell ecto-ADPase responsible for inhibition of platelet function is CD39.J Clin Invest. 1997 Mar 15;99(6):1351-60.

Marcus AJ, Safier LB, Hajjar KA, Ullman HL, Islam N, Broekman MJ, Eiroa AM. Inhibition of platelet function by an aspirin-insensitive endothelial cell ADPase. Thromboregulation by endothelial cells.J Clin Invest. 1991 Nov;88(5):1690-6.

Marcus AJ, Zucker-Franklin D, Safier LB, Ullman HL. Studies on human platelet granules and membranes. J Clin Invest. 1966 Jan;45(1):14-28.

Massberg S, Schulz C, Gawaz M. Role of platelets in the pathophysiology of acute coronary syndrome.Semin Vasc Med. 2003 May;3(2):147-62.

Matter CM, Stuber M, Nahrendorf M.Imaging of the unstable plaque: how far have we got? Eur Heart J. 2009 Nov;30(21):2566-74. Epub 2009 Oct 15.

Mayer A, Vadon M, Rinner B, Novak A, Wintersteiger R, Fröhlich E. The role of nanoparticle size in hemocompatibility. Toxicology. 2009 Apr 28;258(2-3):139-47. Epub 2009 Jan 22.

McGuinnes C, Duffin R, Brown S, L Mills N, Megson IL, Macnee W, Johnston S, Lu SL, Tran L, Li R, Wang X, Newby DE, Donaldson K. Surface derivatization state of polystyrene latex nanoparticles determines both their potency and their mechanism of causing human platelet aggregation in vitro.Toxicol Sci. 2011 Feb;119(2):359-68. Epub 2010 Dec 1.

Michelson A D, Frelinger A L, Furman M I. Resistance to antiplatelet drugs.2006. European Heart Journal.European Heart Journal, Volume8,G53-G58

Miller VM, Hunter LW, Chu K, Kaul V, Squillace PD, Lieske JC, Jayachandran M. Biologic nanoparticles and platelet reactivity. Nanomedicine (Lond). 2009 Oct;4(7):725-33.

Murray CB, Kagan CR, Bawendi MG. Synthesis and characterization of monodisperse nanocrystals and close-packed nanocrystal assemblies. Ann Rev Materials Sci.2000;30:545-610.

Nagalla S, Shaw C, Kong X, Kondkar AA, Edelstein LC, Ma L, Chen J, McKnight GS, López JA, Yang L, Jin Y, Bray MS, Leal SM, Dong JF, Bray PF.Platelet microRNA-mRNA coexpression profiles correlate with platelet reactivity.Blood. 2011 May 12;117(19):5189-97. Epub 2011 Mar 17.

Nemmar A, Hoylaerts MF, Hoet PH, Vermylen J, Nemery B. Size effect of intratracheally instilled particles on pulmonary inflammation and vascular thrombosis. Toxicol Appl Pharmacol. 2003 Jan 1;186(1):38-

Nesbitt WS, Giuliano S, Kulkarni S, Dopheide SM, Harper IS, Jackson SP. Intercellular calcium communication regulates platelet aggregation and thrombus growth.J Cell Biol. 2003 Mar 31;160(7):1151-61.

Nikolas Kipshidze.Nanotechnology in Cardiology.BULLETIN OF THE GEORGIAN NATIONAL ACADEMY OF SCIENCES,2009, vol. 3, no. 165-177

Nyman D.Von Willebrand factor dependent platelet aggregation and adsorption of factor VIII related antigen by collagen.Thromb Res. 1980 Jan 1-15;17(1-2):209-14.

Oberdörster G ,Stone V,Donaldson K. Toxicology of nanoparticles: A historical perspective.Nanotoxicology 2007, 1, 2-25.

Patra HK, Banerjee S, Chaudhuri U, Lahiri P, Dasgupta AK. Cell selective response to gold nanoparticles.Nanomedicine. 2007 Jun;3(2):111-9.

Patscheke H. Role of activation in epinephrine-induced aggregation of platelets.Thromb Res. 1980 Jan 1-15;17(1-2):133-42.

Patscheke H.Correlation of activation and aggregation of platelets. Discrimination between anti-activating and anti-aggregating agents.Haemostasis. 1979;8(2):65-81.

Peng X, Manna L, Yang W, Wickham J, Scher E, Kadavanich A, Alivisatos AP. Shape control of CdSe nanocrystals. Nature. 2000 Mar 2;404(6773):59-61.

Peterman EJ, Gittes F, Schmidt CF. Laser-induced heating in optical traps.Biophys J. 2003 Feb;84(2 Pt 1):1308-16.

Petkar KC, Chavhan SS, Agatonovik-Kustrin S, Sawant KK. Nanostructured materials in drug and gene delivery: a review of the state of the art. Crit Rev Ther Drug Carrier Syst. 2011;28(2):101-64.

Plech, A.; Kotaidis, V.; Grésillon, S.; Dahmen, C.; von Plessen, G. Laser-induced heating and melting of gold nanoparticles studied by time-resolved x-ray scattering. Published 16 November 2004 (7 pages) 195423

Radomski A, Jurasz P, Alonso-Escolano D, Drews M, Morandi M, Malinski T, Radomski MW . Nanoparticle-induced platelet aggregation and vascular thrombosis. British journal of pharmacology 2005 ;146: 882–893

Ramtoola Z, Lyons P, Keohane K, Kerrigan SW, Kirby BP, Kelly JG. Investigation of the interaction of biodegradable micro- and nanoparticulate drug delivery systems with platelets.J Pharm Pharmacol. 2011 Jan;63(1):26-32. doi: 10.1111/j.2042-7158.2010.01174.x. Epub 2010 Nov 16.

Rao W, Deng ZS, Liu J. A review of hyperthermia combined with radiotherapy/chemotherapy on malignant tumors.Crit Rev Biomed Eng. 2010;38(1):101-16.

Roberts DE, McNicol A, Bose R. Mechanism of collagen activation in human platelets. J Biol Chem. 2004 May 7;279(19):19421-30. Epub 2004 Feb 23.

Rowley JW, Oler A, Tolley ND, Hunter B, Low EN, Nix DA, Yost CC, Zimmerman GA, Weyrich AS.Genome wide RNA-seq analysis of human and mouse platelet transcriptomes.Blood. 2011 May 19. [Epub ahead of print]

Rückerl R, Phipps RP, Schneider A, Frampton M, Cyrys J, Oberdörster G, Wichmann HE, Peters A.Ultrafine particles and platelet activation in patients with coronary heart disease--results from a prospective panel study.Part Fibre Toxicol. 2007 Jan 22;4:1.

Shrivastava S, Bera T, Singh SK, Singh G. Ramachandrarao, P.; Dash, D.: Characterization of antiplatelet properties of silver nanoparticles. ACS Nano 2009; 3:1357-1364.

Singha S, Datta H, Dasgupta AK. Size dependent chaperon properties of gold nanoparticles.J Nanosci Nanotechnol. 2010 Feb;10(2):826-32.

Smith AM, Mohs AM, Nie S. Tuning the optical and electronic properties of colloidal nanocrystals by lattice strain. Nat Nanotechnol. 2009 Jan;4(1):56-63. Epub 2008 Dec 7.

Spalding A, Vaitkevicius H, Dill S, MacKenzie S, Schmaier A, Lockette W. Mechanism of epinephrine-induced platelet aggregation. Hypertension. 1998 Feb;31(2):603-7.

Thompson CB.From precursor to product: how do megakaryocytes produce platelets? Prog Clin Biol Res. 1986;215:361-71.

Tschopp TB, Baumgartner HR, Meyer D. Antibody to human factor VIII/von Willebrand factor inhibits collagen-induced platelet aggregation and release.Thromb Res. 1980 Jan 1-15;17(1-2):255-9.

Walkey C, Sykes EA, Chan WC. Application of semiconductor and metal nanostructures in biology and medicine. Hematology Am Soc Hematol Educ Program. 2009:701-7.

Wani M Y, Hashim M A, Nabi F, Malik M A. Nanotoxicity: Dimensional and Morphological Concerns. Advances in Physical Chemistry. Volume 2011 (2011), Article ID 450912, 15 pages. doi:10.1155/2011/450912

Wickline SA, Lanza GM. Nanotechnology for molecular imaging and targeted therapy.Circulation. 2003 Mar 4;107(8):1092-5.

Wickline SA, Neubauer AM, Winter P, Caruthers S, Lanza G. Applications of nanotechnology to atherosclerosis, thrombosis, and vascular biology.Arterioscler Thromb Vasc Biol. 2006 Mar;26(3):435-41. Epub 2005 Dec 22.

Wilson DW, Aung HH, Lame MW, Plummer L, Pinkerton KE, Ham W, Kleeman M, Norris JW, Tablin F.Exposure of mice to concentrated ambient particulate matter results in platelet and systemic cytokine activation.Inhal Toxicol. 2010 Mar;22(4):267-76.

Wilson SR, Sabatine MS, Braunwald E, Sloan S, Murphy SA, Morrow DA. Detection of myocardial injury in patients with unstable angina using a novel nanoparticle cardiac troponin I assay: observations from the PROTECT-TIMI 30 Trial.Am Heart J. 2009 Sep;158(3):386-91. Epub 2009 Jul 15.

Wiwanitkit V, Sereemaspun A, Rojanathanes R. Gold nanoparticles and a microscopic view of platelets: a preliminary observation. Cardiovasc J Afr 2009 ; 20: 141-142.

Wu CC, Teng CM. Comparison of the effects of PAR1 antagonists, PAR4 antagonists, and their combinations on thrombin-induced human platelet activation.Eur J Pharmacol. 2006 Sep 28;546(1-3):142-7.

Wu CC, Wu SY, Liao CY, Teng CM, Wu YC, Kuo SC. The roles and mechanisms of PAR4 and P2Y12/phosphatidylinositol 3-kinase pathway in maintaining thrombin-induced platelet aggregation.Br J Pharmacol. 2010 Oct;161(3):643-58.

Yamawaki H, Iwai N. Mechanisms underlying nano-sized air-pollution-mediated progression of atherosclerosis: carbon black causes cytotoxic injury/inflammation and inhibits cell growth in vascular endothelial cells.Circ J. 2006 Jan;70(1):129-40.

Yamawaki H, Iwai N. Mechanisms underlying nano-sized air-pollution-mediated progression of atherosclerosis: carbon black causes cytotoxic injury/inflammation and inhibits cell growth in vascular endothelial cells.Circ J. 2006 Jan;70(1):129-40.

Yu MK, Kim D, Lee IH, So JS, Jeong YY, Jon S.Image-Guided Prostate Cancer Therapy Using Aptamer-Functionalized Thermally Cross-Linked Superparamagnetic Iron Oxide Nanoparticles.Small. 2011 Jun 7. doi: 10.1002/smll.201100472. [Epub ahead of print].

3

Physiopathology of the Acute Coronary Syndromes

Iwao Emura
Department of Surgical Pathology, Japanese Red Cross Nagaoka Hospital, Japan

1. Introduction

The widespread application of catheter-based interventions, and chronic treatment have contributed to improved long-term prognosis in patients with acute ST-elevation myocardial infarction (STEMI) [1-5]. Despite these indisputable achievements, a large number of individuals remain at substantial risk of severe first attack, recurrent disease and death. Patients with unstable angina were classified into three groups according to short-term risk of death or nonfatal myocardial infarction[6], and the results of noninvasive tests and the corresponding approximate mortality rates were reported [7].

Disruption, fissure, or erosion of an atherosclerotic plaque, with residual mural thrombus (RMT) has a fundamental role in the pathogenesis of acute coronary syndromes (ACS) [8-12]. Most of occlusive thrombi had a layered structure indicating an episodic growth by repeated mural deposits [13, 14]. Morphological studies indicated that plaque complications remained clinically silent days or weeks before the fatal event [15-18]. A RMT predisposes patients to recurrent thrombotic vessel occlusion [15, 16, 17], and plaque disruption, fissure or erosion with thrombus contributes to plaque development and progression [18]. Therefore, a marker that predicts disrupted, fissured or eroded plaque and the coronary thrombus may have practical clinical applications. The diagnosis of these lesions has been tried by several methods [19]. However, plaque disruption itself is asymptomatic, and the associated RMT is usually clinically silent [20]. To the best of our knowledge, markers as a sign of a disrupted, fissured or eroded plaque and a coronary thrombus are not available.

Scavenger receptor-mediated endocytosis of oxidized low-density lipoprotein by macrophages has been implicated in the pathogenesis of atherosclerosis. The differentiation of scavenger receptor A negative (SRA^-) monocytes in peripheral blood (PB) into SRA positive (SRA^+) macrophages was believed to take place in atherosclerotic lesions by stimulation of macrophage-colony stimulating factor (M-CSF) [21-24], and it was reported that freshly isolated blood monocytes were negative for SRA [25]. We surmised that plaque content might be exposed to the blood stream after disruption of plaque, and SRA^- monocytes might differentiate into SRA^+ cells in PB by stimulation of M-CSF contained in plaque content, and that increased SRA^+ cells in PB might be a useful indication of disrupted, fissured or eroded plaque and coronary thrombus.

Although several scavenger receptors, such as SRA, CD36, scavenger receptor-B1, CD68 and Lox-1 have been shown to bind oxidized low-density lipoprotein, SRA and CD36 are responsible for the preponderance of modified low-density lipoprotein uptake in macrophages [26]. In our study, we evaluated the utility of SRA, since SRA antigen is restrictedly expressed on macrophages [26], but CD36 is expressed not only on macrophages and monocytes but also on B lymphocytes.

We reported that the SRA index〔number of SRA^+ cells in 10 high power fields (HPF, x400) of peripheral blood (PB) smear, upper limit: <30〕 greater than 30 was considered to be a useful indication of disrupted, fissured or eroded plaque and coronary thrombus [27, 28]. In this paper, we described the composition of occlusive coronary thrombi obtained from patients with acute ST-elevation myocardial infarction (STEMI), the relationship between the SRA index and these thrombi, and the utility of SRA index as an indication of disrupted, fissured or eroded plaque and coronary thrombus in patients with ACS.

2. Study subjects

Eight autopsy cases with acute myocardial infarction, 393 patients with STEMI and 79 patients with unstable angina (UA) were examined. Patients with STEMI were treated with percutaneous intracoronary thrombectomy during primary angioplasty. High-sensitivity C-reactive protein (h-CRP), creatine kinase (CK) and creatine kinase-MB isozyme (CK-MB) were examined in patients with STEMI. PB from 43 apparently healthy men and women in their 20s was examined as a control.

3. Thrombectomy procedure

On admission, all patients were treated with 162 mg aspirin (Ebis, Osaka, Japan), and they underwent percutaneous coronary intervention of the infarct-related artery through the femoral access route with a 6F guiding catheter. Thrombectomy was performed with a Rescue™ catheter (Boston Scientific, Natick, MA, USA) or a TVAC catheter (NIPRO, Osaka, Japan). Aspirated blood and intracoronary material were collected in a collection bottle, which was equipped with a filter. Stent implantation was performed in 386 patients and all patients were treated with antithrombotic therapy.

4. Tissue processing and histopathological methods

Autopsy was performed 2 or 3 hours after death. Thrombi and organs were fixed in 10 % neutral formalin and embedded in paraffin, and examined using hematoxylin and eosin, and phosphotungstic acid hematoxylin (PTAH) sections. Papanicolaou-stained smears and paraffin-embedded sections were used for the immunohistochemical and immunocytochemical examination, which was performed with the simple stain MAX-PO method (NICHIREI Co., Tokyo, Japan) and with diaminobenzidine as the chromogen using mouse monoclonal anti-human glycoprotein 1b (CD42b, a platelet marker, 1:100; Novo Castra, Newcastle upon Tyne, UK), and mouse monoclonal anti-human SRA (CD204, a macrophage SRA marker, 1:200; Trans Genic Inc., Kumamoto, Japan) antibodies. An antigen retrieval method using citrate buffer and microwave heating was employed. As a negative control, the primary antibody was substituted by phosphate-buffered saline, and a positive stain was not observed in these controls.

5. Cytological methods

I believe that the method of cytological examination of peripheral blood is my original method [29]. Briefly, red blood cells were lysed with lysing reagent (826 mg of NH_4CL + 3.7 mg of EDTA-4Na + 100 mg of $KHCO_3$ in 100 ml H_2O), then nucleated cells were suspended in isotonic sodium chloride solution, and the suspensions containing about $5x10^6$ nucleated cells were smeared on glass slides using Auto smear CF-12 (Sakura Seiki, Tokyo, Japan). Cells that did not adhere to the glass slides were gently washed away with 95% ethanol solution. Smear preparations were fixed in 95% ethanol solution and stained with the Papanicolaou method. A smear preparation of PB is shown in figure 1. About one million and two hundred thousand nucleated cells were smeared in one slide. Nucleated cells are smeared evenly and precise nuclear structures are excellently preserved. About one thousand nucleated cells were observed in one high power field (×400, Figure 2).

Fig. 1. A cytological preparation of peripheral blood stained with the Papanicolaou method. About one million and two hundred thousand nucleated cells are smeared in one slide. Papanicolaou stain.

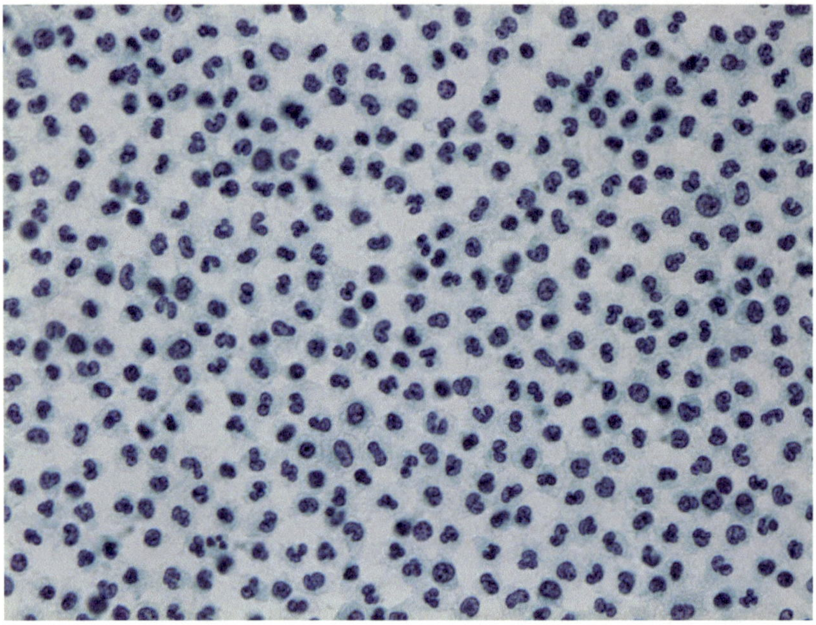

Fig. 2. About one thousand nucleated cells are observed in one high power field (×400). Nucleated cells are smeared evenly and precise nuclear structures are excellently preserved. Papanicolaou stain.

6. Definitions

Thrombi were classified into 4 groups according to previously published definitions considering age and constituents of thrombus[13, 30] : 1) an eosinophilic mass with neo-vascularization (organizing thrombus: OT), 2) a structureless eosinophilic (hyalin) mass (fibrin-rich thrombus: FT), 3) Thrombus containing significant quantities of platelets, erythrocytes, fibrin and leukocytes (mixed thrombus: MT), and 4) tightly packed but individually discernible platelets (platelet thrombus: PT). In this paper, we defined MT and FT as RMT. Plaque components were identified based on the presence of foamy macrophages, cholesterol crystals, collagen tissue, and/or calcification. Since the aspirated material was fragmented, and PT seemed to be the freshest thrombus, contact between PT and other types of thrombus (PT and MT: P-M, PT and FT: P-F,) and contact between PT and plaque content (P-C) were examined in all cases to investigate the process of coronary occlusion. Cases were classified into 3 groups according to the composition of the thrombus: group A, containing PT only and P-C; B, a MT only, P-M and P-C+P-M; C, P-F, P-M+P-F, P-C+P-F, and P-C+P-M+P-F. SRA^+ cells in PB that had the same size and nuclear shape as blood monocytes were defined as SRA^+ cells. The SRA index was defined as the number of SRA^+ cells in 10 HPFs of PB smear samples. Based on the SRA index of apparently healthy people in their 20s, we temporarily set the normal upper limit of the SRA index at 30 [27].

7. Autopsy cases

P-C was observed in 4 autopsy cases, P-M in 3 and P-M + P-F in 1. Numerous emboli of PT were observed in peripheral small arteries and capillaries of the infarct-related artery in 6 cases. SRA index exceeded 30 in 5 cases. A typical case with acute myocardial infarction is presented in figure 3 to 7. This patient is a forty-three year old male. He died suddenly. Postmortem examination revealed disruption of the plaque and occlusive thrombus in the left anterior descending artery (Figure 3). Thrombus is composed of platelet thrombus and mixed thrombus + fibrin-rich thrombus (Figure 4 and 5). Platelet thrombus was adhered on the inner side of mixed thrombus + fibrin-rich thrombus (Figure 4). Immunohistochemistry for CD 42b revealed that platelet thrombus was deeply stained than mixed thrombus + fibrin-rich thrombus (Figure 4). Fibrin mesh is contained in mixed thrombus + fibrin-rich thrombus but not in platelet thrombus (figure 5). SRA^{+} cells are infiltrated in mixed thrombus + fibrin-rich thrombus but not in platelet thrombus (Figure 6). Numerous emboli of fragments of platelet thrombi were observed in small arteries and capillaries at the distal portion of the left anterior descending artery (Figure 7).

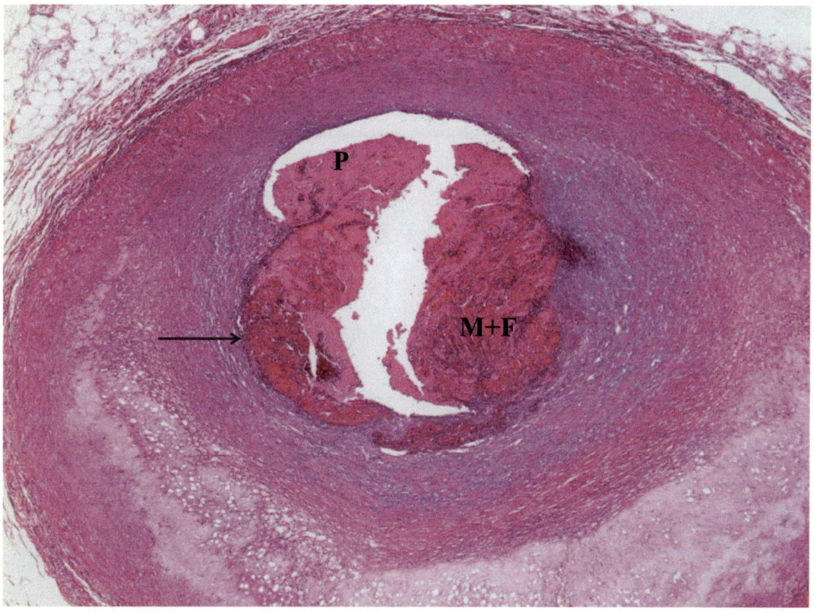

Fig. 3. Plaque disruption (arrow) and thrombus formation in the left anterior descending artery of the patients who died suddenly. Thrombus is composed of platelet thrombus (P) and mixed thrombus + fibrin-rich thrombus (P+M). hematoxylin and eosin.

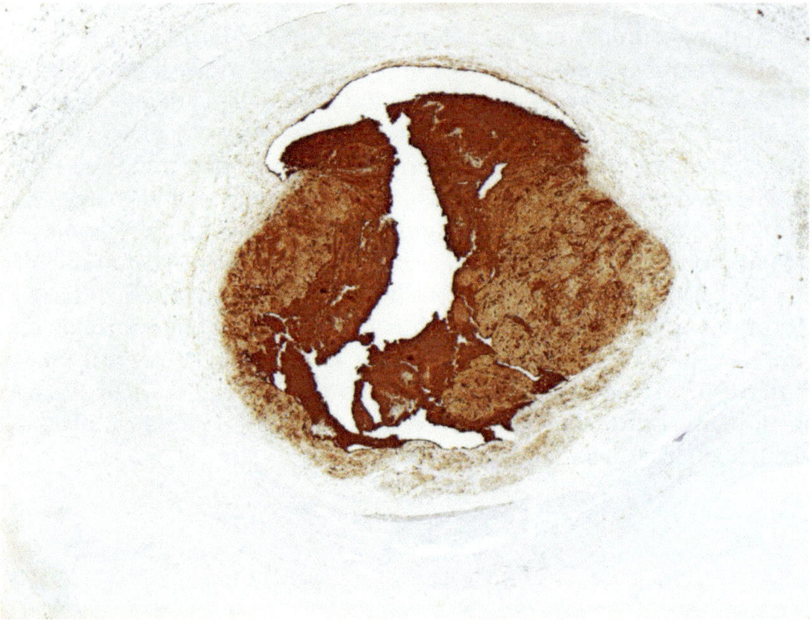

Fig. 4. Serial section of figure 1. Platelet thrombus is deeply stained than mixed thrombus + fibrin-rich thrombus, and adhered on the inner side of mixed thrombus + fibrin-rich thrombus. Immunochemistry for CD42b.

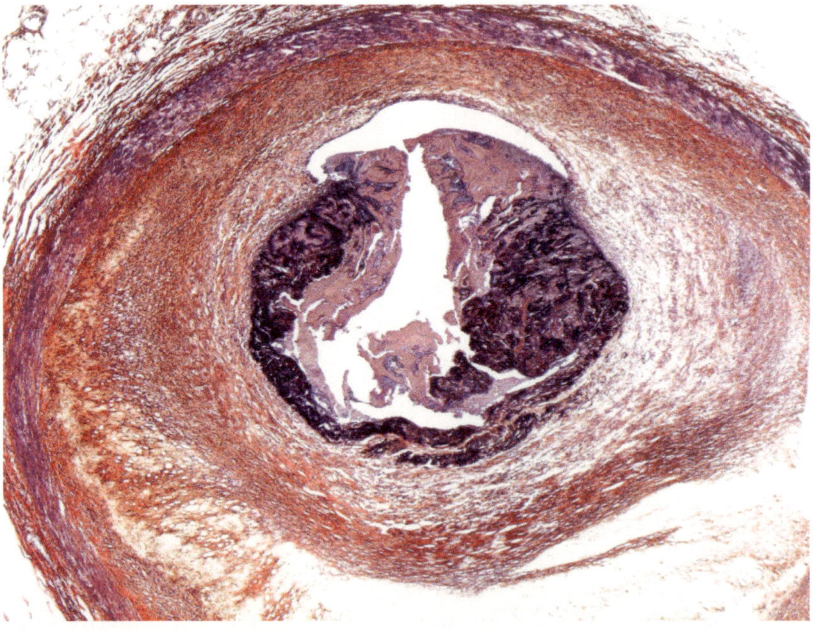

Fig. 5. Serial section of figure 1. Fibrin mesh is contained in mixed thrombus + fibrin-rich thrombus but not in platelet thrombus . phosphotungstic acid hematoxylin stain.

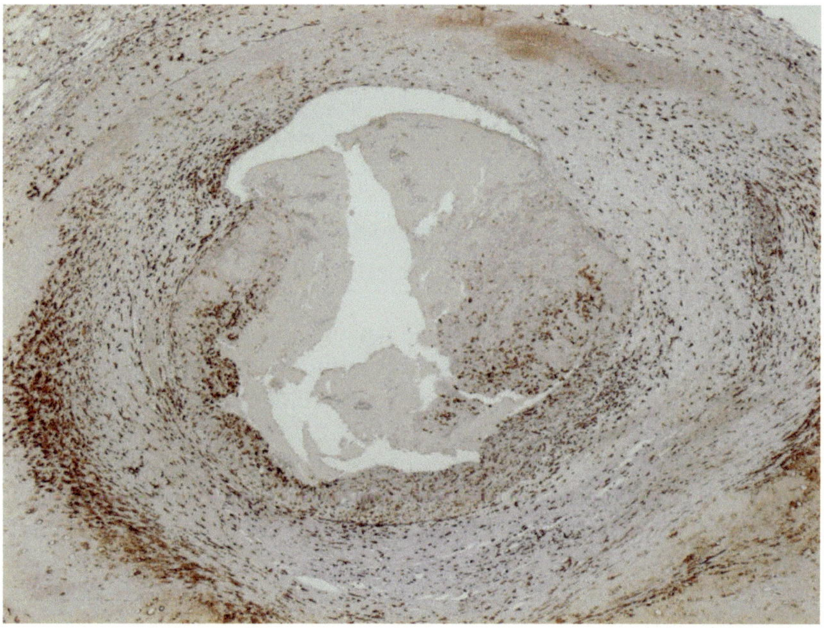

Fig. 6. Serial section of figure 1. Scavenger receptor A positive cells are infiltrated in mixed thrombus + fibrin-rich thrombus but not in platelet thrombus. Immunochemistry for scavenger receptor A.

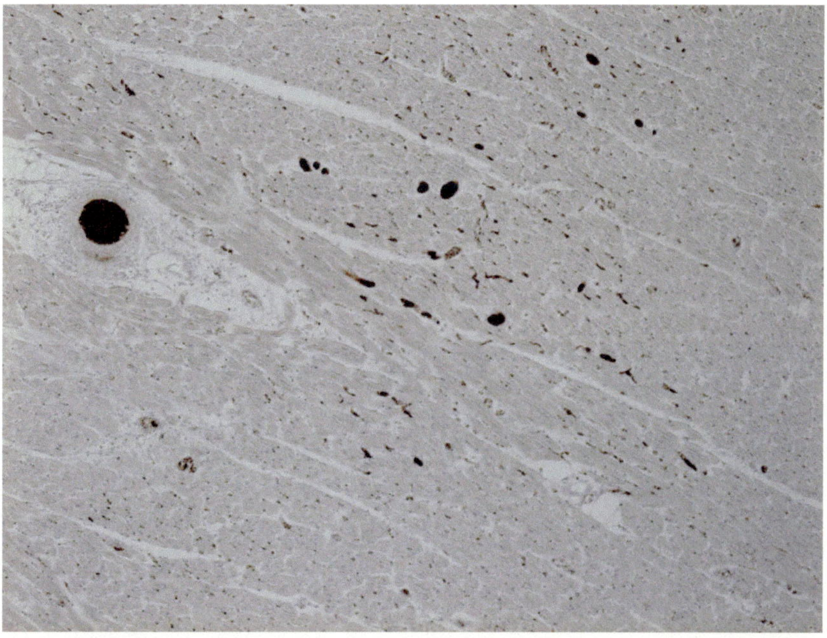

Fig. 7. Numerous emboli of fragments of platelet thrombi are observed in small arteries and capillaries at the distal portion of the left anterior descending artery. Immunohistochemistry for CD 42b.

8. Patients with STEMI

8.1 SRA index and CK, CK-MB, h-CRP

Abnormally increased levels of CK and CK-MB were observed in 53.8 % and 55.6% cases respectively at the hospitalization, and all cases showed abnormally high levels of CK and CK-MB within 24 hours after hospitalization. There was a strong correlation between CK and CK-MB (r=0.986), but no correlation between the SRA index and CK (r=0.025), CK-MB (r=0.005), and h-CRP(r=0.085) were seen (all, Student's t-test).

8.2 Pathological findings of thrombus

Thrombus was observed in 389 (99%) of the 393 patients, plaque contents alone were detected in 2, and neither thrombus nor plaque contents was identified in 2. In 270 patients, only thrombus was found; and both thrombus and plaque content were identified in 119. PT was found in 387 of 389 (99.5%) patients, MT in 269 (69.2%), FT in 57 (14.7%), and OT in 29 (7.5%). Results of the histopathological examination of thrombus are shown in table 1. RMT was detected in 300 (77.1 %) patients (Table 1). One type of contact was detected in 285 (73.3 %) patients, 2 types in 61 (15.7 %) and 3 types in 12 (3.0 %), and PT, or MT alone was found in 29 and 2 patients respectively. Contact between PT and OT was not observed. There was no gradual morphological transition from PT to MT or FT, but there were gradual transitions from MT to FT, and FT to OT in some cases.

Group	Contact Pattern	n	Thrombus n/n (%)	SRA index >30 n/n (%)
A	P	29	89/389(22.9)	46/89 (51.7)
	P-C	60		
B	M	2	243/389(62.5)	181/243(74.5)
	P-M	202		
	P-C+P-M	39		
C	P-F	23	57/389(14.7)	49/57(86.0)
	P-M+P-F	14		
	P-C+P-F	8		
	P-C+P-M+P-F	12		

Table 1. Brief title: Relationships between contact patterns of thrombus and SRA index at hospitalization[1].

[1]P: Platelet thrombus. P-C: Contact between platelet thrombus and plaque content. M: Mixed thrombus. P-M: Contact between platelet thrombus and mixed thrombus. P-F: Contact between platelet thrombus and fibrin-rich thrombus.

Eighty-nine patients were classified into group A, 243 into group B, and 57 into group C (Table 1). Typical findings of group A (P-C) are shown in figure 8. Macrophages in plaque content were positive for SRA, and SRA positive cells were not found in platelet thrombus. Figure 9 to 12 are typical findings of group B (P-M). Platelet thrombus is adhered on the mixed thrombus (Figure 9, 10), and fibrin mesh is not observed in platelet thrombus (Figure 11). SRA positive cells are infiltrated into mixed thrombus along the boundary zone (Figure 12). Typical findings of group C (P-F) are shown in figures 13 and 14. SRA positive cells are diffusely infiltrated in fibrin-rich thrombus (Figure 14). Fragments of PT are frequently found in MT in many cases (Figure 15). SRA^+ cells infiltrated into 147 (54.6%) of 269 MT. These cells and SRA^+ cells in PB were nearly equal in size, and infiltrated into MT along the boundary zone between PT and MT in most cases. SRA^+ cells were diffusely infiltrated into all FT and OT. Some of these SRA^+ cells were large in size. Foam cells in plaque content were positive for SRA. SRA^+ cells were not infiltrated into PT.

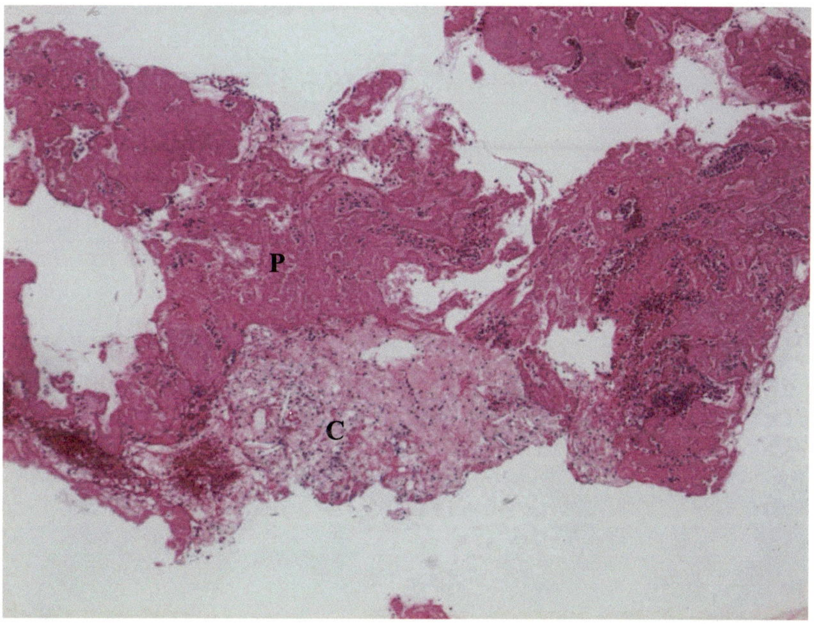

Fig. 8. Contact between platelet thrombus (P) and plaque content (C).

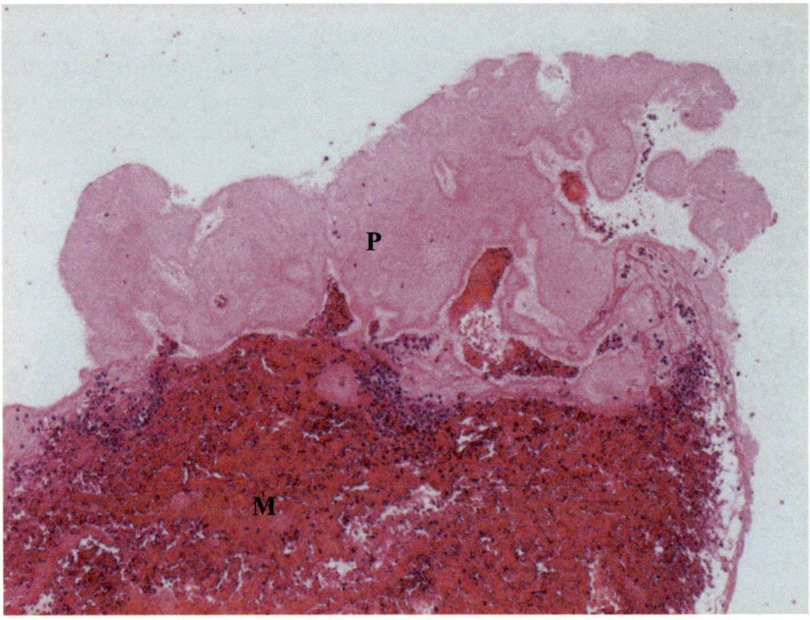

Fig. 9. Contact between platelet thrombus (P) and mixed thrombus (M).

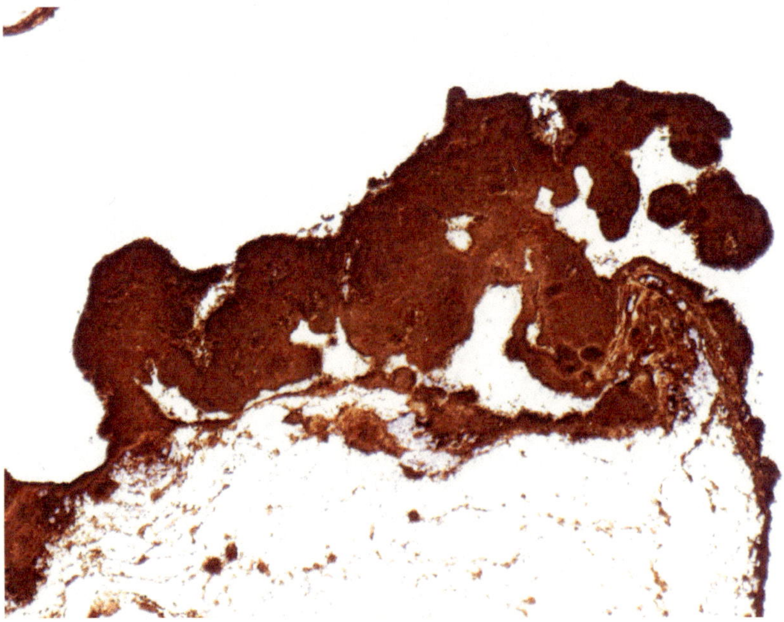

Fig. 10. Serial section of figure 9. Platelet thrombus is strongly stained. Immunochemistry for CD42b.

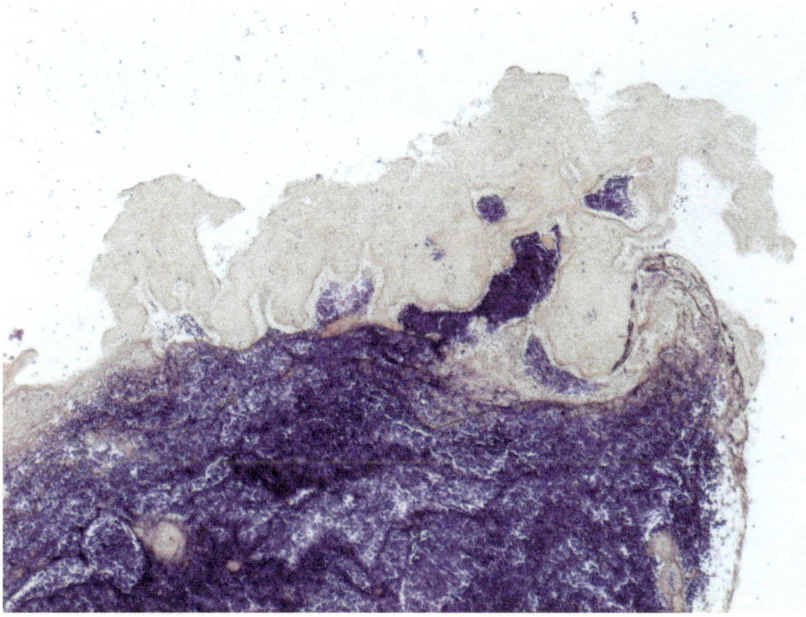

Fig. 11. Serial section of figure 9. Fibrin mesh is not observed in platelet thrombus. phosphotungstic acid hematoxylin stain.

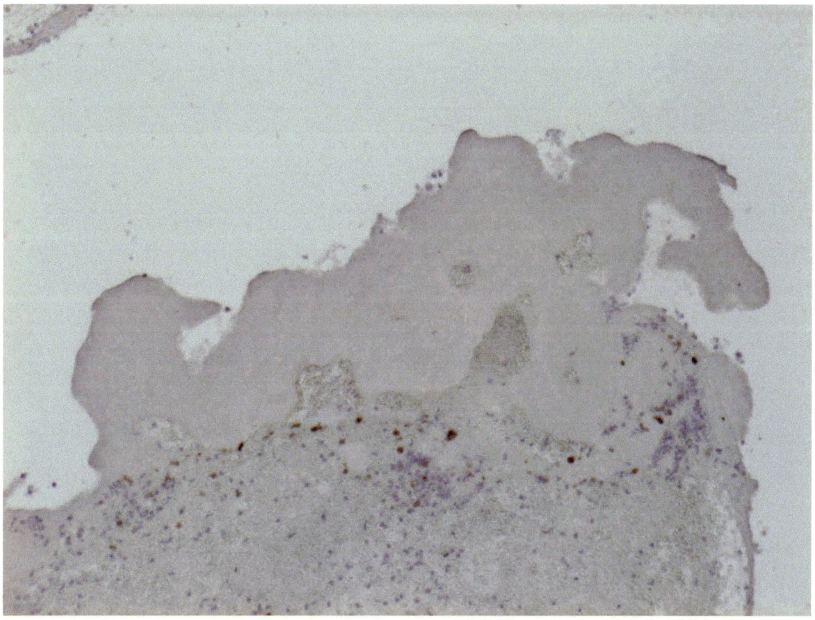

Fig. 12. Serial section of figure 9. Scavenger receptor A positive cells infiltrate into mixed thrombus along the boundary zone. Immunochemistry for CD204.

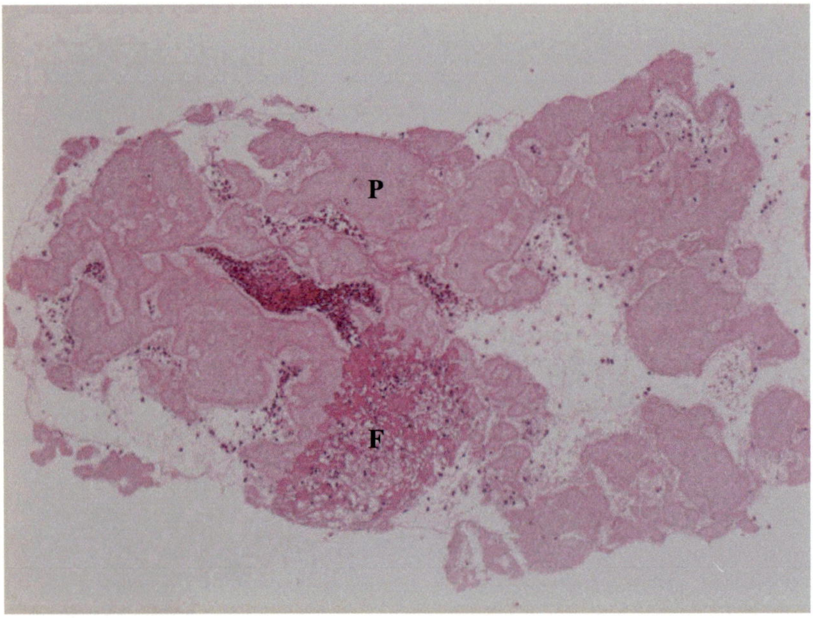

Fig. 13. Contact between platelet thrombus (P) and fibrin-rich thrombus (F).

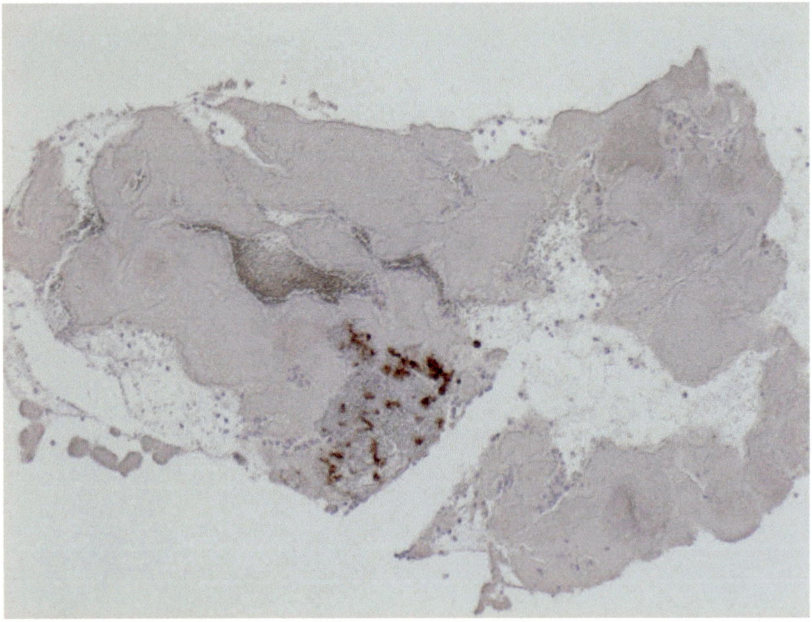

Fig. 14. Serial section of figure 13. Scavenger receptor A positive cells infiltrate into fibrin-rich thrombus. Immunochemistry for CD204.

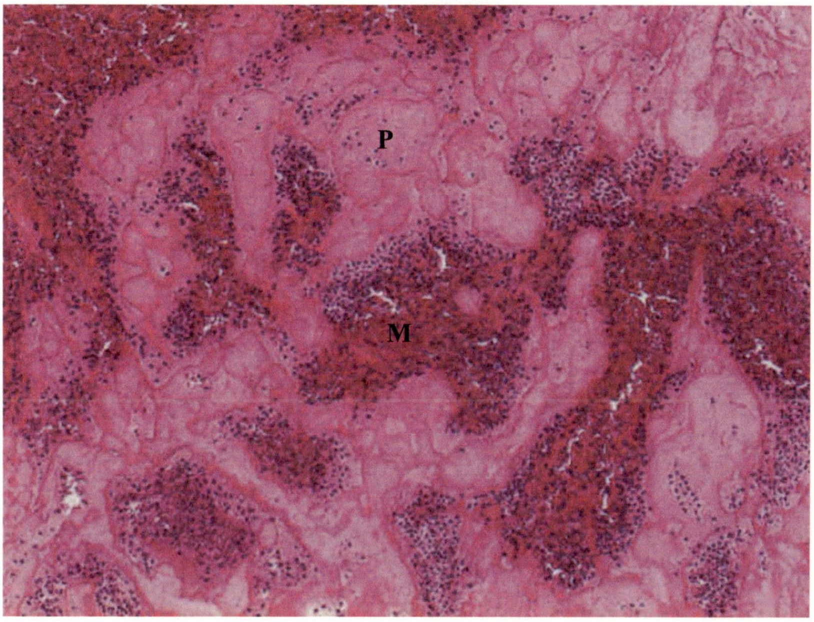

Fig. 15. Small fragments of platelet thrombus (P) are intermingled with mixed thrombus (M).

8.3 SRA⁺ cells in PB

SRA+ cells were observed in all control cases and in all patients with STEMI and UA. Neither SRA+ large macrophages nor foamy cells could be observed in PB of all examined cases. SRA index of control cases ranged 1 to 24 (mean±SD=11.1±7.5). The relationships between SRA index and contact patterns of thrombus at hospitalization were shown in table 1. At hospitalization, SRA index exceeded 30 in 276 of 393 patients with STEMI (Figure 16). Thrombus was identified in all these patients with more than 30 SRA index. PT was identified in 274 (99.3 %), and RMT in 230 (83.3 %) cases. From the viewpoint thrombus, SRA index exceeded 30 in 230 of 300 (76.7 %) cases with RMT and 46 of 89 (51.7 %) cases with PT alone (Table 1). The percentage of patients with a SRA index more than 30 was significantly lower in group A patients than other groups of patients (P<0.001). Significant differences were observed between group A and B, and A and C (both, P<0.001).

Peripheral blood of 109 of 117 patients with less than 30 SRA index at hospitalization were examined repeatedly, and SRA index of all 109 cases exceeded 30 within 2 to 3 days after hospitalization. The maximum SRA indices of STEMI patients during 3 days after hospitalization were significantly higher than those of STEMI patients at hospitalization.

The SRA index of 60 of 79 UA (75.9%) cases were 30 or more at hospitalization. The differences in the SRA index were not significant between STEMI and UA (Table 2, P=0.218, Welch's test).

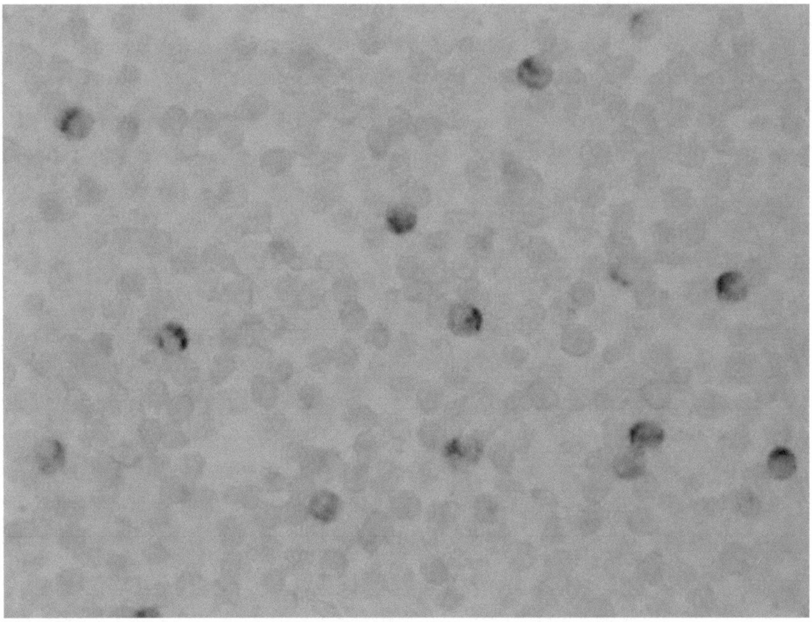

Fig. 16. Scavenger receptor A positive cells in peripheral blood (SRA index: 187/10HPFs).

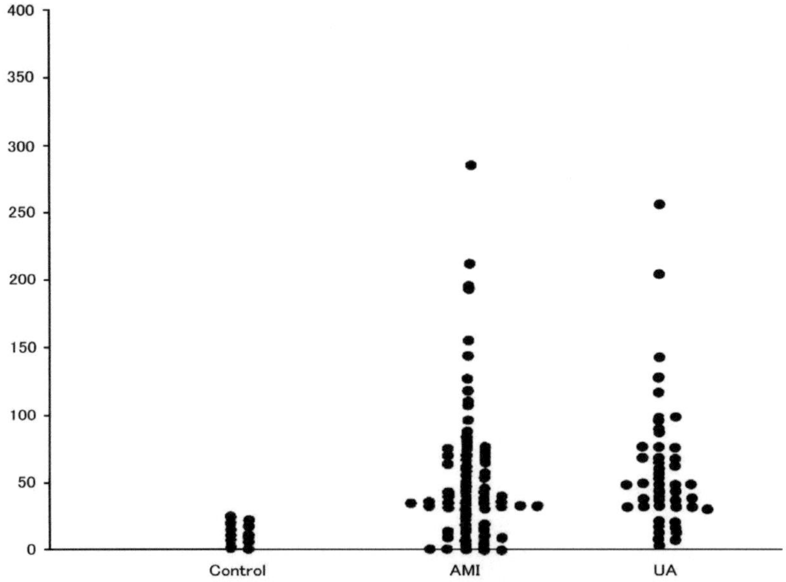

Table 2. The scattered plots of the SRA index of controls, AMI, UA.

9. Differentiation of SRA$^+$ cells in PB

It is reported that freshly isolated blood monocytes were negative for SRA [25]; however, a few reports have indicated that SRA$^-$monocytes can differentiate into SRA$^+$ cells in PB by various stimuli [32, 33, 34]. SRA$^+$ cells were observed in all control cases. We , therefore, surmised that a small number of SRA$^-$ monocytes differentiated into SRA$^+$ cells in PB of healthy men and women by various stimuli. Fuster et al. classified the progression of coronary atherosclerotic diseases into five phases [35]. Phase 1 is represented by a small plaque that is present in most people under the age of 30 years. We set the normal upper limit of the SRA index at 30 [27], since plaque disruption, fissure, or erosion and RMT might not develop in healthy men and women in their 20s, and SRA index of these control cases ranged 1 to 24 (mean±SD=11.1±7.5).
We considered two possibilities on the pathophysiologic mechanisms underlying the differentiation of SRA$^+$ cells in patients with STEMI (myocardial infarction or plaque disruption, fissure or erosion). With the recognition that atherosclerosis is an inflammatory process [36], h-CRP has been evaluated as a potential tool for predicting the risk of AMI [37, 38, 39], and CK and CK-MB are good markers of myocardial injury. Macrophages are known to arise from monocytes, and become larger over twice as large as monocytes with differentiation. SRA$^-$monocytes became positive for SRA after 5 days in culture with M-CSF [40], and differentiated into large macrophages by 10 days [41]. Cytokines elevate in PB after insult [42]. Myocardial infarction is severe insult, so SRA$^+$ cells may increase in PB as a result of myocardial infarction. However, differentiation of SRA$^+$ cells in PB was not considered to result from myocardial injury, because there was no correlation between SRA indices and CK, CK-MB, and h-CRP.
The differentiation of SRA$^-$ monocytes into SRA$^+$ macrophages was believed to take place in atherosclerotic lesions by stimulation of M-CSF [21-24]. Disruption, fissure or erosion of an atherosclerotic plaque is generally recognized as a proximate event responsible for the development of the ACS [8-12]. The SRA index of the patients with less than 30 SRA index at hospitalization rapidly increased, and the SRA index of all these STEMI patients exceeded 30 within 2 to 3 days. We therefore surmised that SRA$^-$ monocytes might differentiate into SRA$^+$ cells as the result of exposure of plaque content that contains M-CSF to the blood stream.

10. Coronary occlusion

Examinations of aspirated material have focused on thrombus age [31, 43, 44]. Rittersma et al. classified thrombi into 3 groups: fresh (< 1 day), lytic (1 to 5 days), and organized thrombus (> 5 days) [31]. However it is hard to understand the constituents of thrombus by this classification. PT and some MT seem to correspond to fresh thrombus, and some MT and FT to lytic thrombus. PT was detected in 387 (99.5 %) of 389 patients, MT in 269 cases (69.2 %) and FT in 57 (14.7 %). SRA$^+$ cells infiltrated into all FT and 147 (54.6 %) of 269 MT, but not PT. These SRA$^+$ cells in PB were thought to be infiltrated into MT, since SRA$^+$ cells infiltrated in MT along the boundary zone between PT and MT (luminal side of the coronary artery). From these findings, PT was considered to be most fresh thrombus, and infarct-related coronary artery was totally and rapidly occluded by the formation of PT.
Using their computer-assisted extracorporeal-perfusion system, Badimon et al.[45] and Lassila et al.[46] found that platelet deposition increased significantly with increased stenosis. Sudden

coronary occlusion was often preceded by a period of plaque instability and thrombus formation, initiated days or weeks before the onset of symptoms [15-18], and total coronary occlusion of the infarct-related artery always results from the growth of RMT [44, 47 - 49]. Considering these reports and the histopathological findings of thrombi, PT was thought to be formed abruptly as a result of severe coronary stenosis due to sudden extrusion of atheromatous debris into vessel lumen in 43 group A patients with a SRA index less than 30 at hospitalization, and due to gradual growth of RMT in group B and C patients. The percentage of patients with SRA index more than 30 at hospitalization was significantly lower in group A patients than other groups of patients. This finding seemed to support the theory, since the SRA index exceeded 30 about 2 days after plaque disruption[27].

11. The fate of platelet thrombus

RMT was observed in 300 of 389 STEMI cases. Meshwork of fibrin was observed in RMT, so RMT was thought not to be fragile. RMT predisposes patients to recurrent thrombotic vessel occulusion[15-17], and plaque disruption, fissure or erosion with thrombus contributes to plaque development and progression[18]. Gradual growth of RMT plays an important role on the increased stenosis of coronary artery, and total occlusion of coronary artery by platelet thrombus.

Meshwork of fibrin was not contained in platelet thrombus. Consequently, platelet thrombus was considered to be very fragile. Fragments of platelet thrombus were frequently observed in mixed thrombus and numerous emboli of fragments of platelet thrombus were observed in small arteries and capillaries at the distal portion of the infarct related artery of autopsy cases. Platelet thrombus was considered to repeat formation and disintegration with the gradual growth and lysis of RMT, and numerous emboli of fragments of platelet thrombus at the distal portion of the infarct related artery may repeatedly injure cardiac myocytes .

12. SRA index and vulnerable plaque

Disruption, fissure, or erosion of an atherosclerotic plaque, with RMT has a fundamental role in the pathogenesis of acute coronary syndromes (ACS) [8-12].

In general, in case of AMI, a direct relationship between the onset of plaque disruption and acute transmural ischemia is assumed; however pathological studies of autopsy [13, 14] and thrombectomy [18, 31, 43] materials indicated that plaque disruption, fissure or erosion with RMT remain clinically silent days or weeks before the fatal event. The SRA index of the patents with less than 30 SRA index at hospitalization exceed normal level within 2 to 3 days. These findings indicated that SRA index rapidly increases in AMI patients after plaque disruption, erosion, or fissure. A SRA index more than 30 was observed in patients with multiple organ dysfunction syndrome[50]. Therefore, SRA index more than 30 was not a specific finding to ACS. SRA index exceeded 30 in 230 of 300 (76.7 %) cases with RMT and 46 of 89 (51.7 %) cases with PT alone, and 276 of all 389 cases at hospitalization. Thrombus was identified in all 276 patients with a SRA index more than 30 at hospitalization. PT was detected in 99.3 % and RMT in 83.3 % of these patients. SRA index did not exceed 30 in healthy control cases. SRA index of these 276 patients was surmised to exceed 30 before the onset of STEMI. The SRA indices of 75.9 % of unstable angina cases were more than 30 at hospitalization [27]. The pathophysiological substrate of the unstable angina is now considered to be common with the acute myocardial infarction. We, therefore, believe that the abnormal increase of SRA^+ cells is considered to be a useful finding to gather the presence of disrupted or fissured or eroded plaque, PT, and probably RMT in patients with UA.

13. References

[1] Keeley EC, Boura JA, Grines CL. Primary angioplasty versus intravenous thrombolytic therapy for acute myocardial infarction: a quantitative review of 23 randomised trials. *Lancet* 2003;361:13-20.

[2] Freemantle N, Cleland J, Young P, Mason J, Harrison J. Beta blockede after myocardial infarction: systematic review and meta regression analysis. *BMJ* 1999;318:1730-1737.

[3] Latini R, Tognoni G, Maggioni AP, et al. For Angiotensin-converting Enzyme Inhibitor Myocardial Infarction Collaborative Group.Clinical sffects of early angiotensin-converting enzyme inhibitor treatment for acute myocardial infarction are similar in the presence and absence of aspirin: systematic overview of indivifual data from96712 randomized patients. *J A Coll Cardiol* 2000;35:1801-07.

[4] Schwartz GG, Olsson AG, Ezekowitz MD, et al. Effects of atovastatin on early recurrent ischemic events in acute coronary syndromes: the MIRACL study: a randomized controlled trial. *JAMA* 2001;285:1711-18.

[5] Antithrombotic trialists' Collaboration. Collaborative meta-analysis of randomized trials of antiplatelet therapy for prevention of death, myocardial infarction, and stroke in high risk patients. *BMJ* 2002;324:71-86.

[6] Gibbons RJ, BaladyGJ, Bricker JT, et al. ACC/AHA 2002 guideline update for exercise testing: summary article: a report of the American College of Cardiology/American Heart Association Task Force on Practice Guidelines (Committee to Update the 1997 Exercise Testing Guidelines). *J Am Coll Cardiol* 2002;40:1531-40.

[7] Kumar A, Cannon CP. Acute coronary syndromes: Diagnosis and management, Part II. *Mayo Clin Proc* 2009;84:1021-36.

[8] Falk E. Plaque rupture with severe pre-existing stenosis precipitating coronary thrombosis : characteristics of coronary atherosclerotic plaques underlying fatal occulusive thrombi. *Br Heart J* 1983;50:127-34.

[9] Davies MJ, Thomas AC. Plaque fissuring— the cause of acute myocardial infarction, sudden ischemic death, and crescendo angina. *Br Heart J* 1985;53:363-73.

[10] Richardson PD, Davies MJ, Born GVR. Influence of plaque configuration and stress distribution on fissuring of coronary atherosclerotic plaques. *Lancet* 1989;2:941-4.

[11] Burke AP, Farb A, Malcom GT, Liang Y-H, Smialek J, Virmani R. Coronary risk factors and plaque morphology in men with coronary disease who died suddenly. *N Engl J Med* 1997;336:1276-82.

[12] Burke AP, Farb A, Malcom GT, Liang Y-H, Smialek J, Virmani R. Effect of risk factors on the mechanism of acute thrombosis and sudden coronary death in women. *Circulation* 1998;97:2110-6.

[13] Falk E. Unstable angina with fatal outcome: Dynamic coronary thrombosis leading to infarction and/or sudden death: autopsy evidence of recurrent mural thrombosis with peripheral embolization culminating in total vascular occlusion. *Circulation* 1985;71:699-708.

[14] Mailhac A, Badimon JJ, Fallon JT, et al. Effect of an eccentric severe stenosis on fibrin(ogen) deposition on severely damaged vessel wall in arterial thrombosis. Relative contribution of fibrin(ogen) and platelets. *Circulation* 1994;90:988-96.

[15] Hackett D, Davie G, Chierchia S, Maseri A. Intermittent coronary occlusion in acute myocardial infarction: value of combined thrombolytic and vasodilatory therapy. *N Engl J Med* 1987;317:1055-9.

[16] Davies SW, Marchant B, Lyons JP, et al. Irregular coronary lesion morphology after thrombolysis predicts early clinical instability. *J Am Coll Cardol* 1991;18:669-74.

[17] Ohman EM, Topol EJ, Califf RM, et al. An analysis of the cause of early mortality after administration of thrombolytic therapy. *Cor Art Dis* 1993;4:957-64.

[18] Burke AP, Kolodgie FD, Farb A, et al. Healed plaque rupture and sudden coronary death. Evidence that subclinical rupture has a role in plaque progression. *Circulation* 2001;103:934-40.

[19] MacNeill BD, Lowe HC, Takano M, Valentin F, Ik-Kyung J. Intravascular modalities for detection of vulnerable plaque. *Arterioscler Thromb Vasc Biol* 2003;23:1333-42.

[20] Davies MJ, Bland JM, Hangartner JRW, Angelini A, Thomas AC. Factors influencing the presence or absence of acute coronary artery thrombi in sudden ischemic death. *Eur Heart J* 1989;10:203-8.

[21] Rajavashisth TB, Andalibi A, Territo MC, et al. Induction of endothelial cell expression of granulocyte and macrophage colony-stimulating factors by modified low-density lipoproteins. *Nature* 1990;344:254-7.

[22] Liao F, Andalibi A, Qiao J-H, Allayee H, Fogelman AM, Lusis AJ. Genetic evidence for a common pathway mediating oxidative stress, inflammatory gene induction, and aortic fatty streak formation in mice. *J Clin Invest* 1994;94:877-84.

[23] Clinton SK, Underwood R, Hayes L, Sherman ML, Kufe DW, Libby P. Macrophage colony-stimulating factor gene expression in vascular cells and in experimental and human atherosclerosis. *Am J Pathol* 1992;140:301-16.

[24] Rosenfeld ME, Ylä-Herttula S, Lipton BA, Ord VA, Witztum JL, Steinberg D. Macrophage colony-stimulating factor mRNA and protein in atherosclerotic lesions of rabitts and humans. *Am J Pathol* 1992;140:291-300.

[25] Takeya M, Tomokiyo R, Jinnouchi K, et al. Macrophage scavenger receptor: Structure, function and tissue distribution. *Acta Histochem. Cytochem* 1999;32:47-51.

[26] Kunjathoor VV, Febbraio M, Poderz EA, et al. Scavenger receptor A-I/II and CD36 are the principal receptors responsible for the uptake of modified low density lipoprotein leading to lipid loading in macrophages. *J Biol Chem* 2002;277:49982-8.

[27] Emura I, Usuda H, Fujita T, Ebe K, Nagai T. Increase of scavenger receptor-A- positive monocytes in patients with acute coronary syndromes. Pathology International 2007;57:502-508.

[28] Emura I, Usuda H, Fujita T, Ebe K, Nagai T. Scavenger receptor A index anfd coronary thrombus in patients with acute ST elevation myocardial infarction. Pathology International 2011;61:351-355.

[29] Iwao Emura. High incidence of apoptosis in peripheral blood of myelodysplastic syndrome patients determined by Papanicolaou-stained preparations. *Laboratory Hematology* 2003;9:42-6.

[30] Rittersma SZH, van der Wal AC, Koch KT, et al. Plaque instability frequently occurs day or weeks before occlusive coronary thrombosis. A pathological thrombectomy study in primary precutaneous coronary intervention. *Circulation* 2005; 111: 1160-5.
[31] Konishi Y, Okamura M, Konishi N, et al. Enhanced gene expression of scavenger receptor in peripheral blood monocytes from patients on cuprophane haemodialysis. *Nephrol Dial transplant* 1997;12:1167-72.
[32] Villanova JG, Lucena JLD, Arcás NF, Engel AR. Increased expression of scavenger receptor type I gene in human peripheral blood from hyperlipidemic patients determined by quantitative additive RT-PCR. *Biochimica et Biophysica Acta* 1996;1300:135-41.
[33] Geng Y-j, Kodama T, Hansson GK. Differential expression of scavenger receptor isoforms during monocyte-macrophage differentiation and foam cell formation. *Arterioscler Thromb* 1994;14:798-806.
[34] Fuster V, Badimon L, Badimon JJ, Cheserbo JH. The pathogenesis of coronary artery disease and the acute coronary syndromes. *N Engl J Med* 1992;326:242-50.
[35] Ross R. Atherosclerosis —an inflammatory disease. *New Engl J Med* 1999;340:115-26.
[36] Kuller LH, Tracy RP, Shaten J, Meilahn EN. Relationship of C-reactive protein and coronary heart disease in the MRFIT nested case-control study : Multiple Risk Factor Intervention Trial. *Am J Epidemiol* 1996;144:537-47.
[37] Koenig W, Sund M, Frohlich M. et al. C-rfeactive protein, a sensitive marker of inflammation, predicts future risk of coronary heart disease in initially healthy middle-aged men : results from the MONICA(monitoring Trends and Determinants in Cardiovascular Disease) Augsberg Cohort Study, 1984 to 1992. *Circulation* 1999;99:237-42.
[38] Libby P, Ridker PM, Maseri A. Inflammation and atherosclerosis. *Circulation* 2002;105:35-1143.
[39] Naito M, Kodama T, Matsumoto A, Doi T, Takahashi K. Tissue distribution, intracellular localization, and in Vitro expression of Bovine macrophage scavenger receptor. *Am J Pathol* 1991;139:1411-23
[40] Young DA, Lowe LD, Clark SC. Comparison of the effects of IL-3, granulocyte-macrophage colony- stimulating factor, and macrophage colony-stimulating factor in supporting monocytes differentiation in culture. *J Immunol* 1990;145:607-15.
[41] Sakamoto K, Arakawa H, Mita S, et al. Elevation of circulating interleukin 6 after surgery: Factors influencing the serum level. Cytokine 194;6:181-186.
[42] Henriques de Gouveia R, van der Wal AC, van der Loos CM, Becker AE. Sudden unexpected death in young adults.Discrepancies between initiation of acute plaque complications and the onset of acute coronary death. *Eur Heart J* 2002; 23: 1433-40.
[43] Murakami T, Mizuno S, Takahashi Y, et al. Intracoronary aspiration thrombectomy for acute myocardial infarction. *Am J Cardiol* 1998; 82: 839-44.
[44] Badimon L, Badimon JJ. Mechanism of arterial thrombosis in nonparallel streamlines: platelet thrombi grow on the apex of stenotic severely injured vessel wall. Experimental study in the pig model. *J Clin Invest* 1989; 84: 1134-44.
[45] Lassila R, Badimon JJ, Vallabhajosula S, Badimon L. Dynamic monitoring of platelet deposition on severely damaged vessel wall in flowing blood. Effects of different stenoses on thrombus growth. *Arteriosclerosis* 1990; 10: 306-15.

[46] Nagata Y, Usuda K, Uchiyama A, Uchikoshi M, sekiguchi Y, Kato H, Miwa A, Ishikawa T. Characteristics of the Pathological images of coronary artery thrombi according to the infarct-related coronary artery in acute myocardial infarction. *Circ J* 2004; 68: 308-14.
[47] Ruggeri ZM. Platelets in atherothrombosis. *Nat Med* 2002; 8: 1227-34.
[48] Gawaz M. Role of platelets in coronary thrombosis and reperfusion of ischemic myocardium. *Cardiovasc Res* 2004; 61: 498-511.
[49] Emura I, Usuda H. Histopathological and cytological examination of autopsy cases with multiple organ dysfunction syndromes. *Pathology International* 2010;60:443-51.

4

Evolution of Biochemical Diagnosis of Acute Coronary Syndrome – Impact Factor of High Sensitivity Cardiac Troponin Assays

Amparo Galán[1], Josep Lupón[2] and Antoni Bayés-Genis[2]
[1]Biochemical Service
[2]Cardiology Service,
España

1. Introduction

In patients with acute thoracic pain and non-conclusive acute myocardial infarction electrocardiogram (non-STEMI), the biochemical diagnosis is an essential tool for its correct treatment. The study of the chosen biomarker for cardiac injury has raised interest during decades. The appearance of immunoassays to assess cardiac troponin I or T has reached great improvements in the diagnosis, evolution and prognosis of the Acute Coronary Syndrome (ACS), as well as in risk stratification of these patients and in patients with chronic cardiac diseases as heart failure or cardiomyopathies. Regarding the analytical sensitivity of the methods that evaluate cardiac troponin I or T these improvements have made possible to measure accurately very tiny seric concentrations of the protein (high sensitivity troponin) (hs-Tn). This fact, being positive in principle sometimes induces to reconsider if tiny seric concentrations of isolated troponin I or T are not due to acute myocardial infarction but to a less severe source which affects the myocardiocite, this will oblige us to assess the clinical presentation in depth.

2. Diagnostic criteria of acute coronary syndrome – Biochemical markers – History background and evolution

Thoracic pain is one of the most frequent reasons for attending the emergengy room at hospitals. About 10% of these patients will be diagnosed Acute Myocardial Infarction. The clinical syntoms and the electrocardiogram can not always differentiate between a patient suffering from acute myocardial infarction or an angina. Electrocardiogram is only diagnostic in 40% of the patients. That is why in processes of acute coronary ischemia different from infarction with rising of segment ST, (infarction no Q or without rising of ST, unstable angina), the use of biochemical markers can be the only criteria to identify the existence of myocardial necrosis, being necessary for infarction diagnosis, treatment, evolution and prognosis.
The biochemical diagnosis of acute coronary syndrome has had remarkable changes over the last few years. During years the enzymatic profile (creatine kinase, activity of the isoenzime CKMB, aspartate aminotransferase and lactate deshidrogenase) has been the

biochemical method chosen for the diagnosis of acute coronary ischemia. The criteria of the WHO (WHO 1979) was followed until 1999, being the catalytic activity of creatine kinase MB isoenzyme (CKMB) the marker chosen. In fact, according to the WHO to reach the diagnosis of acute myocardial infarction (AMI) two of the following three criterias must be fulfilled: precordial pain with evolution longer than 30 minutes, specific electrocardiograph changes and elevation of catalityc activity of creatine kinase (CK) and its isoenzime MB (CKMB).

However, during the 1990s more sensitive and specific cardiac markers are marketed and beginning to be used in order to detect the disease, such as the protein concentration of isoenzime MB (CKMBmass) or Troponin.

In September 2000 the criteria which defines acute myocardial infarction (AMI) was reviewed and a consensus document was published *(European Society of Cardiology/ American College of Cardiology Committe 2000)* between The Joint European Society of Cardiology and The American College of Cardiology where they give great importance to the alterations of cardiac markers: Troponin or CKMBmass (no activity) for the diagnosis of the disease, together with symptoms of ischemia or alterations in the electrocardiogram (ECG). In fact, the main criteria to establish the diagnosis of acute myocardial infarction is to verify the gradual release of troponin or CKMBmass, (typical curve of fast rising-descent), together with at least one of the following alterations: a) ischemic syntoms; b) development of pathological Q waves in ECG; c) indicative changes of ischemia (variations of the segment ST,T)

2.1 Cardiact troponin: Biochemical bases

Troponin is one of the myofibrilar proteins of the skeletal muscle and its function is to regulate muscular contraction in relation with calcium ion (Figure 1). The thick filament of the muscle is formed by myosin and the thin filament by actin, troponin and tropomyiosin. Only actin and myosin are contractile proteins; troponin and tropomyosin are regulatory. Troponin is composed by three peptides called troponin T, troponin I and troponin C. Troponin T is regulatory of tropomyosin; troponin I (inhibitory), inhibits the union actin-myosin; troponin C is the receptor of calcium so when linking calcium disappears the inhibition of troponin I on tropomyosin forming the shuttles actin-myosin and activating the contraction.

The theory currently accepted for the mechanism of muscular contraction involves the ATP-asic activity (two molecules of ADP and inorganic phosphorus) present in the heads of myosin (figure 1). In repose myosin does not contact actin as the sarcplasm does not have enough calcium to produce the contraction, and calcium regulates the ATP-asic activity. During the contraction when receiving the nervous signal calcium is released to the sarcoplasm, this calcium joins immediately to the centers of union of calcium to troponin, inducing a structure change which allows the heads of actin and myosin to link forming an angle of about 90ºC. The release of the phosphorus molecule of the complex actin-myosin-ADP involves a structure change which makes actin slide (power strike) and adopt a 45ºC angle on myosin. This movement produces at the same time a release of ADP. For each actin myosin union provoked by the union of two calcium molecules to troponin C, at least two ATP molecules are needed and to carry two calcium molecules from the cytosol to reticule an ATP molecule is required (Galán A. 2000).

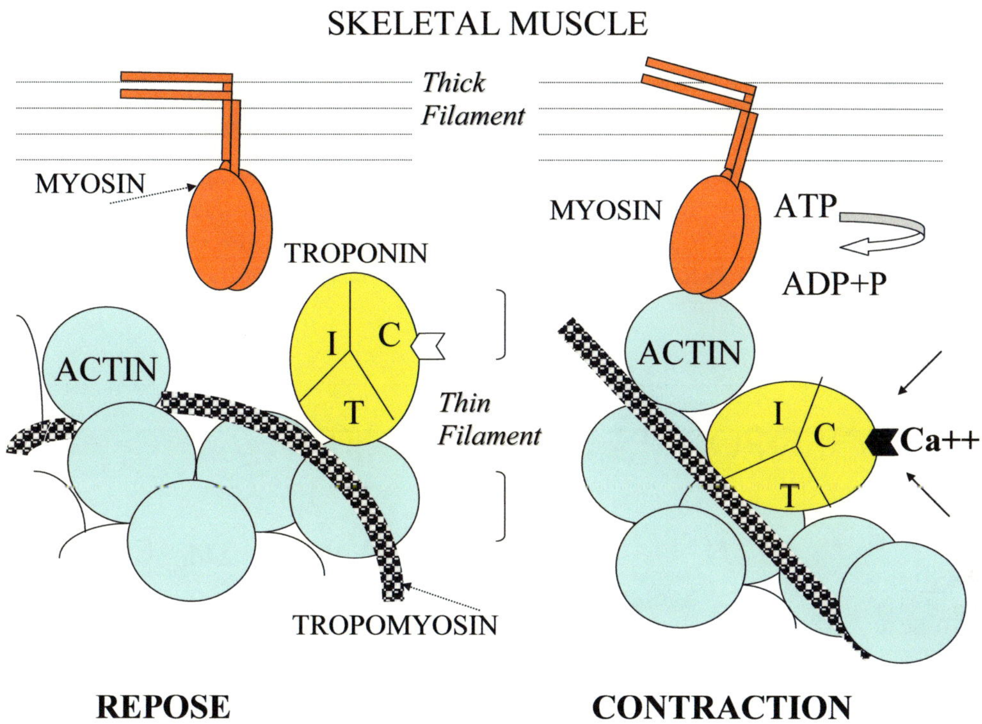

ADP: Adenosin diphosphate
ATP: Adenosin Triphosphate

Fig. 1. Scheme of the process of muscular contraction and involvement of myofibrilar and contractile proteins of the skeletal muscle (Galán A. 2000).

The different kinds of muscles of the organism present different characteristics of contraction, this is due to the structural differences genetically determined in some myofibrilar proteins. Three isoforms have been described for troponin I and T which present structural differences codified by genes located in three different crhomosomes. So for troponin I (figure 2) there are two isoforms of the skeletal muscle one of slow contraction and another one fast and a specific shape of the cardiac muscle. The cardiac isoform has 31 suplementary aminoacids at the N-terminal end of the polypeptide chain and besides it differs from skeletal isoforms as it shows in the tracts of the primary sequences of the protein, a heterogeneity of 69% for the central tract (residues 30 to 110) and 44% for the terminal tract (110-215) which seems to be more stable because of the protection carried out by the subunit C terminal. Troponin T also shows three isoforms codified by genes located in three different chromosomes, one of them is specific for myocardium. The myocardial isoform has an elevated polymorphism provoking isoforms which express in injured myocardial tissue, adult and fetal. Troponin C, however, is identical in both kinds of muscle. (Galán A. 2004).

This fact confers troponin the qualification of cardiac marker of maximum cardiospecificity unlike creatine kinase, creatine kinase MB and myoglobine which co-express in the skeletal muscle and in the myocardium. Some specific anti-bodies have been patented in opposition to troponin T and cardiac Troponin I so that they can be recognised by specific immunoassays. Troponin forms (I and T) of skeletal and cardiac muscle: a) Are codified by different genes; b) Have structures which are clearly differentiated; c) Are recognised by specific immunoassays.

That is why the assessment of troponin T or troponin I favours the specific recognition of myocardial damage even in the presence of concomitant skeletal muscle damage. Therefore only troponin molecules fulfil the cardiospecificity criteria. This cardiospecificity guarantees that the detection of a cardiac troponin molecule in plasma is indicative of myocardial injury.

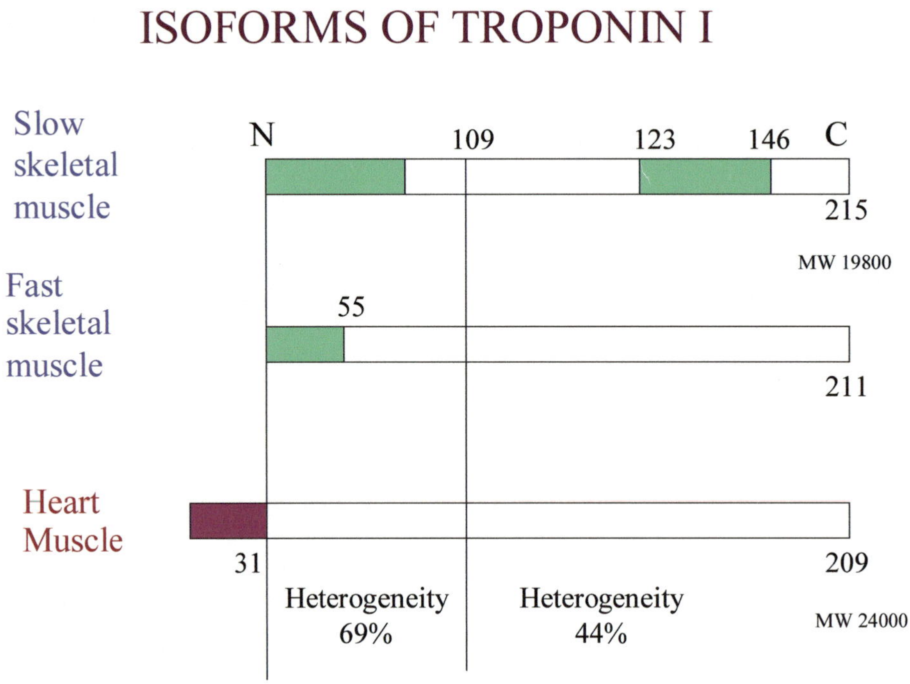

Fig. 2. Isoforms of Troponin I: In the figure we can see two isoforms of skeletal muscle, one of slow contraction and another one fast and a specific form of cardiac muscle. The cardiac isoform has 31 suplementary aminoacids at the end N-terminal of the polypeptide chain, besides it differs from skeletal isoforms as it shows in the tracts of the primary sequence of the protein a heterogeneity of 69% for the central tract (residues 30 to 110) and 44% for the terminal tract (110-215) which seems to be more stable because of the protection carried out by the subunit C terminal (Galän A 2004).

We confirmed the absence of crossed reactions (Galán A. 2002) for an Immunoassay Troponin I (cat. nº RF421 Dade Behring) using the Dimension RxL automatic analyzer (Dade Behring, Newark, Delaware, USA). The cardiospecificity of troponin I was verified using myocardial and skeletal muscle (quadriceps, biceps) tissue. Troponin I was measured in myofibrillar and cytosolic fraction. The absence of troponin I in skeletal muscle was corroborated: the concentration of troponin I in biceps and quadriceps was not detected (< 1% of the values obtained in myocardial tissue). The troponin I concentration in the myofibrillar fraction of cardiac tissue was 7.2 mg/g protein and only 4% of total troponin content was found in the soluble fraction (figure 3).

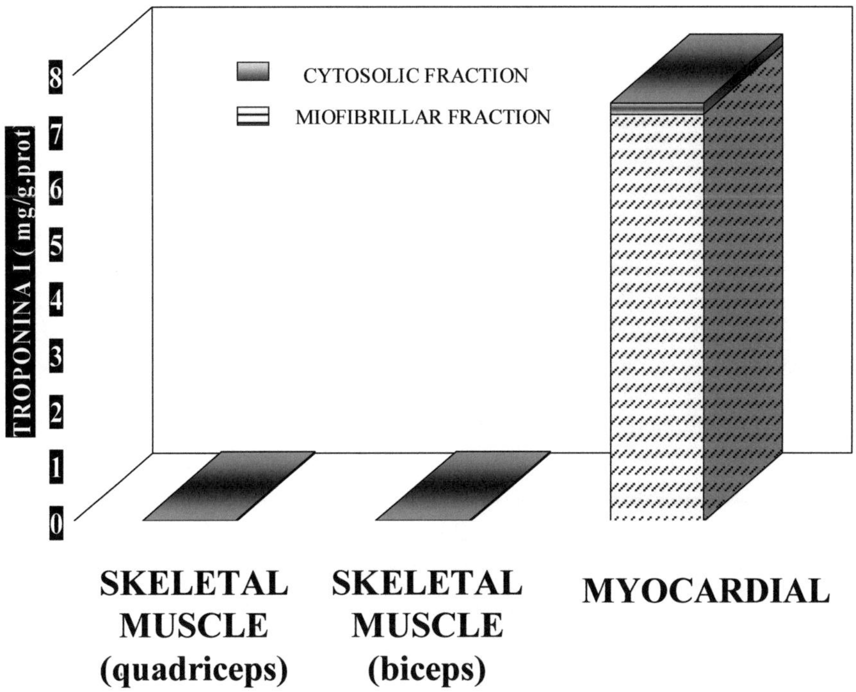

Fig. 3. Tissue specificity for the troponin I method. The figure shows the lack of crossreactivity of troponin I with skeletal muscle. No troponin I concentrations in the crude extract of biceps and quadriceps were detected. The troponin I concentration in the myofibrillar fraction of cardiac tissue was 7.2 mg/g protein and in the cytosolic fraction 0.3 mg/g protein. (Galán A. 2002)

This fact helps to understand the double diagnostic window of troponin: The small fraction dissolved in cytoplasma of the cardiomyocites, which has relative precociousness (>6 hours) in the detection of cellular injuries (similar to other cytoplasmatic proteins) and the majority fraction which is the one linked to tropomyosin complex in structure and only appears in plasma after cellular irreversible damage and after 40 hours from occurring and remains elevated till 10-15 days after the injury, being then used as late marker of myocardial necrosis (figure 4)

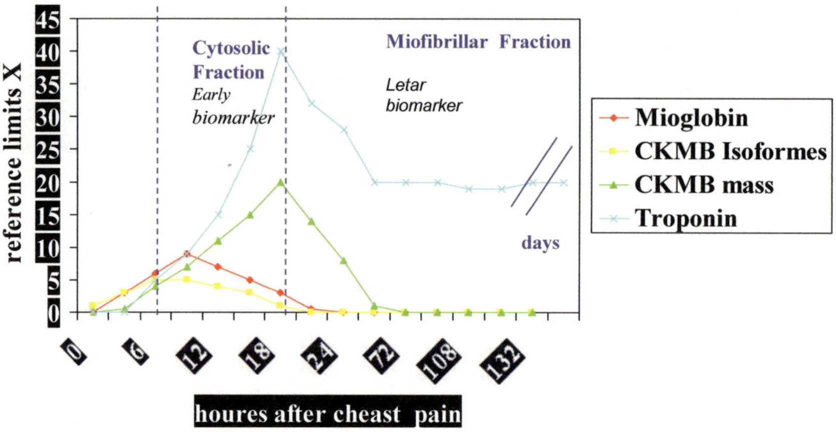

Fig. 4. Plasmatic levels of cardiac markers after ischemic process: Double diagnostic window of Troponin

2.2 Comparative characteristics of troponin with other cardiac markers

Myoglobine and CKMB are located in the cellular cytoplasma which favours a fast exit of the molecule out of the cell and therefore an early appearance in systemic circulation. Troponin has a small fraction in cellular cytoplasma but most of it is found in deep tissue, as part of tropomyosin complexes. On the other hand either myoglobin or CK-MB co-express in skeletal muscle so they do not have the cardiospecificity which troponin shows (Table 1).

CARDIAC BIOMARKER	TISSUE LOCATION	MOLECULA R WEIGHT (dalton)	CELLULAR LOCATION
MIOGLOBIN	Heart muscle *Skeletal muscle*	17.800	Cytosol
CK-MB	Heart muscle *Skeletal muscle*	80.000	Cytosol
Cardiac TROPONIN I	Heart muscle	23.500	3% Cytosol 97% Tropomyosin Complex
Cardiac TROPONIN T	Heart muscle	33.000	6 % Cytosol 94% Tropomyosin Complex

Table 1. Molecular Weight and cellular and tissue location.

Myoglobin and CK isoforms are the earliest markers and with the fastest elimination. CKMB is cytosolic but it has higher PM than Myoglobin so it takes it longer to appear and clear the plasma. Troponin, due to its double location has a wide diagnostic window (from 6 hours to 10-12 days) (Table 2)

CARDIAC MARKER	Home elevation after AMI (houres)	peak elevation (houres)	Return Normal Value (houres)
CKMB ISOFORMS	2-4	6-8	18-24houres
MIOGLOBIN	2-3	6-9	18-24houres
CK-MB	4-6	10-18	1-2 days
TROPONIN I	>6	10-24	5-10 days
TROPONIN T	>6	10-24	5-12 days

Table 2. Cardiac marker Kinetics.

Cardiac troponin has a small fraction (6% for T and 3% for I) dissolved in cytoplasma of the cardiomyocites. This confers the early detection of cellular damage similar to that of other cytoplasmatic proteins, even better than the isoenzime MB of creatine kinase because its molar mass is lower (33.000 g/mol para la T y 23.500 g/mol para la I). Nevertheless, the majority fraction, approximately 90%, is linked in structure to the tropomyosin complex and only appears in plasma after irreversible cellular damage and 40 hours after occurring. Besides, as it remains in plasma for a long time it can also be used as late marker of myocardial necrosis.

Because of all of this, the excellent cardiospecificity and sensitivity of troponin for the detection of myocardial necrosis, together with its wide diagnostic window (from 6-12h to 5-10 days for troponin I and from 6-12 hours to 5-15 days for troponin T) have revolutionised in the latest years the approach of patients with acute coronary syndrome as a lot of studies have demonstrated its usefulness in the diagnosis of myocardial necrosis as well as in the prognostic stratification of these patients in the first hours of evolution.

2.3 Problem of the methods to assess troponin. Solutions taken. Guidelines for clinical practice 1999 and 2001

In the beginning of working with troponin, either physician or biochemists wondered : Is troponin so useful?, Which troponin method is the right one? (Troponin T or Troponin I), What cut-off must we choose?, What marker or markers must be selected?, What intervals must be used?

At present there are black spots in the analytical management of the methods which assess troponin as the election for cut-off or the lack of standardization of the different methods available in the market (Wu Alan HB 2001), (Apple FS, 2001) and the low analytical sensitivity of the methods among others. These factors may cause confusion in the election of the method as well as in the clinical interpretation of the results (Table 3).

- **The choice of cutoff**
- **Lack of Tn I method's estandarization**
- **Low sensitivity of methods**

↓

These factors may cause confusion in the interpretation of results

Table 3. Technical problems in management troponin methods.

To try to help and encourage us to use troponin, in 1999 appeared the first Guidelines for Clinical Practice in the use of troponin published by the National Academy of Clinical Biochemistry (NACB) to establish analytical and clinical recommendations (Wu AHB 1999) and in 2001 the standardization committee of cardiac markers of the International Federation of Clinical Chemistry (IFCC) opted for troponin as election marker for myocardial necrosis and establishes recommendations of analytical and pre-analitical quality for the assays of Tn, (Panteghini M 2001), encouraging the clinical laboratories to use it and inducing the manufacturers to improve the analytical quality of the methods of assessment of the protein.

An example of the problems was the discrepancy arisen when establishing the cut-offs according to the criteria of the different scientific societies: The NACB suggests using the ROC curves of sensitivity and diagnostic specificity choosing two cut-offs (AMI and myocardial damage) or just one cut-off of myocarid damage. Another alternative is to establish Reference Values in normal population and apply 95th percentile as the National Academy of Clinical Biochemistry (NACB) suggests or 99th percentile as the American College of Cardiology suggests (ACC).

Another important problem is the election of the method (table 4). There is only one method in the market to measure TnT and innumerable methods to measure Tn I. The results of the different methods which measure Tn I are not overlapping, which generates doubts about its election. This variability of results does not occur with TnT methods as there is only one TnT immunoanalisis marketed. However, TnT values are not overlapping either with the methods which measure Troponin I. The molecular structure of TnI favours its heterogeneity. In serum there is variability of forms of TnI by oxidation, phosphorilation or protelisis affecting the interaction with anti-bodies in the assays. Besides, the heterogeneity in plasma of the different forms of troponin is another reason that makes it difficult to select the method. In blood we can find tissular forms of troponin making binary or ternary troponin complexes and free cytosolic forms (Figure 5). Therefore the anti-bodies used in the immunoassays of TnI detect different epitopes in free and complexed forms.

- Heterogeneity in plasma of the different forms of troponin
  - Tissular forms:
    binary troponin complexes (I +C)
    ternary troponin complexes (T+I+C)
  - Free cytosolic forms (I and T)
- There is any reference material to standardize marketed troponin methods
- The antibodies used in the immunoassays of TnI detect different epitopes in free and complexed forms.

Table 4. Reasons difficult the election of the method.

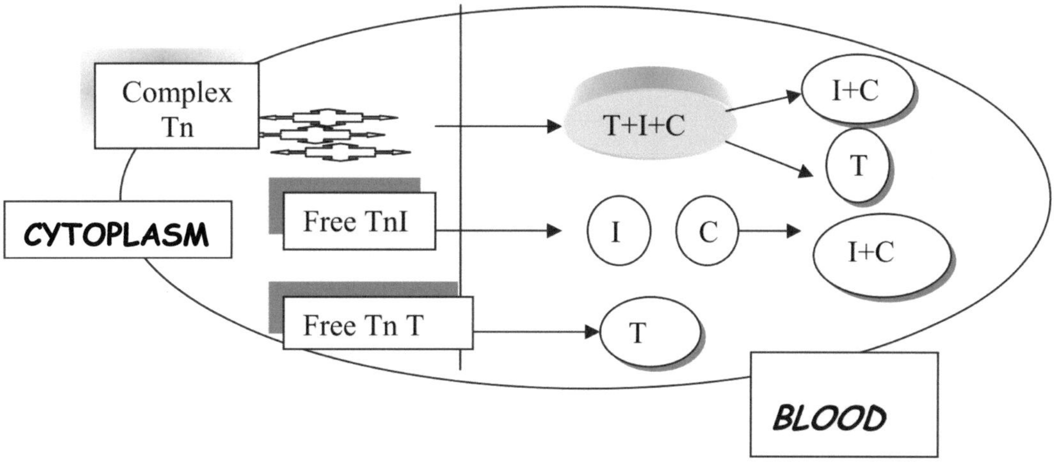

Fig. 5. Scheme of the release in blood of cardiac sub-units of troponin after acute myocardial infarction (according to Wu y cols.) (Galan2004).

So the main problem regarding the methods that assess troponin is the lack of standardization (Figure 6). As a consequence of that there is no transferring of the results among the different commercial methods which assess this protein, what creates confusion due to the analytical and clinical variability of the results. This makes it difficult to choose the best method.

The absence of a material of reference which standardizes the methods means that the results obtained can not be transferred. The methods will have a different cut-off, variations in the limit of the cut-off, as well as imprecisions. On the other hand at low levels close to the reference values the coefficients of variation are elevated.

The most suitable solution in the long run, as it is a difficult matter, to solve this problem is to obtain international reference material, a topic in which scientific societies as IFCC and AACC (American Society of Clinical Chemistry) among others have been working on since 2001. This would standardize the methods and the transferring of the results would be achieved. What would not be unified is the variation of anti-bodies every manufacturer uses. The problem is not completely solved as the reference material obtained, more suitable, was elaborated by a sub-committee of standardization of the AACC in collaboration with the National Institute of Standards and Technology (NIST) and certified in 2006 as standard reference material SRM # 2921. This reference material achieves commutability only with 50% of the commercial methods which assess troponin. In any case, the standardization of the measurement methods of troponin is not finished yet, which involves wide analytical variations noticed among the different immunoassays marketed and appoved by the FDA. (Wu Alan HB 2001).

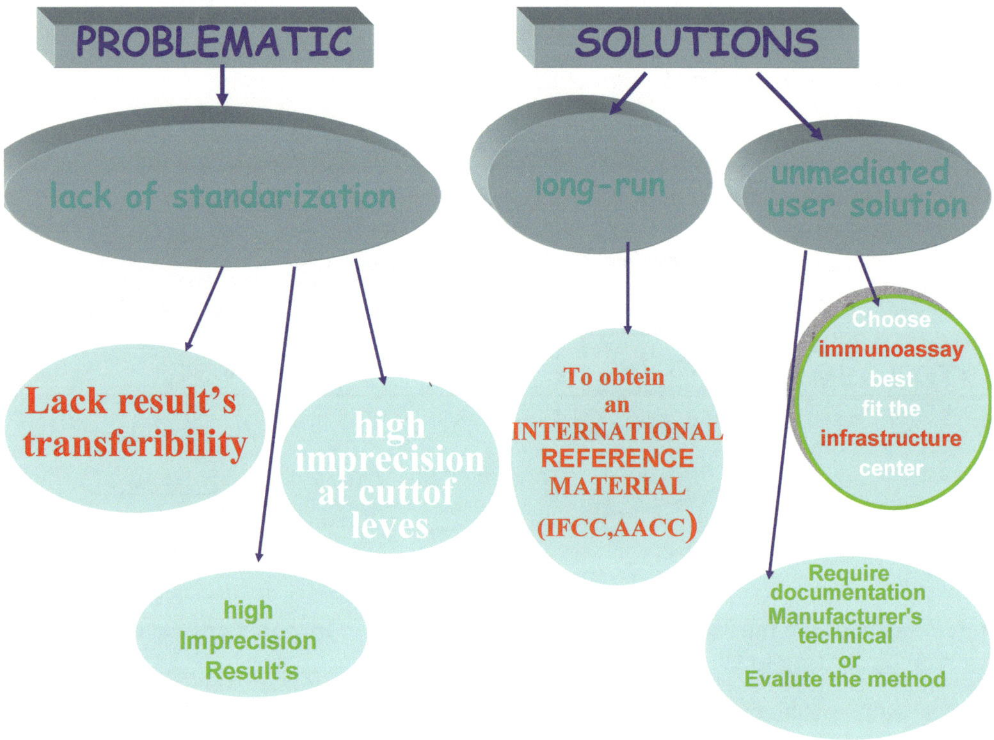

Fig. 6. Analitical problems of the methods which assess troponin: Absence of standardization of the methods.

The immediate solution the user must opt is: Choose the immunoassay which best adapts the infrastructure of the centre (central laboratory, emergency laboratory, or at the patients' side) (bear in mind the analytic system available) and demand the manufacturers the technical documentation about what their method measures. The black spots must be evaluated by the user itself. In case that the imprecision of the chosen method does not fulfil the NABC indications at the point of diagnostic decision, the improvement of the method must be claimed to the manufacturer.

Another important shortage of the initial methods of quantification of troponin is its relative sensitivity (figure 7)

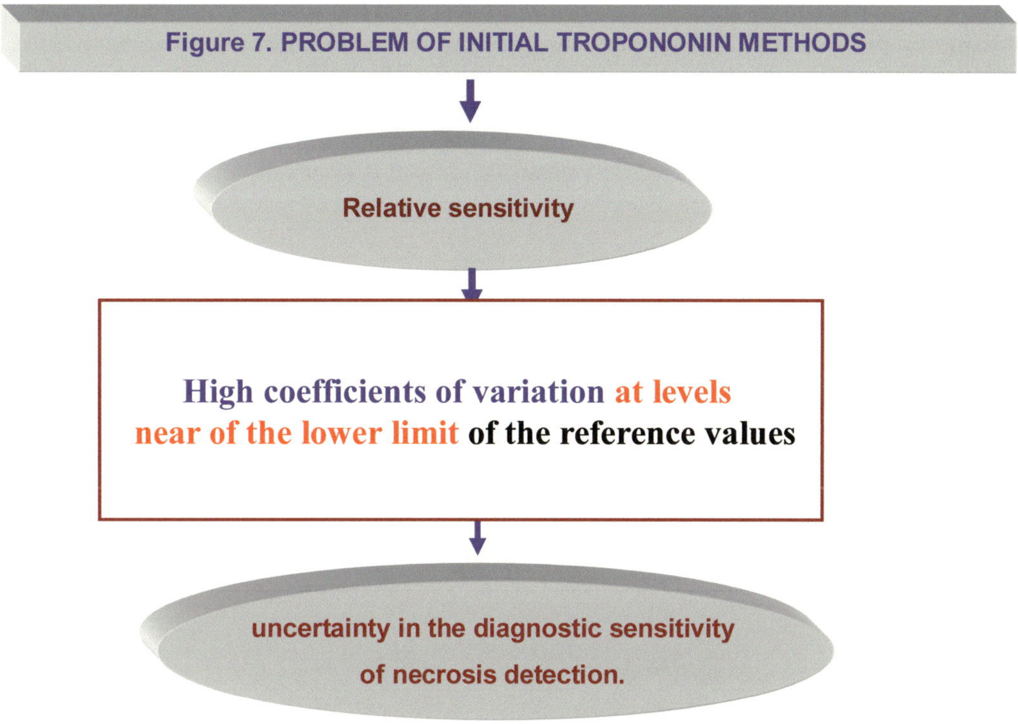

Fig. 7. Problem of initial troponin methods.

In general the methods of assessment of troponin showed elevated values in the limits of detection, limits of quantification far from the reference values, high imprecisions in the limits of quantification, cut-off and reference values, which provokes uncertainty in the diagnostic sensitivity of necrosis detection.

That is why the goals of analytic quality of the different scientific societies have been: Recommend the use of methods to assess troponin with the maximum analytical sensitivity to increase the diagnostic sensitivity of the test in myocardial necrosis as well as avoiding the problems arising because of the lack of standardization of methods.

2.4 Guidelines of clinical practice 2007

In 2007, The Joint ESC/ACF/AHA/ WHF Task Force 2007 (Thygesen 2007) published the last Guidelines of Clinical Practice on the recommendations of the biochemical diagnosis of the detection of ACS and re-define the criteria for Myocardial Infarction establishing a universal definition of AMI. The recommendation (class I) state: In presence of clinical evidence (symptoms or alterations in ECG), concentrations of seric troponin higher than 99th percentile of the interval of reference of the method (with optimal analytic precision CV<10%), are indicative of myocardial necrosis. If troponin is not available the measurement of CKMB-mass is another acceptable alternative. The extraction of blood must be carried out at patient's admission and 6 - 9 hours after admission.

These Guidelines are in accordance with the latest analytic recommendations for the use of troponin published in 2007 by the National Academy of Clinical Biochemistry (NACB) and the Committee of standardization of Cardiac Markers of the IFCC (NACB 2007) which state that: To establish reference values 99th percentile must be applied on a population of at least 120 subjects exempt from myocardial damage. It is required that the imprecision of the method in the 99th percentile chosen is lower or equal to a coefficient of variation of 10%.

3. Methods of new generation: High-sensitivity assays

The recommendations of these Clinical Guidelines have induced the manufacturers to market methods which assess the protein with higher reliability. This has provoked the appearance in the market of a new generation of immunoassays which assess troponin.

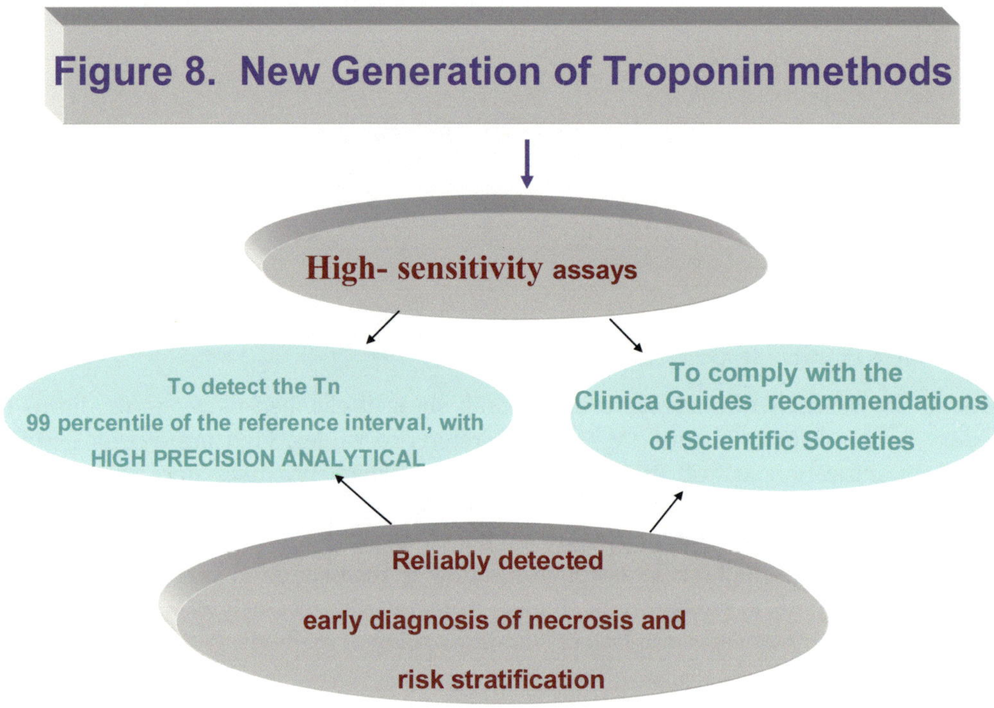

Fig. 8. New generation of troponin methods.

(Figure 8) They are methods with elevated analitic sensitivity and their goal is to detect the 99th percentile of the limit of the detection, quantification limit and normal population with high analitic precision being able to fulfil the recommendations of the scientific societies. The goal of these methods is to be able to know with reliability the early diagnosis of the necrosis and the stratification of myocardial risk. There is a recent publication of Jaffé 2010 which collects the characteristics of analytic sensitivity of all the methods of troponin in the market (table 5, ref Jaffé 2010).

Company-Instrument-Assay (generation)	Detection limit (ug/L)	cTn at 99th percentile (ug/L)	CV at 99th percentile (%)	cTn at 10% CV (ug/L)
Abbott AxSYM ADV (2nd)	0.02	0.04	15.0	0.16
Abbott ARCHITECT	<0.01	0.028	15.0	0.032
Abbott i-STAT	0.02	0.08#	16.5	0.10
Beckman Coulter Access Accu (2nd)	0.01	0.04	14.0	0.06
bioMerieux Vidas Ultra (2nd)	0.01	0.01	27.7	0.11
Innotrac Aio! (2nd)	0.006	0.015	14.0 (at 19 ng/L)	0.036
Inverness Biosite Triage	0.05	<0.05	NA	NA
Inverness Biosite Triage (r)	0.01	0.056	17.0	NA
Mitsubishi Chemical PATHFAST	0.008	0.029	5.0	0014
Ortho Vitros ECi ES	0.012	0.034	10.0	0.034
Radiometer AQT90	0.0095	0.023	17.7	0.039
Response Biomedical RAMP	0.03	<0.1	18.5	0.21
Roche E170	0.01	<0.01	18.0	0.03
Roche Elecsys 2010	0.01	<0.01	18.0	0.030
Roche Cardiac Reader	<0.05	<0.05	NA	NA
Siemens Centaur Ultra	0.006	0.04	10.0	0.03
Siemens Dimension RxL	0.04	0.07	20.0	0.14
Siemens Immulite 2500 STAT	0.1	0.2	NA	0.42
Siemens Immulite 1000Turbo	0.15	NA	NA	0.64
Siemens Stratus CS	0.03	0.07	10.0	0.06
Siemens VISTA	0.015	0.045	10.0	0.04
Tosoh AIA II	0.06	<0.06	8.5	0.09

NA= not assayed 99th = 99th percentile; 10% CV = Concentration measured with a 10% of total imprecision measured as coefficient of variation (CV); (r) = revised assay submitted to FDA per Inverness. Table can be consulted at http://www.ifcc.org/PDF/ScientificActivities/Committees/C-SMCD/cTn_Assay_Table_v091209.pdf. Version updated September 12, 2009

Table 5. Analytical characteristics of the current cardiac troponin I and T assays. (source) Troponinas ultrasensibles en el dolor torácico y los síndromes coronarios agudos. ¿un paso hacia delante? A.S. Jaffé y J.Ordoñez-Llanos. Rev Esp Cardiol, 2010; 63(7)763-68

There are only 4 of them which fulfil the recommendations of the Guidelines for Clinical Practice into effect at present (Thygesen 2007) , (NCB 2007) (CV< 10% in 99th percentile). However, at present there is no recommendation in any Clinical Guideline which classifies high sensitivity methods. Apple et al 1999 have suggested a classification to differentiate such methods. They use two criterias a) coefficient of variation in 99th percentile and b) percentege of values detected in reference population. For a method to be ultra-sensitive must have CV<10% in 99th percentile and detect troponin in less than 50% of the reference population.

Table 6 (from Jaffé 2010) holds the classification of the methods available in the market to assess troponin according to the criteria of Apple 1999. None of the 16 methods mentioned in the table fulfil the two conditions Apple demands in their criteria of high sensitivity method

	99th percentile (in ng/L)	Imprecision at 99th percentile (%)	Classification according imprecision	% of detectable values in reference subjects
Current available assays (generation)				
Abbott AxSYM ADV (2nd)	40	15.0	Clinically	<50%
Abbott ARCHITECT	28	15.0	Clinically	<50%
Abbott i-STAT	80	16.5	Clinically	<50%
Beckman Coulter Access Accu (2nd)	40	14.0	Clinically	50-75%
bioMerieux Vidas Ultra (2nd)	10	27.7	Not acceptable	<50%
Innotrac Aio! (2nd)	15	14.0 (at 19 ng/L)	Clinically	<50%
Inverness Biosite Triage	<50	NA	NA	<50%
Inverness Biosite Triage (r)	56	17.0	Clinically	Unknown
Mitsubishi Chemical PATHFAST	29	5.0	Guideline	<50%
Ortho Vitros ECi ES	34	10.0	Guideline	<50%
Radiometer AQT90	23	17.7	Clinically	<50%
Response Biomedical RAMP	<100	18.5	Clinically	<50%
Roche E170	<10	18.0	Clinically	<50%
Roche Elecsys 2010	<10	18.0	Clinically	<50%
Roche Cardiac Reader	<50	NA	NA	<50%
Siemens Centaur Ultra	40	10.0	Guideline	<50%
Siemens Dimension RxL	70	20.0	Clinically	<50%
Siemens Immulite 2500 STAT	200	NA	NA	<50%
Siemens Immulite 1000 Turbo	NA	NA	NA	<50%
Siemens Stratus CS	70	10.0	Guideline	<50%
Siemens VISTA	45	10.0	Guideline	<50%
Tosoh AIA II	<60	8.5	Guideline	<50%
Research high-sensitive assays				
Beckman Coulter Access hs-cTnI	8.6	10.0	Guideline	>95%
Roche Elecsys hs-cTnT	13	8.0	Guideline	>95%
Nanosphere hs-cTnI	2.8	9.5	Guideline	75-95%
Singulex hs-cTnI	10.1	9.0	Guideline	>95%

Table 6. Classification of the current and the high-sensitive cTn assays according criteria of Apple 2009.(source) Troponinas ultrasensibles en el dolor torácico y los síndromes coronarios agudos. ¿un paso hacia delante? A.S. Jaffé y J.Ordoñez-Llanos. Rev Esp Cardiol, 2010; 63(7)763-68

From these results it is important to point out that the most sensitive methods (research high-sensitivity assays) that is, with concentration values under 99th percentile and with better imprecisions in such percentile, are the ones which show higher proportion of healthy subjects (between 75-95% or >95%) which exceed the value of normality established for the method

4. Repercussion of high sensitivity troponin methods in the management of patients with ACS – Proposal of interpretation in clinical practice

The appearance of this new generation of high sensitivity troponin methods is going to modify the classical diagnostic interpretation of precordial pain we have been making until now as their goal is to be able to measure much smaller protein concentrations than the ones conventional methods are able to measure now. So it will be necessary to learn again and become familiar with the management of the marker. These new myocardial necrosis biomarkers going to appear in the blood stream hours earlier than if the marker is measured using conventional methods. These ones can only detect troponin 6-9 hours after clinical symptoms whereas using high sensitivity troponin the necrosis can be diagnosed earlier, as it starts being detected in blood three hours after pain. In a similar way the exclusion of acute myocardial infarction will also be earlier and considering the negligible amount of troponin which can be detected it will also increase the prediction of adverse clinical events. There are studies which confirm this fact. As the sensitivity of the methods has increased, it has been found a remarkable increase of the diagnostic sensitivity in the early detection of AMI using all, methods of high sensitivity troponinT and conventional Tn T methods (Giannitsis E,2010, Giannitsis E,2010 b) or troponin I (Kavasak PA 2009. Wilson 2009).

These characteristics which theoretically just show benefits can cause diagnostic confusion of an acute coronary syndrome because ultrasensitive troponin elevations are not only due to an acute process as they are also found in sub-acute processes and other cardiac diseases. High sensitivity troponin methods detect a minimum injury of the non-ischemic cardiomiocites, due to cardiac disorders (myocardial injuries such as myocarditis, pericarditis among others or the increase of the cardiac size as in cardiac insufficiency, left ventricular hypertrophia among others) or to other sort of diseases as for example pulmonary edema , sepsis or ictus can cause the release of hsTn into the systemic circulation. That is why not only the ischemic injury but also a wide range of other alterations can be associated with elevated high sensitivity troponin values. Besides, most of these elevations predict an adverse evolution in these patients, being , in this case, the clinic criterias the only way to reach a diagnosis. This causes confusion in the interpretation of troponin, which has traditionally been associated with the acute coronary syndrome being its elevation essential when the patient has acute thoracic pain, having or not elevation of the ST segment in electrocardiogram. Using conventional methods the finding of troponin values over the reference interval, in processes which do not fit with an acute coronary syndrome, induced us to look into the cause, which habitually was not explained. The appearance of high sensitivity methods make us change our criteria as although the reason for the output into the bloodstream of small amounts of the protein, which were not detected by conventional methods, is not known exactly, in processes which do not fit with acute ischemia its find represents a very useful data for the prognosis of the patient.

The appearance of this new generation of methods to assess troponin induces us to continue with the research in the management of these biomarkers, whose future is promising, in order to optimize and learn its management, and until new Guidelines in Clinical Practice appear and reach a consensus on the best way to use and interpret the results, we must be cautious in the application of high sensitivity troponin in clinical practice methods.
That is why the best thing to do (table 7) before implementing a method in clinical practice is to assess comprehensively and establish the reference values in better defined populations, using more strict inclusion criteria, setting up patterns of evolution changes to differentiate an ischemic patient from a patient with troponin elevations due to stable disease or underlying to new pathologic entities different from acute coronary syndrome. The knowledge this data for each of the methods assessing ultrasensitive troponin is an essential tool for the correct use and clinical interpretation of the results. Not to have such data well defined and established makes the diagnostic interpretation difficult and can cause confusion

1.	Establishing reference values (99 th percentil discriminator at CV <10%)
2.	Establishing the increase value of high sensitivity troponin discriminator of Acute Coronary Syndrome (**Δ** Tn discriminator).

Table 7. Mandatory requirements for the use of a high sensitivity troponin method in clinical practice

4.1 Establishing reference values of the method

As it can be seen in table 7 when there is an increase in the analytical sensitivity of the troponin tests, there are more people with troponin concentration over the 99th percentile. So, individuals with cardiovascular risk as hypertension, dislipemia, diabetes, renal insufficiency, cardiac insufficiency among others. This fact can make the clinical interpretation of the test difficult. That is why when evaluating a high sensitivity troponin method we must be especially cautious when establishing the reference values (table 8). The selection of the individuals to be included as reference population must be much more selective, considering much more strict inclusion criteria. The most important exclusion criteria to bear in mind are: pregnancy, current cold or infection, chronic inflammatory disease, patients treated for cardiac disease or lipid management, diabetes, family history of cardiovascular disease, smoking, high blood pressure or treated for high blood pressure, increased C-reactive protein, o interleukin-6 among others. The number of subjects to study must be at least 120 and 99th percentile will be applied. The imprecision of the method in the 99th percentil chosen must be lower or equal to a coefficient of variation of 10% (NACB 2007). We must bear in mind that the value of the 99th percentile chosen must be higher than the value measured by the method with an imprecision lower than 10% (**99th percentil discriminator**). We could expect that if we carried out again reference values in the methods mentioned in tables 5 and 6, with more restrictive inclusion criteria applied , especially in the ones called (research high-sensitivity assays), the percentage of detectable troponin in normal subjects, exempt from cardiovascular pathology, would decrease.

Number of patients	Mínimum de 120 subjects
Exclusion criteria	- pregnancy - infection - chronic inflammatory disease - subjets treated for cardiac disease or lipid management - diabetes - subjects with family history of cardiovascular disease - smoking - high blood pressure - increased C-reactive protein or interleukin-6
statistic	99th percentile
Precision	CV< 10% in 99th percentile

Table 8. Requirements to establish reference values of high sensitivity troponin methods

4.2 Establish the value of increase of high sensitivity troponin discriminator of acute coronary syndrome

As a result of all the above mentioned it is easy to understand the difficulty in interpreting a value of basal high sensitivity troponin in patients who go to the emergency room with precordial pain and without conclusive alterations in the electrocardiogram. From the biochemical point of view, the only way to help to distinguish if a high sensitivity troponin elevation is due to an acute ischemia process or if the origin is a sub-acute cardiac disease or chronic, as it happens with congestive cardiac insufficiency or cardiomyiopaties among others, is to perform serial troponins, as the Guidelines for Clinical Practice in 2007 recommended (Thygesen 2007, NACB 2007). Nevertheless, given the early of the appearance of high sensitivity troponin (3 hours after pain) as well as its high sensitivity in detection, the basal determination and the determination 6-9 after pain would not be the protocol to choose. With these new generation of troponins, the advisable to distinguish if we are facing an acute necrosis process or an underlying ischemia of a chronic process, is to establish a value of the increase of troponin discriminator of acute coronary syndrome **(Δ Tn discriminator)**. To obtain this data the increase in the variation of troponin should be assessed for a 3-hour interval, in a group of patients who suffer from an acute coronary syndrome and in another group patients who suffer a chronic process. In the acute ischemia there will be a significant increase of basal troponin compared with the one carried out between 3 and 6 hours later. In chronic processes the increase in troponin between 3 and 6 hours compared with basal troponin will be much lower. Once the Tn discriminator for a determined method is obtained, in clinical practice the scheme in figure I could be applied, which will help us confirm an acute myocardial infarction, at an earlier stage than with traditional methods, or to look for other causes of the increase in troponin.

The correct establishment of the increase evolution of high sensitivity troponin for an acute coronary syndrome, together with the strict study of normality values will clarify the advantages of this new generation of methods for the early diagnosis of acute coronary syndrome, as well as it will significantly benefit in the stratification of the risk, not only in patients with acute coronary syndrome but also patients who suffer from other myocardial injuries or increase of cardiac size among other causes.

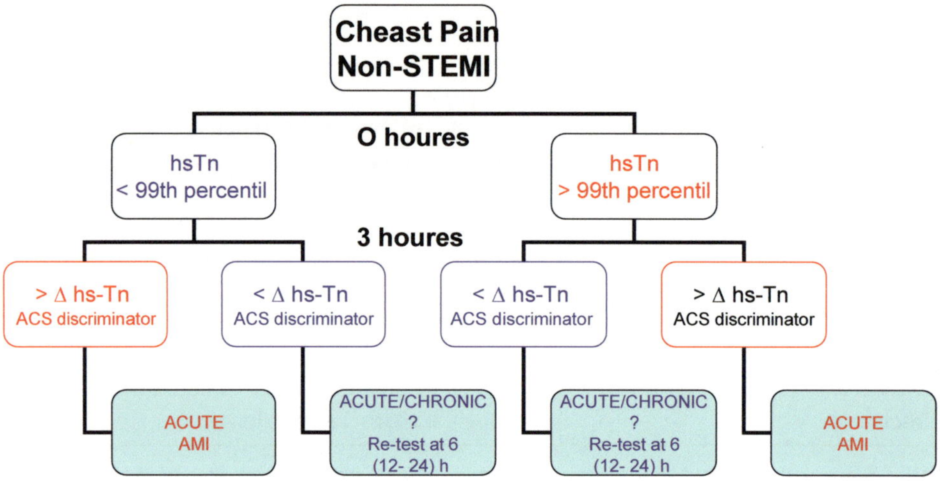

Δ hs-Tn ACS discriminator: troponin increase ACS discriminator
AMI: Acute myocardial infarction
ACS: Acute coronary syndrome

Fig. 9. Clinical significance of hsTn using troponin increase ACS discriminator. Proposal for the use of high sensitivity troponin in clinical practice.

5. High sensitivity troponin in patients with heart failure

Heart failure (HF) is a growing public health problem with high morbidity and mortality (Rosamond W 2008) . Natriuretic peptides are the election markers for diagnosis and risk stratification of patients with Heart failure (Braunwald E 2008) . Cardiac troponin are detected in an important proportion of patients suffering from acute or chronic HF. The mechanism of cardiac damage and appearance in Tn plasma, acute or chronic HF is not exactly known. The levels of troponin in plasma are associated with the increase of the risk of morbility and mortality either in acute or chronic HF giving prognostic information (Parentini 2008). Cardiac troponin is detected in a significant portion of patients with acute and chronic Heart Failure. However, the incidence of detection depends on the sensitivity of the assay used. Latini et al (Latini 2007) ,. measured Plasma troponin T in 4053 patients with chronic HF enrolled in the Valsartan Heart Failure Trial (Val-HeFT). Troponin T was detectable in 10.4% of the population with the conventional cTnT assay (detection limit < or = 0.01 ng/mL) compared with 92.0% with the new hsTnT assay (< or = 0.001 ng/mL). Detectable cTnT predicts adverse outcomes in chronic HF. (High sensitivity Troponin T (hsTnT) is a novel biomarker that provides prognostic information in several clinical settings as heart failure.

6. Conclusions

In view of all the above mentioned we can conclude that the biochemical diagnosis of ACS continues being a current affair and continues envolving. The process of troponin has not finished yet. The appearance of high sensitivity methods seems to be promising. They help to diagnose ACS much earlier and obtain higher stratification of the risk than convencional methods. Besides, it will let us know about the prognostic evolution of other pathologies such as chronic cardiac insufficiency as well as cardiovascular events in stable coronary disease. Nevertheless, to achieve the efficiency that the test deserves we have to learn, again to use and interprete the results of ultra-sensitive troponin. It is necessary to consolidate and establish firmly the dynamic changes of troponin concentrations to interprete the results accurately.

7. References

Apple FS, Adams JE, Wu Alan HB, Jaffe AS. Report on a survey of analytical and clinical characteristics of commercial cardiac troponin assays. In Markers in cardiology: current and future clinical applications. Armonk, NY 2001,4,31

Apple FS. A new season for cardiac troponin assays: It's time to keep a scorecard. Clin Chem 2009; 55:1303-6.

Braunwald E Biomarkers in heart failure.. N Engl J Med. 2008 (20):2148-59

The Joint European Society of Cardiology/ American College of Cardiology Committe. Consensus Document. Myocardial infarction redefined. A consensus document of the Joint European Society of Cardiology/American College of Cardiology Committe for the Redefinition of Myocardial Infarction. Eur Heart J 2000;21:1502-13.

Galán A. Diagnóstico Bioquímico de la Isquemia Coronaria Aguda Medicina Clínica 2000; 115(17) :671-676

Galán, A, Curos, J Durán. A.Corominas ,V.Valle Analytical evaluation of two automatic methods to measure blood CK-MB mass an Troponin I Journal of Automated Methods and Management in Chemistry 2002;24(2):51-57

Galán, A. Curós y A. Corominas. Interés de las troponinas en el síndrome coronario agudo en pacientes con insuficiencia renal. Medicina Clínica, 2004;123:551-6

Giannitsis E, Katus AH. Myocardial infarction. Current recommendation for interpretation of highly sensitive troponin T assay for diagnostic, therapeutic and pronostic puposes in patients with a non-ST-segment - elevation acute coronary Syndrome. European Cardiology 2009; 5(2): 44-47

Giannitsis E, Kurz K, Hallermayer K, Jarausch J, Jaffe AS, Katus AH. Analytical validation of a high-sensitivity cardiac troponin T assay. Clin Chem 2010; 56:254-61.

Giannitsis E, Becker M, Kurz K, Hess G, Zdunek D, Katus HA. High-sensitivity cardiac troponin T for early prediction of evolving non-ST-segment elevation myocardial infarction in patients with suspected acute coronary syndrome and negative troponin results on admission. Clin Chem 2010; 56:642-50.

Jaffé A.S. J.Ordoñez-Llanos J. Troponinas ultrasensibles en el dolor torácico y los síndromes coronarios agudos. ¿un paso hacia delante? Rev Esp Cardiol, 2010; 63(7)763-68

Kavsak PA, MacRae AR, Yerna MJ, Jaffe AS.Analytic and clinical utility of a next-generation, highly sensitive cardiac troponin I assay for early detection of myocardial injury. Clin Chem 2009 ;55(3):573-7

Latini R, Masson S, Anand IS, Missov E, Carlson M, Vago T, Angelici L, Barlera S, Parrinello G, Maggioni AP, Tognoni G, Cohn JN; Val-Heft Prognostic value of very low plasma concentrations of troponin T in patients with stable chronic heart failure. Circulation 2007;116(11):1242-9.

(NACB) National Academy of Clinical Biochemistry. National Academy of Clinical Biochemistry Laboratory medicine practice guidelines: clinical characteristics and utilization of biochemical markers in acute coronary syndromes. Clin Chem 2007; 53: 552-574.

Panteghini M, Gerhardt W, Apple FS, Dati F, Ravkilde J, Wu AH. Quality specifications for cardiac troponin assays. Clin Chem Lab Med. 2001;39:174-8.

Parenti N, Bartolacci S, Carle F, Angelo Cardiac troponin I as prognostic marker in heart failure patients discharged from emergency department. Intern Emerg Med. 2008 Mar;3(1):43-7.

Rosamond W Lloyd-Jones D, Adams R, Carnethon M, De Simone G, Ferguson TB, Flegal K, Ford E, Furie K, Go A, Greenlund K, Haase N, Hailpern S, Ho M, Howard V, Kissela B, Kittner S, Lackland D, Lisabeth L, Marelli A, McDermott M, Meigs J, Mozaffarian D, Nichol G, O'Donnell C, Roger V, , Sacco R, Sorlie P, Stafford R, Steinberger J, Thom T, Wasserthiel-Smoller S, Wong N, Wylie-Rosett J, Hong Y; American Heart Association Statistics Committee and Stroke Statistics Subcommittee. Heart disease and stroke statistics--2009 update: a report from the American Heart Association Statistics Committee and Stroke Statistics Subcommittee Circulation. 2010 Jul 6;122(1):e11.

Thygesen K, Alpert JS, White HD. White on behal of the Joint ESC/ACF/AHA/ WHF Task Force for the Redefinition of Myocardial Infarction. Universal definition of myocardial infarction. European Heart J. 2007;28:2525-2538

WHO Report of the Joint International Society and Federation of Cardiology / World Health Organization Task Force on Standardization of Clinical Nomenclature.Circulation 1979;59:607-609

Wilson SR, Sabatine MS, Braunwald E, Sloan S, Murphy SA, Morrow D. Detection of myocardial injury in patients with unstable angina using a novel nanoparticle cardiac troponin I assay: Observations from the PROTECT-TIMI 30 Trial. Am Heart J 2009; 158:386-91.

Wu AHB, Apple FS, Gibler WB, Jesse RL, Warshaw MM, Valdes R, Jr. National Academy of Clinical Biochemistry Standards of Laboratory Practice: recommendations for use of cardiac markers in coronary artery diseases. Clin Chem 1999;45:1104-1121

Wu Alan HB Analytical issues affecting the clinical performance of cardiac troponin assays. In Markers in cardiology: current and future clinical applications. Armonk, NY 2001,1,1

5

Pathogenesis of Acute Coronary Syndrome, from Plaque Formation to Plaque Rupture

Hamdan Righab[1], Caussin Christophe[1], Kadri Zena[2] and Badaoui Georges[2]
[1]*Marie Lannelongue Hospital, Cardiology Department, Plessis Robinson,*
[2]*Hotel Dieu de France Hospital, Cardiology Department, Beirut,*
[1]*France*
[2]*Lebanon*

1. Introduction

Cardiovascular diseases remain the leading cause of morality in the western world. The aim of this chapter is to understand the pathogenesis of acute coronary syndromes from atherosclerotic plaque formation, to plaque progression and vascular remodeling, to plaque destabilization, to ultimately plaque rupture or erosion and thrombus formation.
A cascade of interacting factors leads to plaque formation, progression, fraglisation, and rupture.
Features associated with plaque rupture are: large eccentric soft lipid core, thin fibrous cap, inflammation in the cap and adventitia, increased plaque neovascularity, and outward or positive vessel remodeling.
Vasospasm is a separate mechanism for developing ACS without plaque rupture or erosion will not be discussed in this chapter.

2. Atherosclerosis

Atherosclerosis is a chronic disease that can remain asymptomatic through decades. It is enhanced by modifiable and non modifiable risk factors and consists of intra intimal accumulation of intra cellular and extracellular oxidized LDL, macrophages, T cells, smooth muscle cells, proteoglycan, collagen, calcium, and necrotic debris. Low endothelial shear stress can contribute to atherosclerotic plaque formation, vulnerabilisation, and rupture. Intimal accumulation of oxidized LDL-C, called fatty streaks constitutes the earliest histopathologic stage of atherosclerosis.
Adhesion molecules expressed by endothelial cells mediate the rolling and adhesion of circulating leukocytes on the endothelial surface. Chemoattractant chemokines promote transmigration of leukocytes into the intima. Monocytes infiltrate beneath the endothelium, differentiate to macrophages, phagocytose the oxidized LDL-C and transform into foam cells. Foam cells produce cytokines, growth factors, reactive oxygen species and matrix-degrading enzymes, sustaining atherosclerosis progression. The intensity of oxidized LDL-C accumulation in the subendothelial space is a major stimulus for the ongoing inflammatory process. The accumulation of lipid-laden foam cells constitute the intermediate lesions or pathologic intimal thickening, which evolve through several stages of progression.

3. Arterial remodeling

Arterial remodeling involves a cascade of structural and morphological changes of a vessel wall in response to various stimuli including changes in blood flow and pressure, and acute injury; all three are common findings in atherosclerotic plaques.
Two types of coronary arterial remodeling have been described:

- Negative remodeling: defined as local shrinkage, negative remodeling is more often seen in patients with stable angina and is associated with smaller plaque areas. It might be seen in arterial wall healing after injuries such as balloon injury, that could be mainly related to vascular wall contracture and consequent luminal narrowing. The biological events involved in this wound healing involve complex series of interacting growth factors, integrins and proteases.
- Positive or outward remodeling: defined by a compensatory increase in local vessel size in response to increasing plaque burden minimizing the degree of luminal stenosis. Positive remodeling characterizes unstable vulnerable plaques.

There are studies demonstrating that plaque rupture occurs in insignificant, mildly occlusive plaques, this could be explained by positive remodeling: the increase in total arterial area that accompanies plaque accumulation. Large positive remodeled plaques while paradoxically protecting against luminal narrowing, are more susceptible to mechanical forces that lead to plaque rupture and an unstable clinical presentation.
The pathogenesis of arterial remodeling is not fully understood and remains debated. Many hypotheses have been advanced.
Arterial wall neovascularisation of atherosclerotic plaques seems to have a potential role in modulating lesion formation and structural changes of the arterial wall, by nourishing the growing plaque. Various angiogenic growth factors and receptors are implicated in coronary wall angiogenesis such as VEGF/VPF, estrogen, interleukin 8, bFGF, and aFGF; the role of TNF-α and TGF-β remains controversial.
Angiotensine II via AT1 receptors is another trigger of plaque neovascularisation and remodeling.
Activation of NADPH oxidase by various triggers such as Angiotensine II and mechanical stretch promotes ROS production and ROS-mediated pathways leading to vascular remodeling.
In addition Low ESS leads to inflammation of the wall beneath the plaque and shift of the extracellular matrix balance toward degradation. Within such an environment the internal elastic lamina undergoes severe fragmentation, and the atherosclerotic process extends into the media degrading the collagen and elastin fibers, thereby promoting arterial expansion and outward remodeling.
Human studies using intravascular ultrasound confirmed that outward or positive remodeling is more common at culprit lesion sites in patients with unstable angina, whereas inward or negative remodeling is more common in patients with stable angina.

Pathogenesis of positive arterial remodeling
Arterial wall neovascularisation
Angiotensine II
ROS
Low ESS

Table 1. This table summarizes factors contributing to positive plaque remodeling that is associated with unstable plaque.

4. Plaque destabilisation

Typically a vulnerable plaque is described as having a thin fibrous cap and a rich superficial lipid core. Weakening of the fibrous cap is due mainly to accelerated degradation of collagen and other matrix components.
Many factors contribute to plaque vulnerabilisation:

4.1 Inflammation

Inflammation cells such as activated monocytes and macrophages and, to a lesser degree, T cells play a crucial role in destabilizing the fibrous cap tissue and, therefore, enhance the risk of plaque rupture.
Adhesion molecules such as VCAM-1 as well as chemokines such as MCP-1 recruite inflammatory cells into the atherosclerotic plaques. Inflammatory cells are activated in the vessel wall by oxidized lipids and cytokines such as M-CSF.
Adventitial neovasculature also enhances inflammatory cells entry and recruitement inside the atherosclerotic lesion.
Many mediators secreted by plaque macrophages could be involved in fibrous cap weakening including:

- Interleukin (IL)-18: also called interferon gamma-inducing factor, is a proinflammatory cytokine secreted by plaque macrophages. Increased serum IL-18 may be an independent predictor of cardiovascular mortality.
- Matrix Metalloproteinases (MMP): mainly MMP-2 (Gelatinse A), MMP-9 (Gelatinase B), and MMP-8 (Collagenase), released from activated macrophage foam cells, directly mediate matrix degradation of the plaque fibrous cap. Oxidized LDL containing arachidonic and linoleic acid upregulates the expression of metalloproteinase, while HDL reverses this effect.
- Tissue factor: expressed by macrophages is the main initiator of thrombogenesis.

Inflammation usually concerns the entire coronary circulation not only the culprit lesion. This fact explains why patients with acute coronary syndrome may have multiple vulnerable plaques.

Mechanisms of Angiotensine II mediated plaque weakening
Upregulation of IL6 gene
Upregulation of MMP genes
Activation of mitogen-activated protein kinase cascades
Activation of tyrosine kinases
Stimulation of neovascularisation

Table 2. This table summarizes the leading mechanisms of Angiotensine II mediated atherosclerotic plaque weakening

4.2 Renin-angiotensin system

There is evidence of angiotensin converting enzyme (ACE), angiotensine II, and AT1 receptors within the plaque. An increased activity of ACE was found within culprits lesions in the setting of acute coronary syndromes, probably related to a local secretion. Angiotensine II increases the likelihood of plaque progression and rupture via AT1 receptors by regulating the gene expression of various bioactive substances mainly interleukine 6 (IL6), metalloproteinases, and other growth factors and cytokines. Angiotensine II also activates multiple intracellular signaling cascades (mitogen-activated protein kinase cascades, tyrosine kinases, and various transcription factors) in coronary endothelial and smooth muscle cells.

In addition Angiotensine II enhances plaque neovascularisation.

4.3 Hemodynamical factors mainly shear stress

4.3.1 Definitions

- Endothelial shear stress (ESS): tangential force derived by the friction of the flowing blood on the endothelial surface. It is the product of the shear rateat the wall and the blood viscosity.
- Shear rate: The spatial gradient of blood velocity from areas at the arterial wall toward areas at the center of the lumen (dv/dy, where dv is change in flow velocity and dy is change in radial distance from the wall).

  Physiologically, the shear rate decreases at the center of the lumen and gradually increases toward the wall.
- Blood viscosity: A principal property of blood related to its internal friction that causes blood to resist flow. Hematocrit is the major determinant of blood viscosity.

Although the entire vasculature is exposed to the atherogenic effects of the systemic risk factors such as hyperlipidemia, cigarette smoking, hypertension, diabetes mellitus, and genetic predisposition, atherosclerotic lesions form at specific regions of the arterial tree, such as in the vicinity of branch points, the outer wall of bifurcations, and the inner wall of curvatures, where disturbed flow occurs and ESS is low.

Low ESS induces endothelial dysfunction by reducing the bioavailability of nitric oxid via a decrease in eNOS messenger ribonucleic acid and protein expression, thereby exposing the endothelium to the atherogenic effect of local and systemic risk factors. Nitric oxide is a key component of normal vascular tone, characterized by strong anti-inflammatory, antiapoptotic, anti-mitogenic, and anti-thrombotic properties. In addition, low ESS downregulates prostacyclin, another endothelial vasodilatory substance and upregulates endothelin-1, a potent vasoconstrictive and mitogenic molecule.

Low ESS also promotes subendothelial deposition and accumulation of LDL-C by increasing mitotic and apoptotic activity of endothelial cells and inducing conformational changes of endothelial cells from fusiform to polygonal shape, widening thereby the junctions between endothelial cells.

Gene expression as well as post-transcriptional activity of the major oxidative enzymes at endothelial cell membranes are enhanced by low ESS, leading to the production of reactive oxygen species within the intima.

In addition gene expression of several adhesion molecules, chemoattractant chemokines and proinflammatory cytokines are upregulated by low ESS.

Mechanisms of low ESS mediated plaque weakening
Endothelial dysfunction: • Decreases eNOS • Downregulates Prostacycline synthesis • Upregulates Endotheline-1 synthesis
LDL-C sub-intimal uptake and accumulation
Promotes inflammation
Promotes oxidative stress

Table 3. This table summarizes the contribution of low ESS to plaque weakening.

4.4 Strenuous exercise

Strenuous exercise especially among those who exercise infrequently and have multiple cardiac risk factors, is associated with increased temporary risk of plaque rupture and myocardial infarction via increase wall stress due to rapid increase in heart rate and blood pressure, coronary vasospasm, increased flexing of epicardial coronary arteries, deepening of existing plaque fissures, and catecholamine induced platelet aggregation.

4.5 In vivo detection of vulnerable plaque with optical coherence tomography

Optical coherence tomography (OCT) is recently developed imaging modality, using infra red light and characterized by the higher existing resolution (axial resolution: 10-15µm) allowing a microscopical description of the atherosclerotic plaque in vivo within the coronary arteries. OCT is validated for the detection of vulnerable plaque wich is typically characterized by:

- Thin fibrous cap < 65 µm
- Rich lipid core: when lipid is present within two or more quadrants of the plaque.
- Microchannels in case of plaque neovascularisation.

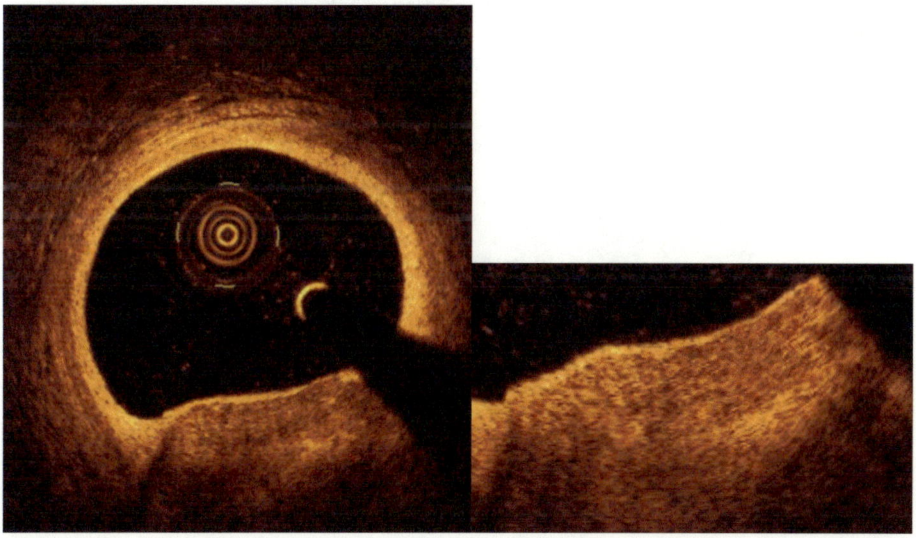

Fig. 1. Fibrous cap assessment with OCT: fibrous cap is a signal rich layer separating the lumen from the signal poor underlying lipid core. Fibrous cap is measured at its thinest segment.

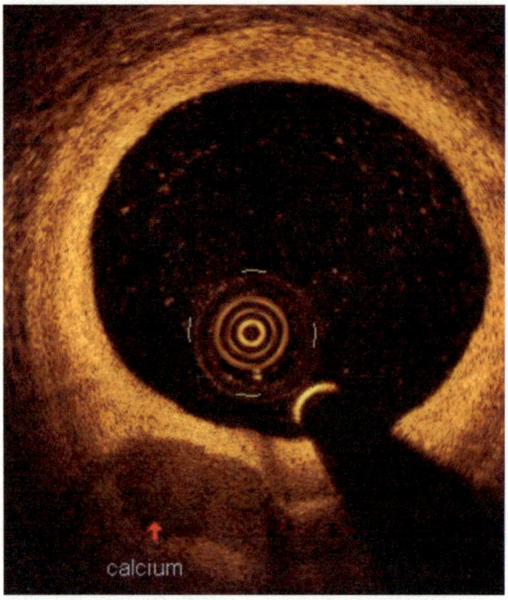

Fig. 2. OCT showing a thick fibrous cap, calcified plaque. Calcium is seen as a homogeneous signal poor region with sharply demarcated edges.

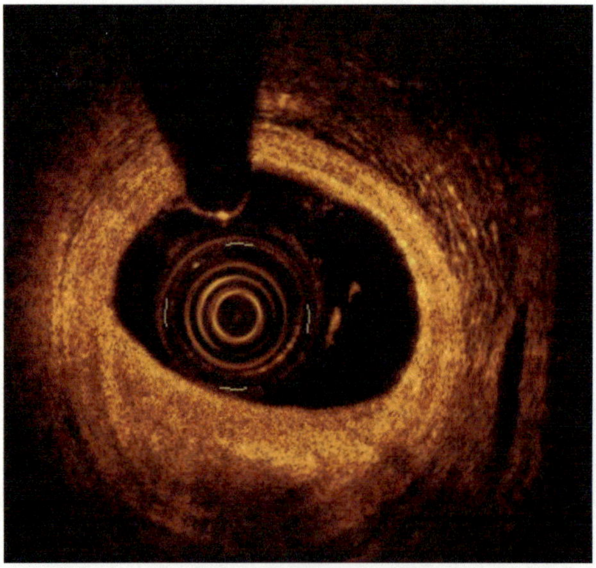

Fig. 3. OCT showing a lipid rich plaque. Lipid is seen as a heterogeneous signal poor region with irregular edges.

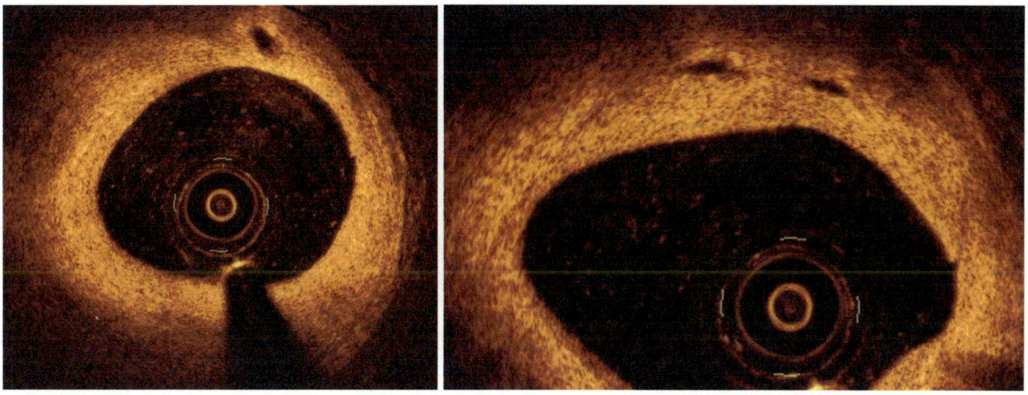

Fig. 4. Adventicial and subintimal increazed neovascularization characterizes unstable plaque and can be detected in vivo with OCT. Neovessels or microchannels are seen as no-signal tubulo-luminal structure without a connection to the vessel lumen and recognized on ≥ 3 consecutive cross sectional OCT images.

5. Plaque rupture

As previously explained the fibrous cap rupture results from an imbalance between synthesis and breakdown of extracellular matrix collagen and other matrix components leading to thinning of the cap, predisposing the cap to spontaneous rupture or rupture in response to a variety of triggers. Plaque rupture primarily occurs in yellowish plaques with an increased lipid core and thin fibrous cap. Rupture of the thin fibrous cap exposes blood flow to the lipid core. The lipid core is believed to be highly thrombogenic when exposed to circulating blood. The enhanced thrombogenicity of the lipid core has been attributed to the high levels of functionally active tissue factor most likely derived from the death of macrophages inside the plaque. In addition to tissue factor, oxidized lipids in the lipid core may also directly stimulate platelet aggregation.

The thrombus is usually occlusive in STEMI and nonocclusive in NSTEMI. Episodes of plaque disruption and thrombosis may be subclinical and do not always result in acute coronary syndrome. Healing process may play an integral role in the progression of atherosclerosis, having the potential to cause sudden plaque growth.

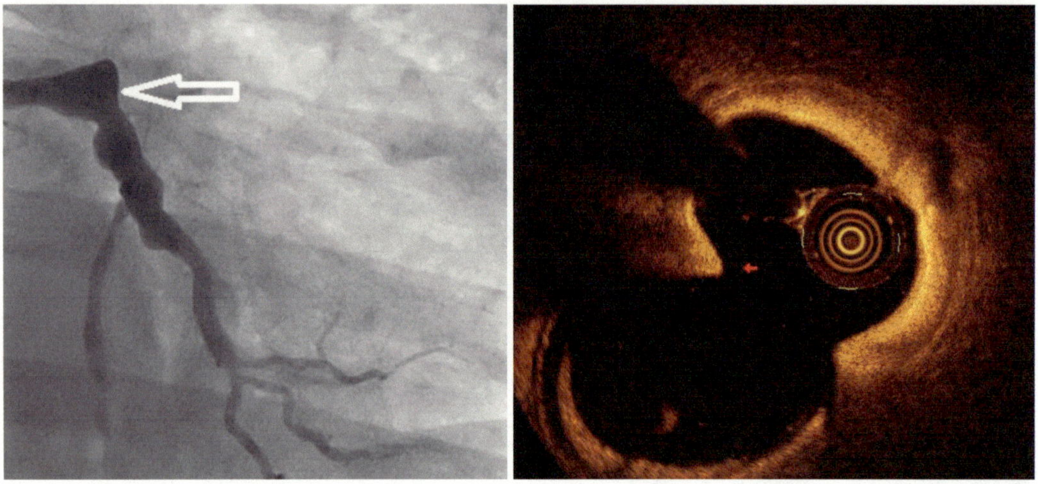

A B

Fig. 5. (A)- Coronary angiogram showing ostial occlusion (TIMI 0 flow) of the left ascending artery responsible of acute STEMI; (B)- OCT performed in the same patient after thrombo-aspiration and restauration of a TIMI 3 flow, shows the site of plaque rupture, defined by a discontinuation of the fibrous cap and cavity formation within the plaque.

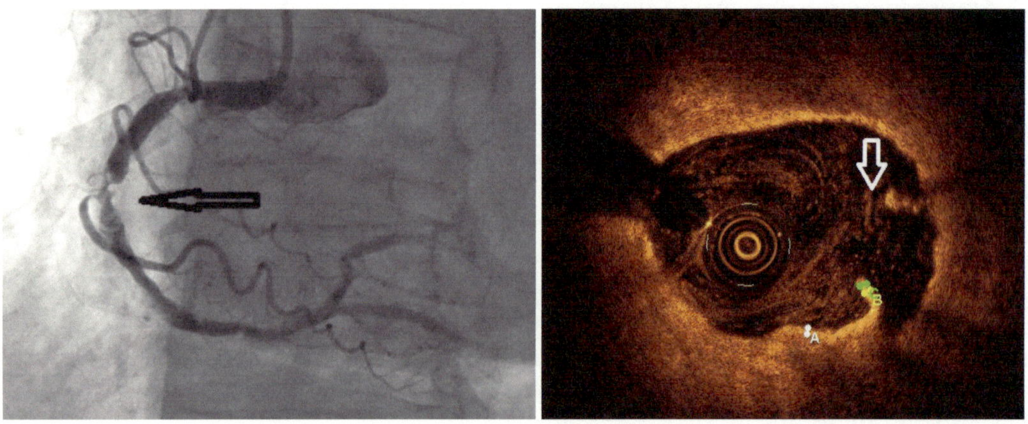

Fig. 6. Rupture site detected with OCT (right) in the setting of NSTEMI. The coronary angiogram (left) shows a subocclusion of the segment 2 of the right coronary artery.

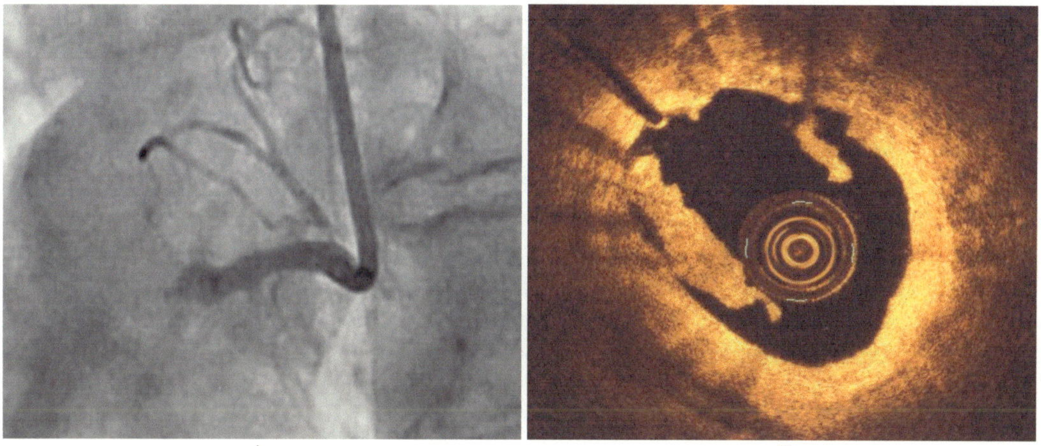

A B

Fig. 7. (A)- Coronary angiogram showing occlusion of the segment 1 of right coronary artery in a patient presenting with STEMI; (B)- OCT performed after thrombo-aspiration showed residual white thrombus seen as a hypersignal protrusion within the lumen.

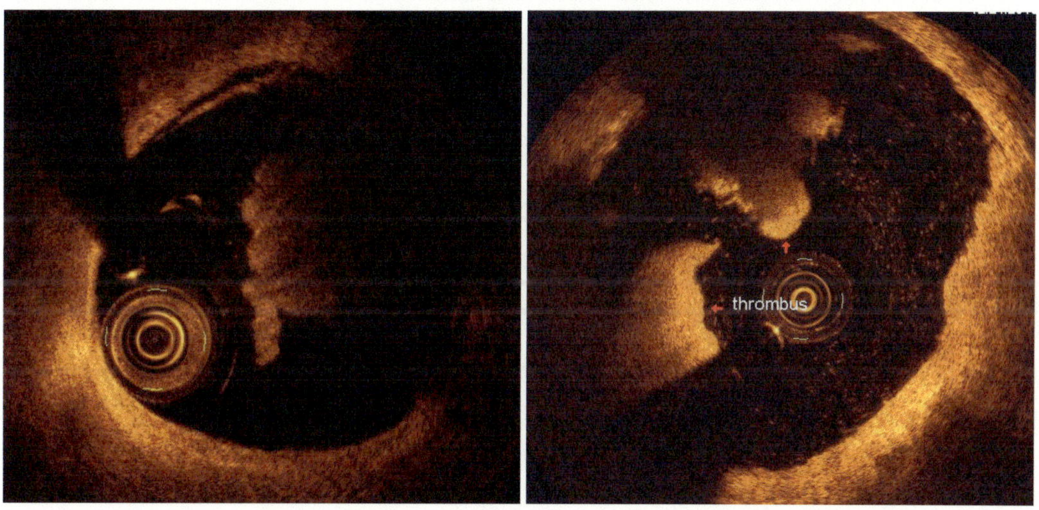

Fig. 8. Red thrombus in the setting of ACS is seen with OCT as hypersignal protusion within the lumen, however, unlike white thrombus, red thrombus is characterised by a signal attenuation and posterior signal free shadowing due to the backscatering properties of the red blood cells wich are highly present in red thrombus.

6. Plaque erosion

Plaque erosion usually occurs in younger patients, women and smokers.

Culprit lesion do not have a large lipid core but instead have a proteoglycan-rich matrix, a deep lipid core, the prevalence of inflammation is lower with less macrophages and T cells and more smooth muscle cells compared to culprit lesions in plaque ruptures. Plaque erosion is defined as acute thrombus in direct contact with the intimal plaque without rupture of a lipid pool. The plaque luminal surface is irregular and eroded.

Thrombus resulting from plaque erosion has been reported to be 20% to 40% of all coronary thrombi. The precise mechanisms of thrombosis in this entity are not known.

Thrombosis in such cases might be triggered by an enhanced systemic thrombogenic state such as enhanced platelet aggregability, increased circulating tissue factor levels, and depressed fibrinolytic state. In addition activated circulating leucocytes may transfer active tissue factor by shedding microparticles and transferring them onto adherent platelets. Virmani et al have also identified yet another pathological variant where a calcified nodule within the plaque erodes through the surface of the plaque leading to thrombosis.

7. Abbreviations

ACS	Acute coronary syndrome
LDL-C	Low density lipoprotein cholesterol
ESS	Endothelial shear stress
VEGF	Vascular endothelial growth factor
VPF	Vascular permeability factor
FGF	Fibroblast growth factor
TNF	Tumor necrosis factor
TGF	Transforming growth factor
AT1	Angiotensine type 1
IL	Interleukine
MMP	Matrix metalloproteinase
NADPH	Nicotinamide Adenosine Dinucleotide Phosphate
VCAM	Vascular cellular adhesion molecule
ROS	Reactive oxygen species
MCP	Monocyte Chemotactic Protein
CSF	Colony stimulating factor
ACE	Angiotensine converting enzyme
HDL	High density lipoprotein
eNOS	Endothelial nitric oxide synthase
OCT	Optical coherence tomography
TIMI	Thrombolysis In Myocardial Infarction
STEMI	ST elevation myocardial infarction
NSTEMI	Non ST elevation myocardial infarction

8. References

[1] Molecular bases of the acute coronary syndrome. Libby, P. Circulation 1995; 91:2844.

[2] Evidence for increased collagenolysis by interstitial collagenases-1 and -3 in vulnerable human atheromatous plaques. Sukhova GK, Schonbeck U, Rabkin E, et al. Circulation 1999; 99:2503.

[3] Site of intimal rupture or erosion of thrombosed coronary atherosclerotic plaques is characterized by an inflammatory process irrespective of the dominant plaque morphology. Van der Wal AC, Becker AE, Van der Loos CM, Das PK. Circulation 1994; 89:36.

[4] Focal and multi-focal plaque macrophage distributions in patients with acute and stable presentations of coronary artery disease. MacNeill BD, Jang IK, Bouma BE, et al.. J Am Coll Cardiol 2004; 44:972.

[5] Increased expression of membrane type 3-matrix metalloproteinase in human atherosclerotic plaque: role of activated macrophages and inflammatory cytokines. Uzui H, Harpf A, Liu M, et al. Circulation 2002; 106:3024.

[6] Oxidized low density lipoprotein regulates matrix metalloproteinase-9 and its tissue inhibitor in human monocyte-derived macrophages. Xu X-P, Meisel SR, Ong JM, et al. Circulation 1999; 99:993.

[7] Expression of angiotensin II and interleukin 6 in human coronary atherosclerotic plaques: potential implications for inflammation and plaque instability. Schieffer B, Schieffer E, Hilfiker-Kleiner D, et al. Circulation 2000; 101:1372.

[8] Distribution of inflammatory cells in atherosclerotic plaques relates to the direction of flow. Dirksen MT, van der Wal AC, van den Berg FM, et al.Circulation 1998; 98:2000.

[9] Association between myocardial infarction and the mast cells in the adventitia of the infarct-related coronary artery. Kaartinen M, Penttila A, et al. Circulation 1999; 99:361.

[10] Prevalence of total coronary occlusion during the early hours of transmural myocardial infarction. DeWood MA, Spores J, Notske R, et al. N Engl J Med 1980; 303:897.

[11] Coronary arteriographic findings in acute transmural myocardial infarction. DeWood MA, Spores J, Hensley GR, et al. Circulation 1983; 68:I39.

[12] The non-Q wave myocardial infarction revisited: 10 years later. Liebson PR, KleinLW et al. Prog Cardiovasc Dis 1997; 39:399.

[13] Elevations in troponin T and I are associated with abnormal tissue level perfusion: a TACTICS-TIMI 18 substudy. Treat Angina with Aggrastat and Determine Cost of Therapy with an Invasive or Conservative Strategy-Thrombolysis in Myocardial Infarction. Wong GC, Morrow DA, Murphy S, et al. Circulation 2002; 106:202.

[14] A Prospective Natural-History Study of Coronary Atherosclerosis. Stone G, Maehara A, Lansky A, de Bruyne B, Cristea E, Mintz G, Mehran R, McPherson J, Farhat N, Marso S, Parise H, Templin B, White R, Zhang Z, Serruys P, for the PROSPECT Investigators. N Engl J Med 2011;364:226-35.

[15] Coronary plaque erosion without rupture into a lipid core a frequent cause of coronary thrombosis in sudden coronary death. Farb A, Burke AP, Tang AL, Liang TY, Mannan P, Smialek J, Virmani R. Circulation. 1996 Apr 1;93(7):1354-63.

[16] Exercise and acute cardiovascular events placing the risks into perspective: a scientific statement from the American Heart Association Council on Nutrition, Physical

Activity, and Metabolism and the Council on Clinical Cardiology.Thompson PD, Franklin BA, Balady GJ, Blair SN, Corrado D, Estes NA 3rd, Fulton JE, Gordon NF, Haskell WL, Link MS, Maron BJ, Mittleman MA, Pelliccia A, Wenger NK, Willich SN, Costa F; American Heart Association Council on Nutrition, Physical Activity, and Metabolism; American Heart Association Council on Clinical Cardiology; American College of Sports Medicine.Circulation. 2007 May 1;115(17):2358-68.

[17] Shed membrane microparticles with procoagulant potential in human atherosclerotic plaques: a role for apoptosis in plaque thrombogenicity. Mallat Z, Hugel B, Ohan J, Lesèche G, Freyssinet JM, Tedgui A. Circulation. 1999 Jan 26;99(3):348-53

[18] Pathophysiology of Coronary Thrombosis: Role of Plaque Rupture and Plaque Erosion. Shah P K, Progress in Cardiovascular Diseases, Vol. 44, No. 5, 2002: pp 357-368.

[19] Role of Endothelial Shear Stress in the Natural History of Coronary Atherosclerosis and Vascular Remodeling Molecular, Cellular, and Vascular Behavior. Chatzizisis Y S, Coskun A U, Jonas M, Edelman E R, Feldman C L, Stone P H, JACC Vol. 49, No. 25, 2007;June 26, 2007:2379–93.

[20] Forum Review Article Cyclic Stretch, Reactive Oxygen Species,and Vascular Remodeling. Birukov K G. antioxidant and signaling;Volume 11, Number 7, 2009.

[21] Relationship Between Coronary Artery Remodeling and Plaque Composition in Culprit Lesions An Intravascular Ultrasound Radiofrequency Analysis. Higashikuni Y,Tanabe K, Yamamoto H, Aoki J, Nakazawa G, MD; Onuma Y, Otsuki S, Yagishita A, Yachi S,Nakajima H, Hara K. Circ J 2007; 71: 654 -660.

[22] Morphological Predictors of Arterial Remodeling in Coronary Atherosclerosis. Burke A, Kolodgie F D, Farb A,Weber D, Virmani R. Circulation 2002;105;297-303.

[23] Proteolysis of the Pericellular Matrix: A Novel Element Determining Cell Survival and Death in the Pathogenesis of Plaque Erosion and Rupture. Lindstedt K, Leskinen M, Kovanen P. Arterioscler Thromb Vasc Biol 2004; 24; 1350-1358.

[24] Differential Accumulation of Proteoglycans and Hyaluronan in Culprit Lesions: Insights Into Plaque Erosion. Kolodgie F, Burke A, Farb A, Weber D, Kutys R,Wight T, Virmani R. Arterioscler Thromb Vasc Biol 2002;22;1642-1648

[25] Clinical Classification and Plaque Morphology Determined by Optical Coherence Tomography in Unstable Angina Pectoris. Mizukoshi M, Imanishi T, Tanaka A, Kubo T, Liu Y, Takarada S, Kitabata H, Tanimoto T, Komukai K, Ishibashi K, Akasaka T. Am J Cardiol 2010;106:323–328.

[26] Diagnostic accuracy of optical coherence tomography and integrated backscatter intravascular ultrasound images for tissue characterization of human coronary plaques. Kawasaki M, Bouma BE, Bressner J, Houser SL, Nadkarni SK, MacNeill BD, Jang IK, Fujiwara H, Tearney GJ. J Am Coll Cardiol. 2006 Jul 4; 48(1):81-8.

[27] Assessment of Coronary Arterial Thrombus by Optical Coherence Tomography. Kume T, Akasaka T, Kawamoto T, Ogasawara Y, Watanabe N, Toyota E, Neishi Y, Sukmawan R, Sadahira Y, Yoshida K; Am J Cardiol, 2006;97:1713–1717.

[28] Relation of microchannel structure identified by optical coherence tomography to plaque vulnerability in patients with coronary artery disease. Kitabata H, Tanaka A, Kubo T, Takarada S, Kashiwagi M, Tsujioka H, Ikejima H, Kuroi A, Kataiwa H, Ishibashi K, Komukai K, Tanimoto T, Ino Y, Hirata K, Nakamura N, Mizukoshi M, Imanishi T, Akasaka T. Am J Cardiol. 2010 Jun 15;105(12):1673-8.

6

Plaque, Platelets, and Plug – The Pathogenesis of Acute Coronary Syndrome

Anggoro B. Hartopo[1,2] et al.*
[1]*Department of Cardiology and Vascular Medicine, Faculty of Medicine Universitas Gadjah Mada*
[2]*Pusat Jantung Terpadu / Heart Centre Dr. Sardjito Hospital, Yogyakarta Indonesia*

1. Introduction

Acute coronary syndrome is a clinical condition of partial or total obstruction of blood flow in the coronary artery due to acute thrombus formation. Culprit vessel, coronary artery segment within which the site of origin of thrombus formation lies, is occupied by eroded or ruptured atherosclerotic plaque. Direct contact between circulating blood constituent and atherosclerotic plaque content owing to loss of endothelial cell barrier orchestrates the haemostasis events, i.e. thrombus formation and coagulation activation. Evolved within years of human life span, atherosclerotic undergoes three main steps: initiation, progression and finally complication (Libby, 2002).

Atherosclerotic plaque development involves cellular and molecular interactions as well as blood flow dynamic alterations in the affected area. Although these steps affect all individual, some gather the risk factors to develop progression and complication of coronary atherosclerotic lesion faster and more prominent than others. Given the dynamic nature of these steps, understanding several mechanisms engage in every step will provide insight into therapeutic approach. Here, we review the last two steps of coronary atherosclerotic plaque development, with the focus in the role of platelets, anucleated cells being the target for therapeutic advancement in atherosclerosis and acute coronary syndrome.

2. Formation of atherosclerotic plaque

The earliest event of atherosclerosis formation is the retention of apolipoprotein B-containing lipoproteins from circulation into subendothelial of the arterial wall (Tabas et al., 2007). This particular lipoprotein interacts with subendothelial proteoglycan through ionic affinity and hence instigates lipoprotein retention in the intimal layer, the innermost part of the arterial wall (Borén et al., 1998; Skalen et al., 2002). During this stage, the tendency of

---

*Budi Y. Setianto[1,2], Hariadi Hariawan[1,2], Lucia K. Dinarti[1,2], Nahar Taufiq[1,2], Erika Maharani[1,2], Irsad A. Arso[1,2], Hasanah Mumpuni[1,2], Putrika P.R. Gharini[1,2], Dyah W. Anggrahini[1,2] and Bambang Irawan[1,2]
[1]*Department of Cardiology and Vascular Medicine, Faculty of Medicine Universitas Gadjah Mada, Indonesia*
[2]*Pusat Jantung Terpadu / Heart Centre Dr. Sardjito Hospital, Yogyakarta, Indonesia*

retention of lipoprotein depends greatly on sustained plasma level of apolipoprotein B-containing lipoproteins and, in the lesser degree, lipoprotein size, charge, and composition as well as endothelial permeability (Tabas et al., 2007). Three classes of lipoproteins have apolipoprotein B as integral constituent: very low density lipoproteins (VLDL), intermediate density lipoproteins (IDL), and low density lipoproteins (LDL) (Sniderman et al., 1991). Among them, LDL has the biggest apolipoprotein B proportion and is the most likely to interact with subendothelial proteoglycan (Sniderman et al., 1991).

Modification of LDL apolipoprotein B entrapped in intimal layer by oxidative mechanism results in oxidative LDL (oxLDL) (Stocker & Keaney, 2004). Smooth muscle cells, endothelial cells and macrophages are capable to modify LDL via oxidative modification (Diaz et al., 1997). OxLDL is susceptible to scavenging macrophages and gives rise to the generation of cholesterol-laden foam cells (Stocker & Keaney, 2004). OxLDL continuously activates adjacent endothelial cells. Activated endothelial cells express adhesion molecules on their luminal surfaces which attract inflammatory cells from circulation, mainly monocytes and lymphocytes which transmigrate to intimal layer. The blend of inflammatory and resident vascular cells promotes the formation of atherosclerotic plaque. Arterial smooth muscle cells proliferate and migrate to the intimal layer in response to several growth factors releasing from chronic inflammation microenvironment in the intimal layer (Libby, 2002). Smooth muscle cells form a layer which envelopes the core of "inflammatory nidus" at the endothelial site, produce and release collagen and thus shape the so called fibrous cap. Below the cap, "inflammatory nidus" continuously attracts circulating LDL, modifies it and recognizes it as antigen which attracts more inflammatory cells.

Atherosclerotic plaque mainly composes of two constructions which undergo dynamic changes: fibrous cap and lipid-rich core. The theories of how plaque originated have been proposed. Response-to-injury theory proposes the initial step in atherogenesis is endothelial denudation due to injurious substance or forces leading to alteration of normal vascular homeostatic properties (Ross, 1993). Injury to endothelial cells enhances endothelial permeability and adhesiveness for leukocytes to attach and migrate into subendothelial. Here inflammation occurs and macrophage recruitment and platelet adhesion and aggregation take place, which promote procoagulant tendency of the plaque. Response-to-retention theory suggests LDL retention into subendothelial is the initial event and the prerequisite for plaque to form (Tabas et al., 2007). Endothelial injury does not play important role in this process, since plasma LDL is capable to cross normal endothelial cells through transcytosis mechanism and retains in subendothelial (Simionescu & Simionescu, 1993). Subsequent events are monocyte recruitment and lipid-laden macrophage formation which initiate subendothelial inflammation (Tabas et al., 2007). Oxidative modification theory indicates that to initiate plaque formation, subendothelial LDL should be modified chemically in order to attract macrophages' scavenger receptor and be internalized to form foam cells (Stocker & Keaney, 2004). Native plasma LDL can enter subendothelial and is taken up by resident vascular cells via LDL receptor-mediated endocytosis. This native LDL does not initiate an inflammatory response and is not phagocytosed by monocytes, thus does not induce atherosclerosis (Torzewsky & Lackner, 2006).

As the plaque progress, fibrous cap is thinner and turn out to be fragile due to the imbalance of extracellular matrix metabolism, the infiltration of the fibrous cap by macrophages and foam cells, and the calcification process (Burnier et al., 2009). All of these contribute to fibrous cap weakening and lost its protective role. Once fibrous cap lose its integrity, it exposes thrombogenic plaque to circulation. Platelets, around 150,000 until 450,000 per millilitre circulate in the blood without contacting endothelial cells, adhere to exposed site, are activated and initiate the event to seal the broken plaque surface. Unfortunately, this process gives rise to thrombus formation and acute coronary syndrome.

3. Activated platelet promotes progression of the plaque

Putative notion that platelets have role merely in the complicating stage of atherosclerosis has recently been challenged by several evidence indicating the wider involvement of platelets in both early and late atherosclerosis steps (Ruggeri, 2002; Gawaz et al., 2005). In histopathology study of human atherosclerosis, platelets were observed in the lesions, both in the free form and derivative form being phagocytozed by foam cells and macrophages (Sevitt, 1986). Platelet patrols the blood circulation ensuring the integrity of endothelial cells. Once this integrity disrupts, platelets expose to subendothelial component and rapidly undergo activation to form haemostasis thrombus; this is the case of plaque erosion or rupture in acute coronary syndrome. However, intact yet activated endothelial cells can also promote platelet activation, this is the case of progressed atherosclerosis plaque.

3.1 Role of platelet in progressed plaque dynamic

Advanced responses to modified apolipoprotein B-containing LDL through chronic and maladaptive inflammation, macrophage and foam cell apoptotic and plaque necrotic formation are representatives of progressed plaque (Tabas et al., 2007). Endothelial cells lining the plaque are continuosly under activated state and express adhesion molecules and chemoattractant mediator in their surface. Monocytes and lymphocytes are attracted and adhere to these molecules and mediators, enter subendothelial and advance inflammatory state in the "inflammatory nidus" of the plaque (Lusis, 2000).

The histomorphology of progressed plaque is characterized by the presence of large lipid-rich necrotic core, and a thin fibrous cap. Fibrous cap composes mainly of extracellular matrix produced by vascular smooth muscle cells (Lusis, 2000). Supportive function of fibrous cap relies on the integrity of this matrix which is maintained through fine balance between matrix production and degradation (Ross, 1993). In progressed plaque, the matrix degradation activity is increased in line with inflammatory activity in the "inflammatory nidus" of the plaque below the cap. Macrophage-derived proteases degrade extracellular matrix, thus weaken fibrous cap (Ross, 1993).

Necrotic core of progressed plaque is derived from foam cells that endure apoptosis and necrotic. Initially, necrosis core is an acellular lipid-rich core, which predominantly consist of deposited lipids, such as cholesterol esters and free cholesterol derived mostly from retain LDL particles (Lusis, 2000). High toxicity of LDL oxidation and formation of reactive oxygen species damage the surroundings vascular cells, including foam cells (Madamanchi et al., 2005). The death of foam cells discharges extracellular lipids and cell debris into adjacent environments, thus promotes necrotic core formation (Lusis, 2000). Necrotic core enlarges and, in addition to free cholesterol, composes of cholesterol crystals, hyalinized hemorrhage and foam cell necrotic remnants (Virmani et al., 2000). Intimal calcifications, resulting from advance lipid oxidation and inflammatory cytokine reaction which modify osteogenic regulatory genes to promote osteogenesis, scatter in the base of necrotic core adjacent to the medial layer (Virmani et al., 2000; Abedin et al., 2004). Neovascularization in the intimal and medial layer is another hallmark of progressed plaque (Fleiner et al., 2004). Hyperplastic network of vasa vasorum and ectopic neovascularization of the plaque are associated with intimal thickening, lipid contents and the degree of inflammation (Fleiner et al., 2004). The extent of these microvessels delivers a channel for entry of inflammatory cells into the plaque, boosting inflammation even more (Lusis, 2000). This blood vessel networks are fragile and prone to rupture and create an outward expansion of intraplaque hemorrhage that may overwhelm the integrity of the fibrous cap (Dickson & Gottlieb, 2003).

Thrombogenic property of lipid-rich necrotic core is determined by its collagen and tissue factor content. Two important direct platelet agonists dwell in the lipid-rich core, i.e lysophosphatidic acid which mediates platelet shape change during thrombus formation and collagen which induces platelet adhesion and aggregation (Lusis, 2000). Tissue factor, another major thrombogenic subtrate in the lipid-rich core, is released by endothelial cells, smooth muscle cells, monocytes and macrophages or foam cells (Moons et al., 2002). The most abundant tissue factor site is in the necrotic core (Moons et al., 2002). Tissue factor activates coagulation cascade and promotes thrombus stabiliy through fibrin network formation. Platelets are also capable in releasing tissue factor which give a hint of their role in supporting coagulation process (Zillmann et al., 2001).

3.2 Platelet-endothelial interaction promotes progressed plaque

Platelets have two storage granules, alpha and dense granules. Alpha granules contain adhesion molecules, chemokines, coagulation and fibrinolysis proteins, growth factors, and other proteins (Linden & Jackson, 2010). Dense granules contain molecules such as calcium, magnesium, phosphate and pyrophosphate, adenosine and guanosine triphosphate, adenosine and guanosine diphosphate and serotonin (Linden & Jackson, 2010). These granules develop in megakaryocytes, the progenitor cell of platelets. Platelet also contains lysosomes which have ubiquitous lysosomal membrane proteins: LAMP-1, LAMP-2, and CD63 (LAMP-3), acid hydrolases, cathepsins and other proteins (King & Reed, 2002).

In the alpha granules, platelet-specific proteins are synthesized only in megakaryocytes and deliver to platelets which undergo proteolytic upon platelet activation, which include platelet factor 4 (PF-4) and β-thromboglobulin (King & Reed, 2002). Platelet-selective proteins are synthesized principally by megakaryocytes but also in fewer number by few other cells and found in a larger concentration in platelets than plasma. These platelet-selective proteins include coagulation factor V, thrombospondin, P-selectin, and von Willebrand factor (King & Reed, 2002).

It is expected that platelets keep away from contact with vascular walls or other blood cellular components. Under steady laminar blood stream, platelets tend to flow away from endothelial cell surface area, avoiding connection with endothelial cells. Furthermore, intact and inactivated endothelial cell prevent platelet to adhere to its surface. Endothelial cells control platelet activity through inhibitory mechanisms involving cyclooxigenase 2 (Cox-2), prostacyclin or prostanoid synthetic systems (Gawaz, 2006). However, activated endothelial cells are capable to capture platelets and activated them, even without any endothelial damage (intact endothelial cells). Activated platelets will express several molecules, release their granule contents and stimulate surrounding cells, thus promoting plaque progression.

3.2.1 Rolling and adhering of platelet to endothelial cell surface

During inflammation, endothelial cells are activated and change their phenotype becoming prone to be adhesive for platelets (Gawaz, 2006). In vitro experiment showed that platelets adhere to activated human umbilical vein endothelial cells (HUVEC) which is mediated by fibrinogen, fibronectin and von Willebrand factor bound to platelets and endothelial cell receptors, ICAM-1, integrin αvβ3 and GPIb (Bombelli et al., 1998). In vivo experiment discloses that loose contact between platelets and activated endothelial cells precedes a tighter adhesion (Frenette et al., 1995). Rolling of platelets to activated endothelial cell is mediated by endothelial P-selectin and constitutively-expressed platelet P-selectin glycoprotein ligand 1 (PSGL-1) (Frenette et al., 1995; Frenette et al., 2002).

P-selectin is a type-1 membrane glycoprotein with a C-type lectin domain and is stored in the Weibel-Palade bodies of endothelial cells and alpha granules of platelets (Furie & Furie, 1995). It rapidly translocate to cell membrane upon endothelial cell or platelet activation (Frenette et al., 2002). PSGL-1 is an adhesion molecule primarily expressed in myeloid cells and T cells and functions as the main P-selectin ligand which mediates interactions between myeloid cells and endothelial cells as well as between myeloid cells and platelets (Vandendries et al., 2004). In the study of apoE-knock-out and the P-selectin gene deletion mice, atherosclerotic lesion development was significantly delayed, indicating the role of P-selectin as a key adhesion receptor in promoting advanced atherosclerosis (Dong et al., 2000). In early atherogenesis, it is likely that intact endothelial cells activate quiescent platelets through rolling mechanism via endothelial cell P-selectin and platelet PSGL-1 interaction. Endothelial cells coating atherosclerotic plaque are constantly under activated state, thus expressed P-selectin and attract platelets. P-selectin-expressed activated platelets bind to activated endothelial cells in a greater amount than non-activated platelets do.

In addition to platelet PSGL-1, platelet GP1bα is capable to interact with endothelial P-selectin and mediate platelet rolling (Gawaz et al., 2006). GP1bα is a component of GP Ib-IX-V complex which comprises four polypeptides: GP Ibα, GP Ibβ, GP IX, and GP V (Romo et al., 1999). GP Ib-IX-V complex bind to subendothelial von Willebrand factor, exposed when endothelial cell disrupted and initiate thrombosis. GP1α contains von Willebrand factor-binding site and molecular structure nearly similar to PSGL-1 (Romo et al., 1999). Consequently, during endothelial cell activation, in addition to P-selectin, von Willebrand factor are also released from Weibel Palade body to the surface cell membrane. Both endothelial cell P-selectin and von Willebrand factor become the target for platelet GP1bα (Theilmeier et al., 2002). A study using mice deficient of von Willebrand factor showed some level of protection from atherosclerosis thus elucidated the role of von Willebrand factor on plaque formation and progression in intact endothelial cells (Methia et al., 2001).

3.2.2 Tight adhesion of platelet to endothelial cell surface

P-selectin-mediated loose contact is subsequently changed by tighter connection involving endothelial cell integrin, αvβ3 and platelet integrin, αIIbβ3 (Langer & Gawaz, 2008). Ligation of platelet GPIbα to endothelial cell von Willebrand factor during platelet rolling lead to activation of platelet integrin (Kasirer-Friede et al., 2002). Integrins are ubiquitous transmembrane α/β heterodimers that mediate cell-matrix and cell-cell interactions (Bennet, 2005). Platelets express 3 members of the β1 subfamily (αIIβ1, αvβ1, and αvIβ1) and 2 members of the β3 subfamily (αvβ3 and αIIbβ3) (Bennet, 2005). An αIIbβ3 is the most important integrin on platelets (Gawaz et al., 1991). In vitro and in vivo studies show that platelet αIIbβ3 and endothelial cell αvβ3, mediate firm contact between platelets and activated endothelial cells (Bombeli et al., 1998; Maasberg et al, 1999). By forming a bridge to fibrinogen, αIIbβ3 promotes arrest of platelets to adhesion molecules, intercellular adhesion molecule-1 (ICAM)-1, and to αvβ3 on activated endothelial cells (Bombeli et al., 1998; von Hundelshausen & Weber, 2007). Fibrinogen links platelet fibrinogen receptor on the surface of αIIbβ3 to the endothelial cell αvβ3 and forms the firm platelet adhesion to activated endothelial cells (Gawaz et al., 1991).

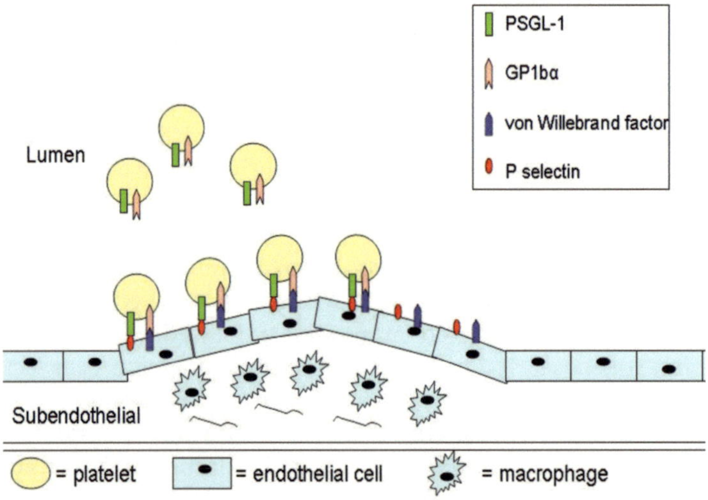

Fig. 1. Rolling of platelets to endothelial cells is mediated by platelet PSGL-1 and GP1bα bind to endothelial cell von Willebrand factor and P selectin.

It is worth mentioning that interaction between platelets and activated endothelial cells is not sufficient to promote thrombus formation. However, platelet adhesion to endothelial cells contributes to the progression of the plaque. Platelets mediate such effects through releasing products following adhesion and activation. The contents of storage granules are liberated upon platelet activation. It is estimated more than 300 proteins are secreted from activated platelets, which act in an autocrine or paracrine manner to modulate cell signaling and mediate the plaque progression (Coppinger et al., 2004).

Endothelial cell chemotactic, adhesion, and proteoliytic capacities are altered by paracrine modulation of substances released by adherent activated platelets. Here are the lists of platelet contents released upon adhesion and activation : (1) adhesion proteins (e.g., P-selectin, vitronectin, fibrinogen, fibronectin, von Willebrand factor, thrombospondin and αIIbβ3), (2) growth factors (e.g., PDGF, TGF-β, EGF and bFGF), (3) chemokines (e.g. RANTES, PF-4 and epithelial-neutrophil activating protein 78 (ENA-78)), (4) cytokine-like factors (e.g. IL-1β, CD40 ligand and β-thromboglobulin) and (5) coagulation factors (e.g. factor V, factor XI, PAI-1, plasminogen and protein S) (Gawaz et al., 2005).

In vitro study revealed that activated platelets coincubated with cultured endothelial cells gave rise to a secretion of MCP-1 and surface expression of ICAM-1 and αvβ3 on endothelial cells, which is mediated by an IL-1-dependent mechanism (Gawaz et al., 2000). MCP-1 is an effectual chemotactic factor for monocytes and ICAM-1 is an adhesion molecule which advocates monocyte and neutrophil recruitment to endothelial cells. This study emphasized the important role of IL-1β on mediating endothelial cell activity upon platelet activation. IL-1 is the prototypic cytokine released by inflammatory cells and three members of the IL-1 gene family have been identified: IL-1, IL-1β, and IL-1 receptor antagonist (IL-1RA) (von Hundelshausen & Weber, 2007). Platelet activation induces rapid and persistent synthesis and release of IL1β and converts endothelial cell phenotype to become more adhesive to circulating neutrophils (Lindemann et al., 2001). Inhibition of β3 integrin attenuated the synthesis of platelet IL-1β, indicating firm adhesion of platelet to endothelial cells is prerequisite for IL-1β sustained secretion (Lindemann et al., 2001).

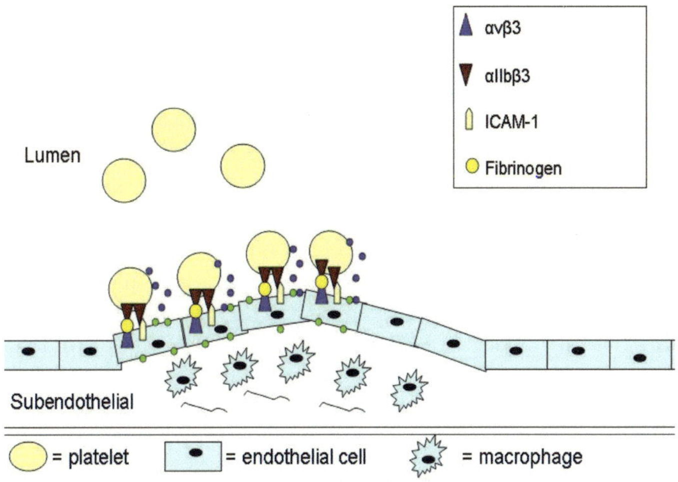

Fig. 2. Tight adhesion of platelets to endothelial cells is mediated by platelet αIIbβ3 bind to endothelial cell αvβ3, bridged by fibrinogen, and ICAM-1. This results in release of platelet contents (blue dots) which mediates endothelial activated molecules (green dots) expression,

Upon activation, platelet expresses CD40 ligand (CD40L) which ligates CD40 expressed by activated endothelial cells (Henn et al., 1998). Platelet CD40L and endothelial cell CD40 interaction amplifies the release of IL-8 and MCP-1 from endothelial cells and enhances the expression of endothelial cell adhesion receptors including E-selectin, VCAM-1, and ICAM-1 (Henn et al., 1998). In vivo study using mice deficient of platelet CD40L shows that platelet CD40L accelerate plaque formation and progression, mainly due to prevention of leukocyte recruitment (Lievens et al., 2010). This study implicates that platelet CD40L is important for recruitment of monocytes, neutrophils and lymphocytes during plaque intitiation and progression. Ligation of CD40L on endothelial cells promotes endothelial cell tissue factor expression, thus enhances a procoagulant phenotype on endothelial cells (Slupsky et al., 1998). Furthermore, it implicates in both the generation and secretion of matrix metalloproteinase-9 (MMP-9) and protease receptor urokinase-type plasminogen activator receptor (uPAR), thus promotes proteolytic activity on endothelial cells (May et al., 2002). Tight adhesion of platelet to endothelial cell via αIIbβ3 binding enhances platelet CD40L upregulation and matrix degradation (May et al., 2002). This endothelial-mediated matrix degradation is important in digestion of fibrous cap, thus promotes imbalance of matrix production and degradation and subsequently weakens the cap. This contributes to loss of cap protection and threatens plaque in rupture-prone condition.

PF-4, stored in platelet alpha granules, is the most abundant protein secreted by activated platelets. In histopathological study on human carotid atherosclerotic, PF-4 accumulates within macrophages of the plaque in the early lesion and continues to accumulate in foam cells and neovascular endothelial cells as lesion progressed (Pitsilos et al., 2003). PF-4 is deposited on the endothelial cell surface and retained by subendothelial proteoglycan (Aidoudi & Bikfalvi, 2010). PF-4 can activate endothelial cells by stimulating E-selectin expression (Yu et al., 2005). In vitro study indicates that PF-4 inhibits apolipoprotein B-containing LDL catabolism and facilitates retension of LDL on cell surface (Sachais et al., 2002). PF-4 blocks LDL uptake by LDL receptor expressed by vascular wall cells, thus increases its retention and prolongs its residence time in the vascular space which allows apolipoprotein-B to be modified and increases ox-LDL deposition (Nassar et al., 2002).

RANTES, secreted by activated platelets, triggers monocyte arrest and recruitment under flow conditions in vitro and in perfused carotid arteries (von Hundelshausen et al., 2001). Platelet P-selectin is important mediator of RANTES upregulation, indicates that RANTES is secreted during platelet rolling to endothelial cells (Schober et al., 2002). In atherosclerotic lesions and injury of apolipoprotein-E deficient mice, RANTES is expressed on endothelial cells (von Hundelshausen et al., 2001). Endothelial cells should have been modified by IL-1β, in order to receive the deposition of RANTES (Weyrich et al., 2002). Taken together, platelet-generated RANTES involves in atherosclerosis early in the beginning and more prominently in the plaque progression by modulating intimal hyperplasia and monocyte recruitment (Schober et al., 2002). Initial knowledge of ENA-78 activity is that this CXC chemokine superfamily member is synthesized and secreted by activated endothelial cells which give a proadhesive activity for neutrophils (Walz et al., 1997). Activated platelet expresses ENA-78 which attract leukocyte to adhere the endothelial cells (Schober et al., 2002). Furthermore, activated platelet-induced IL-1β action can stimulate endothelial cells to secret ENA-78 which encourage endothelial cell adhesiveness (Weyrich et al., 2002).

3.3 Platelet-leukocyte interaction enhances progressed plaque

Migration and recruitment of leukocytes into atherosclerotic plaque are essential steps of atherosclerosis progression. Leukocytes are captured and begin rolling on P-selectin expressing-endothelial cells. Leukocytes express PSGL-1 which engages in leukocyte rolling and attachment to P-selectin. Similar to that of platelet, P-selectin-mediated leukocyte binding to endothelial cells is a loose contact. This connection mediates rolling of leukocytes on the endothelial surface without firm attachment.

In addition to direct contact between leukocytes and endothelial cells, activated platelets interact with leukocyte as well. Among leukocytes, monocytes and lymphocytes are the first to be involved in atherogenesis and plaque progression.

3.3.1 Activated platelets bind and promote monocyte activation and transmigration

Monocytes are predominant leukocytes lodge in atherosclerotic plaque. Adherent platelets efficiently mediate monocyte rolling and arrest, even at high shear rate. Monocyte rolling is mediated by P-selectin on activated platelets and PSGL-1, constitutively expressed on monocytes (Kuijper et al., 1998). CD15, expressed by monocytes, has also been shown to bind platelet P-selectin (Larsen et al., 1990).

The initial connection between platelet P-selectin and monocyte PSGL-1 and CD15 is a loose attachment, and within rapid periode it leads to elevated expression of the monocyte integrin αMβ2 (membrane-activated complex 1 (Mac-1)) and makes tighter adhesion which support binding to platelet (Neumann et al., 1999). Monoctyte Mac-1 has several counter-receptors expressed on activated platelet, such as GP1b, JAM-3 and ICAM-2 (Simon et al., 2000; Santoso et al., 2002; Diacovo et al., 1994).

Platelet junctional adhesion molecule (JAM) supports platelet chemokine deposition and promotes monocyte recruitment (von Hundelshausen & Weber, 2007). JAM-3 is identified as a counter-receptor on platelets for the monocyte Mac-1 and mediates platelet-monocytes interactions (Santoso et al., 2002). Mac-1 is also able to bind indirectly to platelet αIIbβ3 linked by soluble fibrinogen bridge (Gawaz et al., 1991). Furthermore, several protein-receptor complexes mediate platelet-monocyte adhesion, such as thrombospondin which form a bridging of the CD36-CD36 interaction in both monocytes and platelets, CD40L on the platelet which attach to monocyte CD40 and monocyte triggering receptor expressed on myeloid cell 1 (TREM-1) to platelet-expressed TREM-1 ligand (Van Gils et al., 2009).

The attachment of activated adherent platelets to monocytes induces monocyte activation through shedding, expressing and releasing fungsional proteins. Interaction between platelets and monocytes increases the expression and activity of chemotaxis (MCP-1 and MIP-1α), proteolysis (uPAR and MMP), thrombosis (tissue factors), activation (TNF-α and IL-8) and adhesion (Mac-1 and VLA-4) factors on monocytes as well as potentiates monocyte to macrophage differentiation (Gawaz et al., 2005). In this respect, platelet-monocyte interaction provides an atherogenic environment at the vascular wall that supports plaque formation and regression (Gawaz et al., 2005). Similar to adherent platelets, activated platelets circulating in blood stream can affect endothelial cell and leukocyte phenotype (Huo et al., 2003). Circulating activated platelets are detected in the blood of patients with atherosclerotic conditions, such as acute coronary syndromes (Sarma et al., 2002), stable coronary disease (Furman et al., 1998), and diabetes mellitus (Broijersen et al., 1998).

In vitro study shows that platelet P-selectin increases monocytoid cell adhesion to endothelial cells (Theilmeier et al., 1999). In vivo study using apoE-knock-out mice reveals that circulating activated platelets, through platelet P-selectin, promote monocyte recruitment to atherosclerotic plaque and accelerate the formation of atherosclerotic lesions (Huo et al., 2002). Platelet P-selectin-mediated interactions lead to deposition of platelet-derived proinflammatory factors, RANTES and PF-4, to the vessel wall and monocytes, resulting in activation of monocyte integrins, increased monocyte recruitment and accelerate atherosclerosis (Huo et al., 2002). Inversely, at low levels, activated endothelial cells express PSGL-1 and bind P-selectin on platelets and monocytes, thus mediating monocyte tethering and platelet recruitment to the endothelial cells (Da Costa Martins, 2007).

Not only do adherent platelets form tight binding to monocyte, but also circulating activated platelets attach to monocyte and form platelet monocyte complex (PMC). PMC reflected great capacity of platelet activation and in lesser extent, monocyte activation (Van Gils et al., 2009). Activated platelets bind via P-selectin to its receptor on monocytes, PSGL-1, and form complexes (Van Gils et al., 2009). PMCs mediate monocyte tethering and adhering to endothelial cell surface, making adherent monocyte-PMC cluster and promoting monocyte, and probably platelet, transmigration into subendothelial plaque lesion (Da Costa Martins et al., 2004). PMC high adhesive capability to activated endothelial cell is due to increasing integrin activation on monocyte and subsequently, increasing cell adhesion to fibronectin, VCAM-1 and ICAM-1 (Da Costa Martins, 2006). Monocytes transmigrate into the atherosclerotic plaque, and change phenotype, becoming macrophages which express scavenger receptors and digest oxLDL to become foam cells (Libby & Aikawa, 2001).

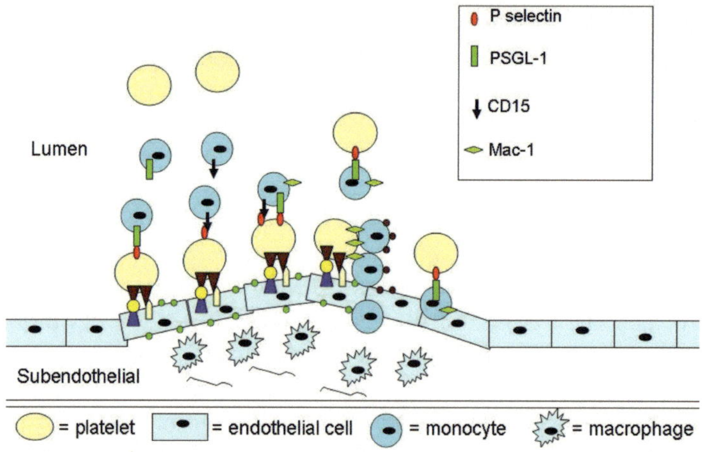

Fig. 3. Activated platelets recruit monocytes via platelet P selectin binding to monocyte PSGL-1 and CD15, subsequently stabilized by monocyte Mac-1 bind to counter receptors in platelets thus promoting monocyte adhesion and transmigration into subendothelial.

Monocytes are the main source of tissue factor, an important determinant of thrombogenic plaque (Lindmark et al., 2000). Along with more monocyte recruitment, macrophage proliferation and tissue factor production intensify, filling the plaque with inflammatory and thrombogenic material which promote plaque progression.

3.3.2 Activated platelets bind and promote lymphocyte activation and transmigration

Lymphocyte transmigration from circulation to atherosclerotic plaque follows three steps: selectin-mediated rolling, integrin-modulated adhesion and transmigration. The transmigration of all lymphocyte populations, i.e. T cells, B cells, and natural killer cells, are enhanced by activated platelets (Li, 2008). Activated platelets interact with lymphocytes through binding between platelet P-selectin and lymphocyte PSGL-1 forming a loose contact, which subsequently induces clustering of αL integrin and enhances lymphocyte firm adhesion via ICAM-1 binding (Atarashi et al., 2005). Among lymphocytes, T cells have stronger adhesive capacity than B cells, indicates that T cells are selectively recruited in mediation of P-selectin expressing cells (Li, 2008) Enhancement of T cell adhesion on subendothelial matrix is mediated by activated platelets through formation of platelet-T cell conjugates and via ligations of P-selectin, CD40L and αIIbβ3 integrins (Li, 2008).

In progressed atherosclerotic plaque, T cells make up nearly 10% to 20% of the cell population and assemble at sites which are prone to rupture and cause fatal thrombosis (Hansson et al., 2002). Most of the T cells in atherosclerotic lesions is T helper (CD3+ and CD4+) and T-cell antigen receptor positive (TCRβ+), which indicate a function of recognition of antigens presented by macrophages or dendritic cells (Hansson et al., 2002). They modulate cell mediated immunity through secretion of interferon (IFN-γ), IL-2, and IL-22 (Hansson et al., 2002). IFN-γ inhibits smooth muscle cell new collagen synthesis, which is essensial in supporting fibrous caps, thus weakens fibrous cap and promotes rupture-prone plaque (Libby et al., 2010). Smooth muscle cells in the rupture-prone plaque express HLA-DR which is susceptible to IFN-γ action (Libby & Aikawa, 2001). Furthermore, activated T cells induce production of MMP and tissue factor, mediated by CD40-CD40L binding, which enhances the thrombogenicity of the plaque lipid-rich core (Libby et al., 2010).

4. Activated platelet plays important role in coronary atherothrombosis

Arterial thrombosis is the acute complication that develops on the chronic atherosclerosis lesion, i.e. atherothrombosis, and in the coronary artery it causes acute coronary syndromes, during which blood flow through coronary segment is partially or totally obstructed. Platelets are prominent constituents of the thrombi that occlude the lumen of arteries. In this regard, atherothrombosis is a term that describes the combination of acute, a complication, and chronic, a progression, events of arterial disease (Ruggeri, 2002). Platelets are involved in both processes, through promoting plaque progression and participating in ruptured plaque-driven thrombus formation (Ruggeri, 2002).

Inducing event of acute coronary syndrome is plaque rupture or erosion. Rupture of fibrous cap lining the plaque is account for 60–65% of occlusive thrombi and erosion of endothelial cells lining the plaque is responsible for the rest 35–40% (Dickson & Gottlieb, 2003). In the rupture-prone atherosclerotic plaque, fibrous cap maintains protective role for the integrity of the plaque and provides a barrier between the thrombogenic material in the necrotic core and circulating blood components, mainly platelets and coagulation factors (Libby & Aikawa, 2001). As plaque progressed, leukocyte-driven inflammation is heightened in the intimal layer. Inflamed leukocytes can hinder biosynthesis of collagen from smooth muscle cells and can themselves overexpress collagen-degrading proteinases which in turn give the condition of the imbalance between collagen synthesis and degradation, thus weakening the fibrous caps and lead to plaque rupture (Libby & Aikawa, 2001). Furthermore, leukocytes participate in augmentation the production of the procoagulant factor, primarily tissue factor, in plaque lesion and give rise to the high thrombogenicity of the plaque's lipid core (Libby et al., 2010). In addition to intrinsic factor within plaque, vessel lumen shear stress contribution for rupture of the plaque is considerate as well, since lumen restricted-area surrounding the plaque causes a local rising in blood flow velocity. Wall shear rate may exceed considerably at the edge of a severe occlusion in a coronary artery. High shear stress may specifically enhance platelet reactivity to matrix extra cellular of plaque (Ruggeri, 2002). The main trigger for the formation of a thrombus is the loss of the endothelial cell barrier and exposure of thrombogenic subendothelial extracellular matrix components with circulating blood. The response of platelets to this event can be divided into three successive but closely integrated phases: adhesion, activation and aggregation (Ruggeri, 2002). Several indices of activated platelets in the circulating blood are increased in patients with coronary artery disease and acute coronary syndromes, such as platelet surface molecule expression, platelet-monocyte aggregates, platelet-neutrophil aggregates and soluble proteins releasing upon platelet activation, mainly soluble CD40L (sCD40L) (Linden et al., 2007; Setianto et al., 2010).

4.1 Platelet tethering and adhesion initiate atherothrombosis

Erosion or rupture of the plaque poses circulating platelets, some of them have already activated, with highly thrombogenic extra cellular matrix components of the lipid core

which contains several adhesive molecules such as collagen, von Willebrand factor, laminin, fibronectin and thrombospondin (Andrews & Berndt, 2004). These molecules, once exposed, provide ligands for various activated platelet surface receptors. Under low shear rate condition, such as in vein and large artery flow, the molecules bind to platelet receptors are collagen, fibronectin and laminin, whereas under higher shear rates, such as in small arteries and atherosclerotic vessel, collagen and von Willebrand factor are principal molecules to mediate platelet slackening, tethering and adhesion (Andrews & Berndt, 2004). The early step of atherothrombosis is tethering of platelets to the surface of rupture plaque and is accomplished through the interaction between platelet GPIbα and collagen-bound von Willebrand factor (Ruggeri, 2002) and platelet GPVI and collagen (Andrews & Berndt, 2004). GPIbα is the major ligand-binding subunit of GPIb-IX–V or von Willebrand factor receptor and, in addition to binding site for von Willebrand factor, contains partially overlapping binding sites for the leukocyte integrin Mac-1, α-thrombin, and P-selectin expressed on activated platelets or activated endothelial cells (Andrews & Berndt, 2004). GPVI is a collagen receptor of the immunoglobulin superfamily that forms a complex with the FcR g-chain at the cell surface in human and mouse platelets (Andrews & Berndt, 2004).
Von Willebrand factor, stored both by alpha granules of platelets or Weibel-Palade body of endothelial cells, is an adhesive glycoprotein found in circulating blood or subendothelial matrix (Andrews & Berndt, 2004). Circulating von Willebrand factor, which amount is much higher than that in subendothelial matrix, can be immobilized in exposed collagen via collagen binding site and become the substrate for platelet GP1bα (Massberg et al., 2003). In addition to collagen-bound, circulating von Willebrand factor can also be immobilized by forming the multimeric connection to matrix-bound, platelet-bound or subendothelial von Willebrand factor (Ulrichts et al., 2005). Immobilized von Willebrand factor is capable to catch circulating platelets via binding with platelet GPIbα (Andrews & Berndt, 2004). Ligation of non-activated platelet GPIbα with collagen-bound von Willebrand factor is not stable enough and is intended mainly to slow down platelets and maintain them in the rupture site, where subsequently platelets will be activated through various receptors, mainly integrin, and stable adhesion is formed.

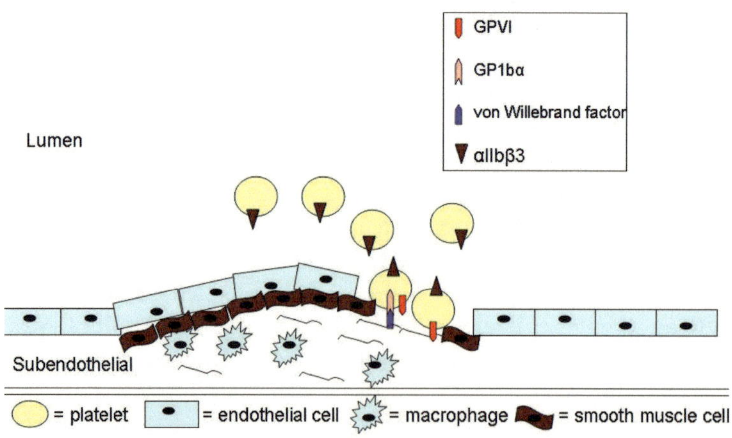

Fig. 4. Plaque rupture exposes platelets to thrombogenic collagen which attract them to adhere via platelet GPVI bind to collagen and GP1bα bind to collagen-bound von Willebrand factor, initiate thrombus formation.

In addition to collagen-bound von Willebrand factor, collagen itself can capture non-activated circulating platelets through platelet GPVI. However, GPVI has only a low affinity for collagen which makes GPVI, same as GPIbα, incapable to mediate stable platelet adhesion. Ligation of GPVI during the initial contact between platelets and subendothelial collagen provides an activation signal through platelet integrins, αIIbβ3 and α2β1, which is essential for subsequent stable platelet adhesion and aggregation (Gawaz, 2004). Although not tightly adherent, this early adhesion of platelets is of adequate affinity to facilitate arrest at high shear rate, leading ultimately to much more stable integrin-mediated adhesion (Andrews & Berndt, 2004).

4.2 Platelet activation and aggregation enhance atherothrombosis

Platelet activation and aggregation are the ensuing steps that occur within minutes, marked by the accumulation of platelets into the haemostatic thrombus (Ruggeri, 2002). Collagen-bound von Willebrand factor and platelet GPIbα interaction convey signal activation of platelet integrin αIIbβ3 to undergo conformational changes which are compulsory for firm, irreversible platelet resting on the subendothelial matrix surface (Gawaz, 2004). Conformational changes of αIIbβ3 enable an exposure of fibrinogen binding site which form cross linking with αIIbβ3 on different platelets by fibrinogen bridge (Andrews & Berndt, 2004). Similarly, ligation of GPVI shifts platelet αIIbβ3 and α2β1 from a low to a high affinity state and contributes to stable platelet adhesion (Gawaz, 2004). Until this step, stable adhesion of platelets is promoted by irreversible binding of platelet αIIbβ3 to collagen-bound von Willebrand factor and platelet α2β1 to uncoated collagen. The integrin-dependent stable adhesion of platelets consequently leads to activation of adherent platelets. Activated platelets are receptive to wide range of agonists or stimulants and adhesive proteins. They express surface receptors, which, upon activation by agonists and adhesive proteins, stimulate internal signaling pathways that lead to further platelet activation, degranulation, and capacity enhancement to bind with other adhesive proteins or platelets. Transmembran receptors are the main agonist-stimulated receptor families and greatly activated during thrombus formation. The important platelet receptors in this class are thrombin receptors (protease activation receptor (PAR-1 and PAR-4), ADP receptors (P2Y1, and P2Y12) and integrins (mainly αIIbβ3) (Freedman, 2005).

Activation of platelets by thrombin through PAR-1 and PAR-4 receptors results in calcium flux, platelet shape change, and stimulation of a variety of platelet-signaling pathways (Freedman, 2005). Importantly, thrombin-PAR receptor interaction leads to activation of integrin αIIbβ3 receptor complex through inside-out signalling (Freedman, 2005).

In non-activated platelets, αIIbβ3, the most abundant platelet integrins, has a very low affinity for its ligands (Cosemans et al., 2008). However, platelet activation remarkably increases the capacity of αIIbβ3 to attach to its ligands, particularly fibrinogen, fibrin, fibronectin and von Willebrand factor (Cosemans et al., 2008). These soluble adhesive proteins are immobilized and are attached to activated αIIbβ3 on the surface of activated adherent platelets and become the substrate for more non-activated circulating platelet recruitment and aggregation (Ruggeri, 2002). The interaction of circulating platelets with adherent platelets carries on through activated αIIbβ3 cross linking between platelets bridged by soluble fibrinogen, thus form the platelet aggregates (Gawaz, 2004). Platelet activation increases the surface density of αIIbβ3, thus more soluble fibrinogen attach and bridge other platelets, makes cross linking and allows continuing platelet aggregation and thrombus growth. The inhibiton of interaction of platelet αIIbβ3 - von Willebrand factor and αIIbβ3 - fibrinogen by αIIbβ3 antagonists, i.e tirofiban, abciximab and eptifibatide, is of potentially benefit in acute settings of coronary atherothrombosis, due to inhibition of platelet aggregation, thrombus growth and stability.

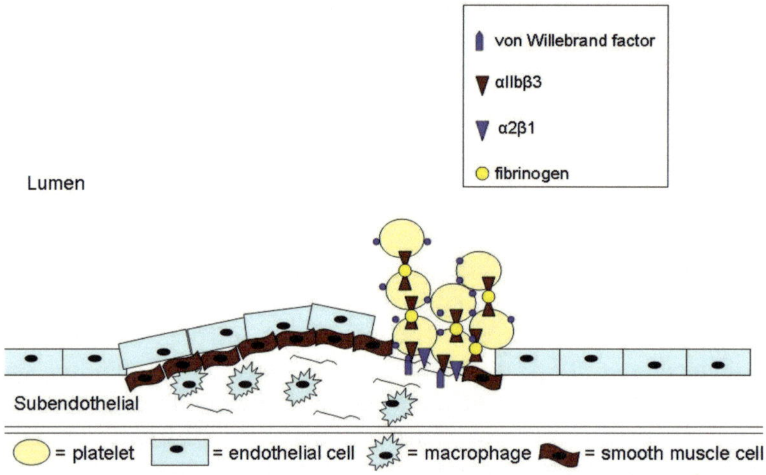

Fig. 5. Adhesion and activation of platelets form stable plug via platelet αIIbβ3 bind to collagen-bound von Willebrand factor and platelet α2β1 bind to collagen, thus stimulate release of platelet surface receptors (blue dots) receptive to agonists and adhesive proteins.

In addition to integrin activation, several means of activation responses of platelets include: mobilization of cytosolic calcium, secretion of ADP, shedding and secretion of CD40L, released of tromboxane A2 (TxA2) and formation of pseudopods which support an effective sealing of the denuded plaque area (Cosemans et al., 2008; Gawaz, 2004). ADP, secreted by dense granules of activated platelets, stimulates platelets in autocrine loop through its receptors, P2Y1 and P2Y12. P2Y1 activation mediates platelet shape change and initiates platelet aggregation by mobilization of intracellular calcium (Andre et al., 2003). P2Y12 activation by ADP signal mediates inhibition of adenylyl cyclase and stabilizes platelet aggregates as well as participates in the firm adhesion by activating αIIbβ3 (Andre et al., 2003). Persistent signal to keep P2Y12 in active state is of paramount important to prevent platelet disaggregation and to maintain αIIbβ3 in its active conformation (Cosemans et al., 2008). In addition to autocrine loop, ADP also works in paracrine mechanism by stimulating and recruiting non activated circulating platelets and inducing them to undergo aggregation with adherent platelets (Gawaz, 2004). Antagonist for P2Y12, i.e ticlopidine and clopidogrel, has already been widely used in acute coronary syndrome.

CD40L, expressed and released by activated platelets, binds to activated αIIbβ3 and contributes in supporting platelet aggregate stability (Andre et al., 2002). Upon platelet activation, the cytosolic CD40L protein is exocytosed to the platelet plasma membrane from where it is also shed and release into circulation in soluble form, sCD40L (Andre et al., 2002). These transmembran and soluble forms are detected to be elevated in patients with acute coronary syndrome (Aukrust et al., 1999; Garlichs et al., 2001; Setianto et al., 2010). Both transmembrane and soluble CD40L can form a cluster with platelet αIIbβ3 and lead to more platelet activation and enhance thrombus formation and stabilization (Andre et al., 2002).

TxA2 is made from arachidonic acid and is secreted by activated adherent platelets. It strengthen the activation process after the release into the extracellular space and create platelet feedback activation by acting as autocrine and paracrine manner on its thromboxane platelet receptor (Gawaz, 2004). TxA2 has a vasoconstricting activity and thus favors formation of the thrombus by slowing down the blood flow (Gawaz, 2004). Aspirin induces a complete and permanent inhibition of platelet TxA2 production through the inactivation of cyclooxygenase. In addition to $\alpha IIb\beta 3$-mediated stability, several other adhesion and signaling receptors contribute to thrombus stability, such as PECAM-1, JAM-A, JAM-C, ESAM, CD226, and Epf kinases/ephrins, which is enable the tight contact of one platelet with receptors on adjacent platelets (Brass et al., 2005).

5. Conclusion

Platelet is a key maker for progression of atherosclerotic plaque. Its ability to interact with activated endothelial cells and leukocytes, provide the milieu of inflammation and thrombus-prone environment in atherosclerotic plaque. Platelet, with relatively similar pattern, captures monocyte and lymphocyte and grants them the path to transmigrate into atherosclerotic plaque. Platelet is a central player during coronary plaque rupture. It starts and nurtures coronary thrombus formation and stabilization. Platelet-based therapeutic modalities for atherosclerosis and acute coronary syndrome are still in progressed studies with some of them yield beneficial effect while others inconclusive.

6. References

Abedin, M.; Tintut, Y.; & Demer, L.L. 2004. Vascular Calcification: Mechanisms and Clinical Ramifications. *Arteriosclerosis, Thrombosis, and Vascular Biology*, Vol.24, No.7, (May 2004), pp.1161-1170, ISSN: 1079-5642.

Aidoudi, S. & Bikfalvi, A. 2010. Interaction of PF4 (CXCL4) With The Vasculature: A Role in Atherosclerosis and Angiogenesis. *Thrombosis and Haemostasis*, Vol.104, No.5, (November 2010), pp.941-948, ISSN:0340-6245.

André, P.; Prasad, K.S.S.; Denis, C.V.; He, M,; Papalia, J.M.; Hynes, R.O.; Phillips, D.R. & Wagner, D.D. 2002. CD40L Stabilizes Arterial Thrombi by A 3 Integrin-Dependent Mechanism. *Nature Medicine*, Vol.8, No.3, (March 2002), pp.247-252, ISSN:1078-8956.

Andre, P.; Delaney, S.M.; LaRocca, T.; Vincent, D.; DeGuzman, F.; Jurek, M.; Koller, B.; Phillips, D.R. & Conley, P.B. 2003. P2Y12 Regulates Platelet Adhesion/Activation, Thrombus Growth, and Thrombus Stability in Injured Arteries. *The Journal of Clinical Investigation*, Vol.112, No.3, (August 2003), pp.398-406, ISSN:0021-9738.

Andrews, R.K. & Berndt, M.C. 2004. Platelet Physiology and Thrombosis. *Thrombosis Research*, Vol.114, No.5-6, (2004), pp. 447-453, ISSN:0049-3848.

Atarashi, K.; Hirata, T.; Matsumoto, M.; Kanemitsu, N. & Miyasaka, M. 2005. Rolling of Th1 Cells Via P-Selectin Glycoprotein Ligand-1 Stimulates LFA-1-Mediated Cell Binding To ICAM-1. *The Journal of Immunology*, vol.174, no.3, (February 2005), pp.1424-1432, ISSN:0022-1767.

Aukrust, P.; Müller, F.; Ueland, T.; Berget, T.; Aaser, E.; Brunsvig, A.; Solum, N.O.; Forfang, K.; Frøland, S.S. & Gullestad, L. 1999. Enhanced Levels of Soluble and Membrane-Bound CD40 Ligand in Patients With Unstable Angina. Possible Reflection of T

Lymphocyte and Platelet Involvement in The Pathogenesis of Acute Coronary Syndromes. *Circulation*, Vol. 100, No.6, (August 1999), pp.614-20, ISSN:0009-7322.

Bennet, J.S. 2005. Structure and Function of The Platelet Integrin αIIbβ3. *Journal of Clinical Investigation*, Vol.115, No.12, (December 2005), pp.3363–3369, ISSN:0021-9738.

Bombeli, T.; Schwartz, B.R. & Harlan, J.M. 1998. Adhesion of Activated Platelets to Endothelial Cells: Evidence For A GPIIbIIIa-Dependent Bridging Mechanism and Novel Roles for Endothelial Intercellular Adhesion Molecule 1 (ICAM-1), Alphavbeta3 Integrin, and GP1balpha. *Journal of Experimental Medicine*, Vol.187, No.3, (February 1998), pp.329-339, ISSN:0022-1007.

Borén, J.; Olin, K.; Lee, I.; Chait, A.;, Wight, T.N. & Innerarity, T.L. 1998. Identification of The Principal Proteoglycan-Binding Site in LDL. A Single-Point Mutation in Apo-B100 Severely Affects Proteoglycan Interaction Without Affecting LDL Receptor Binding. *Journal of Clinical Investigation*, Vol.101, No.12, (June 1998), pp.2658–2664, ISSN:0021-9738.

Brass, L.F.; Zhu, L. & Stalker, T.J. 2005. Minding The Gaps to Promote Thrombus Growth and Stability. *Journal of Clinical Investigation*, Vol.115, No.12, (December 2005), pp. 3385–3392, ISSN:0021-9738.

Broijersen, A.; Hamsten, A.; Eriksson, M.; Angelin, B. & Hjemdahl, P. 1998. Platelet Activity In Vivo in Hyperlipoproteinemia–Importance of Combined Hyperlipidemia. *Thrombosis and Haemostasis*, Vol.79, No.2, (February 1998), pp.268–275, ISSN:0340-6245.

Burnier, L.; Fontana, P.; Angelillo-Scherrer, A. & Kwak, B.R. 2009. Intercellular Communication in Atherosclerosis. *Physiology*, Vol.24, No.1 (February 2009), pp.36-44, ISSN:1548-9213.

Coppinger, J.A.; Cagney, G.; Toomey, S.; Kislinger, T.; Belton, O.; McRedmond, J.P.; Cahill, D.J.; Emili, A.; Fitzgerald, D.J. & Maguire, P.B. 2004. Characterization of The Proteins Released From Activated Platelets Leads to Localization of Novel Platelet Proteins in Human Atherosclerotic Lesions. *Blood*, Vol.103, No.6, (March 2004), pp.2096-2104, ISSN:0006-4971.

Cosemans, J.M.E.M.; Iserbyt, B.F.; Deckmyn, H. & Heemskerk, J.W.M. 2008. Multiple Ways to Switch Platelet Integrins On and Off. *Journal of Thrombosis and Haemostasis*, Vol.6, No.8, (August 2008), pp.1253–1261, ISSN:1538-7933.

Da Costa Martins, P.; van den Berk, N.; Ulfman, L.H.; Koenderman, L.; Hordijk, P.L & Zwaginga, J.J. 2004. Platelet-Monocyte Complexes Support Monocyte Adhesion to Endothelium by Enhancing Secondary Tethering and Cluster Formation. *Arteriosclerosis, Thrombosis, and Vascular Biology*, Vol. 24, No. 1, (January 2004), pp. 193-199, ISSN:1079-5642.

Da Costa Martins, P.A.; van Gils, J.M.; Mol, A.; Hordijk, P.L. & Zwaginga, J.J. 2006. Platelet Binding to Monocytes Increases The Adhesive Properties of Monocytes by Up-Regulating The Expression and Functionality of β1 and β2 Integrins. *Journal of Leukocyte Biology*, Vol. 79, No. 3, (March 2006), pp. 499-507, ISSN:0741-5400.

Da Costa Martins, P.; García-Vallejo, J.; van Thienen, J.V.; Fernandez-Borja, M.; van Gils, J.M.; Beckers, C.; Horrevoets. A.J.; Hordijk, P.L. &; Zwaginga, J.J. 2007. P-Selectin Glycoprotein Ligand-1 Is Expressed on Endothelial Cells and Mediates Monocyte Adhesion to Activated Endothelium. *Arteriosclerosis, Thrombosis, and Vascular Biology*, Vol.27, No.5, (May 2007), pp.1023-1029, ISSN:1079-5642.

Diaz, M.; Frei, B.; Vita, J.A. & Keaney, J.F.Jr. 1997. Antioxidants and Atherosclerotic Heart Disease. 1997. *The New England Journal of Medicine,* Vol.337, No.6, (August 1997), pp.408–416, ISSN:0028-4793.

Diacovo, T.G.; deFougerolles, A.R.; Bainton, D.F. & Springer, T.A. 1994. A Functional Integrin Ligand on The Surface of Platelets: Intercellular Adhesion Molecule-2. *The Journal of Clinical Investigation,* Vol.94, No.3, (September 1994), pp:1243-51, ISSN:0021-9738.

Dickson, B.C. & Gotlieb, A.I. 2003. Towards Understanding Acute Destabilization of Vulnerable Atherosclerotic Plaques. *Cardiovascular Pathology,* Vol.12, No.5, (September 2003), pp.237-248, ISSN:1054-8807.

Dong, Z.M.; Brown, A.A. & Wagner, D.D. 2000. Prominent Role of P-Selectin in the Development of Advanced Atherosclerosis in ApoE-Deficient Mice. *Circulation,* Vol.101, No.19, (May 2000), pp.2290-2295, ISSN:0009-7322.

Fleiner, M.; Kummer, M.; Mirlacher, M.; Sauter, G; Cathomas, G.; Krapf, R. & Biedermann, B.C. 2004. Arterial Neovascularization and Inflammation in Vulnerable Patients Early and Late Signs of Symptomatic Atherosclerosis. *Circulation,* Vol.110, No.18, (November 2004), pp.2843-2850, ISSN:0009-7322.

Freedman, J.E. 2005. Molecular Regulation of Platelet-Dependent Thrombosis. *Circulation,* Vol.112, No.17, (October 2005), pp.2725-2734, ISSN:0009-7322.

Frenette, P.S.; Johnson, R.C.; Hynest, R.O. & Wagner, D.D. 1995. Platelets Roll on Stimulated Endothelium In Vivo: An Interaction Mediated by Endothelial P-Selectin. *Proceedings of the National Academy of Sciences of the United States of America.* Vol.92, No.16, (August 1995), pp.7450-7454, ISSN:0027-8424

Frenette, P.S.; Denis, C.V.; Weiss, L.; Jurk, K.; Subbarao, S.; Kehrel, B., Hartwig, J.H.; Vestweber, D. & Wagner, D.D. 2002. P-Selectin Glycoprotein Ligand 1 (PSGL-1) is Expressed on Platelets and Can Mediate Platelet–Endothelial Interactions In Vivo. *Journal of Experimental Medicine,* Vol.191, No.8, (April 2000), pp.1413–1422, ISSN: 0022-1007.

Furie, B. & Furie, B.C. 1995. The Molecular Basis of Platelet and Endothelial Cell Interaction with Neutrophils and Monocytes: Role of P-Selectin and The P-Selectin Ligand, PSGL-1. *Thrombosis and Haemostasis,* Vol.74, No.1, (July 1995), pp:224-227, ISSN: 0340-6245.

Furman, M.I.; Benoit, S.E.; Barnard, M.R.; Valeri C,R.; Borbone, M.L.; Becker, R.C.; Hechtman, H.B. & Michelson, A.D. 1998. Increased Platelet Reactivity and Circulating Monocyte-Platelet Aggregates in Patients With Stable Coronary Artery Disease. *Journal of American College of Cardiology,* Vol.31, No.2, (February 1998), pp.352–358, ISSN:0735-1097.

Garlichs, C.D.; Eskafi, S.; Raaz, D.; Schmidt, A.; Ludwig, J.; Herrmann, M.; Klinghammer, L.; Daniel, W.G. & Schmeisser, A. 2001. Patients with Acute Coronary Syndromes Express Enhanced CD40 Ligand/CD154 on Platelets. *Heart,* Vol.86, No.6, (December 2001), pp.649-655, ISSN:1355-6037.

Gawaz, M.P; Loftus, J.C.; Bajt, M.L.; Frojmovic, M.M., Plow, E.F. & Ginsberg, M.H. 1991. Ligand Bridging Mediates Integrin Alpha IIbbeta3 (Platelet GPIIB-IIIA) Dependent Homotypic and Heterotypic Cell-Cell Interactions. *The Journal of Clinical Investigation,* Vol.88, No.4, (October 1991), pp.1128-1134, ISSN:0021-9738.

Gawaz, M.; Brand, K.; Dickfeld, T.; Pogatsa-Murray, G.; Page, S.; Bogner, C.; Koch, W.; Schömig, A. & Neumann, F. 2000. Platelets Induce Alterations of Chemotactic and Adhesive Properties of Endothelial Cells Mediated Through an Interleukin-1-Dependent Mechanism. Implications for Atherogenesis. *Atherosclerosis*, Vol.148, No.1, (January 2000), pp.75-85, ISSN:0021-9150.

Gawaz, M. 2004. Role of Platelets in Coronary Thrombosis and Reperfusion of Ischemic Myocardium. *Cardiovascular Research*, Vol.61, No.3 (February 2004), pp.498–511, ISSN:0008-6363.

Gawaz, M.; Langer, H. & May, A.E. 2005. Platelets in Inflammation and Atherogenesis. *The Journal of Clinical Investigation*, Vol.115, No.12, (December 2005), pp.3378-3383, ISSN:0021-9738.

Gawaz, M. 2006. Platelets in The Onset of Atherosclerosis. *Blood Cells, Molecules, and Diseases*, Vol.36, No.2 , (April 2006), pp.206–210, ISSN: 1079-9796.

Hansson, G.K.; Libby, P.; Schönbeck, U. & Yan, Z. 2002. Innate and Adaptive Immunity in the Pathogenesis of Atherosclerosis. *Circulation Research*, Vol.91, No.4, (August 2002), pp.281-291, ISSN:0009-7330.

Henn, V.; Slupsky, J.R.; Gräfe, M.; Anagnostopoulos, I.; Förster, R.; Müller-Berghaus, G.; & Kroczek, R.A. 1998. CD40 Ligand on Activated Platelets Triggers an Inflammatory Reaction of Endothelial Cells. *Nature*, Vol.391, No.6667, (February 1998), pp.517-615, ISSN:0028-0836.

Huo, Y.; Schober, A.; Forlow, S.B.; Smith, D.F.; Hyman, M.C.; Jung, S.; Littman, D.R.; Weber, C. & Ley, K. 2003. Circulating Activated Platelets Exacerbate Atherosclerosis in Mice Deficient in Apolipoprotein E. *Nature Medicine*, Vol.9, No.1 (January 2003), pp.61 - 67, ISSN:1078-8956.

Kasirer-Friede, A.; Ware, J.; Leng, L.; Marchese, P.; Ruggeri, Z.M. & Shattil, S.J. 2002. Lateral Clustering of Platelet GP Ib-IX Complexes Leads to Up-regulation of the Adhesive Function of Integrin $\alpha_{IIb}\beta_3$. *The Journal of Biological Chemistry*, Vol.277, No.14, (April 2002), pp:11949-11956, ISSN:0021-9258.

King, S.M. & Reed, G.L. 2002. Development of Platelet Secretory Granules. *Seminars in Cell & Developmental Biology*, Vol.13, No.4 (August 2002), pp.293–302, ISSN:1084-9521.

Kuijper, P.H.; Gallardo Torres, H.I.; Houben, L.A.; Lammers, J.W.; Zwaginga, J.J. & Kenderman, L. 1998. P-selectin and MAC-1 Mediate Monocyte Rolling and Adhesion to ECM-Bound Platelets Under Flow Conditions. *Journal of Leukocyte Biology*, Vol.64, No.4, (October 1998), pp.467–473, ISSN:0741-5400.

Langer, H.F. & Gawaz, M. 2008. Platelet-vessel Wall Interactions in Atherosclerotic Disease. *Thrombosis and Haemostasis*, Vol.99, No.5, (May 2008), pp.480-486, ISSN:0340-6245.

Larsen, E.; Palabrica, T.; Sajer, S.; Gllbert, G.E.; Wagner, D.D.; Furie, B.C. & Furie, B. 1990. PADGEM-Dependent Adhesion of Platelets to Monocytes and Neutrophils Is Mediated By A Lineage-Specific Carbohydrate, LNF III (CD15). *Cell*, Vol.63, No.3, (November 1990), pp.467-474, ISSN:0092-8674.

Li, N. 2008. Platelet–lymphocyte Cross-talk. *Journal of Leukocyte Biology*, Vol.83, No.5, (May 2008), pp.1069–1078, ISSN:0741-5400.

Libby, P. 2002. Inflammation in Atherosclerosis. *Nature*, Vol.420, No.19/26, (December 2002), pp.868-874, ISSN:0028-0836.

Libby, P. & Aikawa, M. 2001. Evolution and Stabilization of Vulnerable Atherosclerotic Plaques. *Japanese Circulation Journal*, Vol.65, No.6, (June 2001), pp.473 -479, ISSN:0047-1828.

Libby, P.; Okamoto, Y.; Rocha, V.Z. & Folco, E. 2010. Inflammation in Atherosclerosis: Transition from Theory to Practice. *Circulation Journal*, Vol.74, No.2, (February 2010), pp.213-220, ISSN:1346-9843.

Lievens, D.; Zernecke, A.; Seijkens, T.; Soehnlein, O., Beckers, L.; Munnix, I.C.A.; Wijnands, E.; Goossens, P.; van Kruchten, R.; Thevissen, L.; Boon, L.; Flavell, R.A.; Noelle, R.J.; Gerdes, N.; Biessen, E.A.; Daemen, M.J.A.P.; Heemskerk, J.W.M.; Weber, C. & Lutgens, E. 2010. Platelet CD40L Mediates Thrombotic and Inflammatory Processes in Atherosclerosis. *Blood*, Vol.116, No.20, (November 2010), pp.4317-4327, ISSN:0006-4971.

Lindemann, S.; Tolley, N.D.; Dixon, D.A.; McIntyre, T.M.; Prescott, S.M.; Zimmerman, G.A. & Weyrich, A.S. 2001. Activated Platelets Mediate Inflammatory Signaling by Regulated Interleukin 1β Synthesis. *The Journal of Cell Biology*, Vol. 154, No. 3, (August 2001), pp.485-490, ISSN:0021-9525.

Linden, M.D.; Furman, M.I.; Frelinger III, A.L.; Fox, M.L.; Barnard, M.R.; Li, Y.; Przyklenk, S.K. & Michelson, A.D. 2007. Indices of Platelet Activation and The Stability of Coronary Artery Disease. *Journal of Thrombosis and Haemostasis*, Vol.4, No.5, (April 2007), pp.761–765, ISSN:1538-7933.

Linden, M.D. & Jackson, D.E. 2010. Platelets: Pleiotropic Roles in Atherogenesis and Atherothrombosis. *The International Journal of Biochemistry & Cell Biology*, Vol.42, No.11, (November 2010), pp.1762-1766, ISSN:1357-2725.

Lindmark, E.; Tenno, T. & Siegbahn, A. 2000. Role of Platelet P-Selectin and CD40 Ligand in The Induction of Monocytic Tissue Factor Expression. *Arteriosclerosis, Thrombosis, and Vascular Biology*, Vol. 20, No.10, (October 2000), pp.2322-2328, ISSN:1079-5642.

Lusis, J.A. 2000. Atherosclerosis. *Nature*, Vol.407, No.6801, (September 2000), pp.233-240, ISSN:0028-0836.

Madamanchi, N.R.; Vendrov, A. & Runge, M.S. 2005. Oxidative Stress and Vascular Disease. *Arteriosclerosis, Thrombosis, and Vascular Biology*, Vol.25, No.1, (January 2005), pp.29–38, ISSN:1079-5642.

Massberg, S.; Enders, G.; de Melo Matos, F.C.; Tomic, L.I.D.; Leiderer, R.; Eisenmenger, S.; Messmer, K. & Krombach, F. 1999. Fibrinogen Deposition at The Postischemic Vessel Wall Promotes Platelet Adhesion During Ischemia-Reperfusion in Vivo. *Blood*, Vol.94, No.11, (December 1999), pp.3829–3838, ISSN:0006-4971.

Massberg, S.; Gawaz, M.; Grüner, S.; Schulte, V.; Konrad, I.; Zohlnhöfer, D.; Heinzmann, U. & Nieswandt, B. 2003. A Crucial Role of Glycoprotein VI for Platelet Recruitment to the Injured Arterial Wall In Vivo. *The Journal of Experimental Medicine*, Vol.197, No.1, (January 2003), pp.41-49, ISSN:0022-1007.

May, A.E.; Kälsch, T.; Massberg, S.; Herouy, Y.; Schmidt, R. & Gawaz, M. 2002. Engagement of Glycoprotein IIb/IIIa (αIIbβ3) on Platelets Upregulates CD40L and Triggers CD40L-Dependent Matrix Degradation by Endothelial Cells. *Circulation*, Vol.106, No.16, (October 2002), pp.2111-2117, ISSN:0009-7322.

Methia, N.; Andre, P.; Denis, C.V.; Economopoulos, M. & Wagner, D.D. 2001. Localized Reduction of Atherosclerosis in Von Willebrand Factor-Deficient Mice. *Blood*, Vol.98, No.5, (September 2001), pp.1424–1428, ISSN:0006-4971.

Moons, A.H.M.; Levib, M. & Peters, R.J.G. 2002. Tissue Factor and Coronary Artery Disease. *Cardiovascular Research*, Vol. 53, No.2, (February 2002), pp.313-325, ISSN:0008-6363.

Nassar, T.; Sachais, B.S.; Akkawit, A.; Kowalska, M.A.; Bdeir, K.; Leitersdorf, E.; Hiss, E.; Ziporen, L.; Aviram, M.; Cines, D.; Poncz, M. & Higazi, A.A. 2003. Platelet Factor 4 Enhances the Binding of Oxidized Low-density Lipoprotein to Vascular Wall Cells. *The Journal of Biological Chemistry*, Vol.278, No.8, (February 2003), pp.6187-619, ISSN:0021-9258.

Neumann, F. J.; Zohlnhofer, D.; Fakhoury, L.; Ott, I.; Gawaz, M. & Schomig, A. 1999. Effect of Glycoprotein IIb/IIIa Receptor Blockade on Platelet-Leukocyte Interaction and Surface Expression of The Leukocyte Integrin Mac-1 in Acute Myocardial Infarction. *Journal of American College of Cardiology*, Vol.34, No.5, (November 1999), pp.1420–1426, ISSN:0735-1097.

Pitsilos, S.; Hunt, J.; Mohler, E.R.; Prabhakar, A.M.; Poncz, M.; Dawicki, J.; Khalapyan, T.Z.; Wolfe, M.L.; Fairman, R.; Mitchell, M.; Carpenter, J.; Golden, M.A.; Cines, D.B. & Sachais, B.S. 2003. Platelet Factor 4 Localization in Carotid Atherosclerotic Plaques: Correlation With Clinical Parameters. *Thrombrosis and Haemostasis*, Vol.902, No.6, (December 2003), pp.1112-1120, ISSN:0340-6245.

Romo, G.M.; Dong, J.F.; Schade, A.J.; Gardiner, E.E., Kansas, G.S., Li, C.Q., McIntire, L.V., Berndt, M.C. & López, J.A. 1999. The Glycoprotein Ib-IX-V Complex is a Platelet Counterreceptor for P-selectin. *The Journal of Experimental Medicine*, Vol.190, No.6, (September 1999), pp.803-814, ISSN:0022-1007

Ross, R. 1993. The Pathogenesis of Atherosclerosis: A Perspective for The 1990s. *Nature*, Vol.362, No.6423, (April 1993), pp.801-809, ISSN:0028-0836.

Ruggeri, Z.M. 2002. Platelets in Atherothrombosis. *Nature Medicine*, Vol.8, No.11, (November 2002), pp.1227-1234, ISSN:1078-8956.

Sachais, B.S.; Kuo, A.; Nassar, T.; Morgan, J.; Kariko, K.; Williams, K.J.; Feldman, M.; Aviram, M.; Shah, N.; Jarett, L.; Poncz, M.; Cines, D.B. & Higazi, A.A. 2002. Platelet Factor 4 Binds to Low-Density Lipoprotein Receptors and Disrupts The Endocytic Itinerary, Resulting in Retention of Low-Density Lipoprotein on The Cell Surface. *Blood*, Vol.99 , No.10, (May 2002), pp.613-3622, ISSN:0006-4971.

Santoso, S.; Sachs, U.J.H.; Kroll, H.; Linder, M.; Ruf, A.; Preissner, K.T. & Chavakis, T. 2002. TheJunctional Adhesion Molecule 3 (JAM-3) on Human Platelets is A Counter receptor for The Leukocyte Integrin Mac-1. *The Journal of Experimental Medicine*, Vol.196, No.5, (September 2002), pp.679-691, ISSN:0022-1007.

Sarma, J.; Laan, C.A.; Alam, S.; Jha, A.; Fox, K.A.A. & Dransfield, I. 2002. Increased Platelet Binding to Circulating Monocytes in Acute Coronary Syndromes. *Circulation*, Vol. 105, No.18, (May 2002), pp.2166-2171, ISSN:0009-7322.

Schober, A.; Manka, D.; von Hundelshausen, P.; Huo, Y.; Hanrath, P.; Sarembock, I.J.; Ley, K. & Weber, C. 2002. Deposition of Platelet RANTES Triggering Monocyte Recruitment Requires P-Selectin and is Involved in Neointima Formation After Arterial Injury. *Circulation*, Vol.106, No.12, (September 2002), pp.1523-1529, ISSN: 0009-7322.

Setianto, B.Y.; Hartopo, A.B.; Gharini, P.P.; Anggrahini, D.W. & Irawan, B. 2010. Circulating soluble CD40 ligand mediates the interaction between neutrophils and platelets in acute coronary syndrome. *Heart Vessels*, Vol.25, No.4, (July 2010), pp.282-287, ISSN: 0910-8327.

Sevitt, S. 1986. Platelets and Foam Cells in the Evolution of Atherosclerosis Histological and Immunohistological Studies of Human Lesions. *Atherosclerosis*, Vol.61, No.2, (August 1986), pp.107-115, ISSN:0021-9150.

Simionescu, M. & Simionescu, N. 1993. Proatherosclerotic Events: Pathobiochemical Changes Occurring in The Arterial Wall Before Monocyte Migration. *The FASEB Journal*, Vol.7, No.14, (November 1993), pp.1359-1366, ISSN:0892-6638.

Simon, D.I.; Chen, Z.; Xu, H.; Li, C.Q.; Dong, J.; McIntire, L.V.; Ballantyne, C.M.; Zhang, L.; Furman, M.I.; Berndt, M.C. & López, J.A. 2000. Platelet Glycoprotein Ib Alpha Is A Counterreceptor for The Leukocyte Integrin Mac-1 (CD11b/CD18). *The Journal of Experimental Medicine*, Vol.192, No.2, (July 2000), pp.193-204, ISSN:0022-1007.

Skålén, K.; Gustafsson, M.; Rydberg, E.K.; Hultén, L.M.; Wiklund, O.; Innerarity, T.L. & Borén, J. 2002. Subendothelial Retention of Atherogenic Lipoproteins in Early Atherosclerosis. *Nature*, Vol.417, No.13, (June 2002), pp.750-754, ISSN:0028-0836.

Slupsky, J.R.; Kalbas, M.; Willuweit, A.; Henn, V.; Kroczek, R.A. & Müller-Berghaus, G. 1998. Activated Platelets Induce Tissue Factor Expression on Human Umbilical Vein Endothelial Cells By Ligation of CD40. *Thrombrosis and Haemostasis*, Vol.80, No.6, (December 1998), pp.1008–1014, ISSN:0340-6245.

Sniderman, A.; Vu, H. & Cianflone, K. 1991. Effect of Moderate Hypertriglyceridemia on The Relation of Plasma Total and LDL Apo B Levels. *Atherosclerosis*, Vol.89, No.2-3, (August 1991), pp.109-116, ISSN: 0021-9150.

Stocker, R. & Keaney, J.F.Jr. 2004. Role of Oxidative Modifications in Atherosclerosis. *Physiological Review*, Vol.84, No.4, (October 2004), pp.1381-1478, ISSN: 0031-9333

Tabas, I.; Williams, K.J., & Borén, J. 2007. Subendothelial Lipoprotein Retention As the Initiating Process in Atherosclerosis: Update and Therapeutic Implications. *Circulation*, Vol.116, No.16, (October 2007), pp.1832-1844, ISSN:0009-7322.

Theilmeier, G.; Lenaerts, T.; Remacle, C.; Collen, D.; Vermylen, J. & Hoylaerts, M.F. 1999. Circulating Activated Platelets Assist THP-1 Monocytoid/Endothelial Cell Interaction Under Shear Stress. *Blood*, Vol.94, No.8, (October 1999), pp.2725-2724, ISSN:0006-4971.

Theilmeier, G.; Michiels, C.; Spaepen, E.; Vreys, I.; Collen, D.; Vermylen, J. & Hoylaerts, M.F. 2002. Endothelial von Willebrand Factor Recruits Platelets To Atherosclerosis-Prone Sites in Response To Hypercholesterolemia. *Blood*, Vol.99, No.12, (June 2002), pp.4486-4493, ISSN:0006-4971.

Torzewski, M. & Lackner, K.J. 2006. Initiation and Progression of Atherosclerosis—Enzymatic or Oxidative Modification of Low-Density Lipoprotein? *Clinical Chemistry and Laboratory Medicine*, Vol.44, No.12, (December 2006), pp.1389–1394, ISSN: 1434-6621.

Ulrichts, H.; Vanhoorelbeke, K.; Girma, J.P.; Lenting, P.J.; Vauterin, S. & Deckmyn, H. 2005. The Von Willebrand Factor Self-Association is Modulated By a Multiple Domain Interaction. *Journal of Thrombosis and Haemostasis*, Vol.3, No.3, (March 2005), pp. 552–556, ISSN:1538-7933.

Vandendries, E.R.; Furie, B.C. & Furie, B. 2004. Role of P-selectin and PSGL-1 in Coagulation and Thrombosis. *Thrombosis and Haemostasis*, Vol.92, No.3, (September 2004), pp.459-466, ISSN:0340-6245.

Van Gils, J. M.; Zwaginga, J. J. & Hordijk, P. L. 2009. Molecular and Functional Interactions Among Monocytes, Platelets, and Endothelial Cells and Their Relevance for

Cardiovascular Diseases. *Journal of Leukocyte Biology*, Vol.85, No.3, (February 2009), pp.195–204, ISSN:0741-5400.

Virmani, R.; Kolodgie, F.D.; Burke, A.P.; Farb, A. & Schwartz, S.M. 2000. Lessons From Sudden Coronary Death: A Comprehensive Morphological Classification Scheme for Atherosclerotic Lesions. *Arteriosclerosis, Thrombosis, and Vascular Biology*, Vol.20, No.5, (May, 2000), pp.1262–1275, ISSN: 1079-5642.

Von Hundelshausen P, Weber KS, Huo Y, Proudfoot, A.E.I.; Nelson, P.J.; Ley, K. & Weber, C. 2001. RANTES deposition by platelets triggers monocyte arrest on inflamed and atherosclerotic endothelium. *Circulation*. Vol.103, No.13, (April 2001), pp.1772–1777, ISSN:0009-7322.

Von Hundelshausen, P. & Weber, C. 2007. Platelets as Immune Cells Bridging Inflammation and Cardiovascular Disease. *Circulation Research*, Vol.100, No.1, (January 2007), pp. 27-40, ISSN:0009-7330.

Walz, A.; Schmutz, P.; Mueller, C. & Schnyder-Candrian, S. 1997. Regulation and Function of The CXC Chemokine ENA-78 Inmonocytes and Its Role in Disease. *Journal of Leukocyte Biology*, Vol.62, No.5 (November 1997), pp.604-611, ISSN:0741-5400.

Weyrich, A.S.; Prescott, S.M. & Zimmerman, G.A. 2002. Platelets, Endothelial Cells, Inflammatory Chemokines, and Restenosis Complex Signaling in the Vascular Play Book. *Circulation*, Vol. 106, No. 12, (September 2002), pp.1433-1435, ISSN:0009-7322.

Yu, G.; Rux, AH.; Ma, P.; Bdeir, K. & Sachais, B.S. 2005. Endothelial Expression of E-Selectin is Induced By The Platelet-Specific Chemokine Platelet Factor 4 Through LRP in An NF-Kappa b-Dependent Manner. *Blood*, Vol.105, No.9, (May 2005), pp. 3545–3551, ISSN:0006-4971.

Zillmann, A.; Luther, T.; Müller, I.; Kotzsch, M.; Spannagl, M.; Kauke, T.; Oelschlägel, U.; Zahler, S. & Engelmann, B. 2001. Platelet-Associated Tissue Factor Contributes to the Collagen-Triggered Activation of Blood Coagulation. *Biochemical and Biophysical Research Communications*, Vol. 281, No. 2, (February 2001), pp.603–609, ISSN: 0006-291X.

7

Acute Coronary Syndrome Secondary to Acute Aortic Dissection – Underlying Mechanisms and Possible Therapeutic Options

Kazuhito Hirata[1], Tomoya Hiratsuji[2], Minoru Wake[1] and Hidemitsu Mototake[3]
[1]*Okinawa Chubu Hospital, Division of Cardiology*
[2]*Okinawa Hokubu Hospital,Division of Cardiology*
[3]*Okinawa Chubu Hospital, Cardiovascular Surgery*
Japan

1. Introduction

Acute coronary syndrome(ACS) and acute aortic dissection(AAD) are life-threatening conditions which can be difficult to differentiate in the emergency room because of the similarity of clinical presentations. In addition, ACS can be caused in AAD as a complication of the dissecting process. Usual form of ACS is caused by an obstruction of the epicardial coronary arteries, which is initiated with the rupture of an unstable atherosclerotic plaque complicated with subsequent thrombus formation(Libby , 2001). On the other hand, ACS secondary to AAD is caused by malperfusion of the coronary artery by an obstruction of the orifice as a complication of the dissecting process. If AAD is compicated with ACS, prognosis becomes worse and the treatment of choice may be totally different from usual ACS. Medications and procedures which are usually used in cases of ordinary ACS, such as Heparin, antiplatelets, thrombolytic agents and catheter interventions, may be harmful in ACS secondary to AAD. So it is of great importance to make a correct diagnosis of ACS secondary to AAD for better treatment and survival.

2. Acute coronary syndrome in patients with acute type A aortic dissection

2.1 Incidence

Incidence of coronary involvement in AAD has been reported to be 1.8-11.3%(Hirst, 1958 ; Hagan, 2000 ; Kawahito, 2003 ; Neri, 2001 ; Spittel, 1993) . Incidence may vary according to the different study population(autopsy, surgical patients or non-selected patients in the emergency room). We recently evaluated the incidence of coronary malperfusion in 159 patients with type A AAD who presented to the emergency room within 12 hours from the onset and found that 9.4 % had coronary malperfusion(Hirata, 2010). On the contrary, the incidence of the AAD in ACS is not so frequent. In the large studies dealing with prehospital thrombolysis, 0.3-0.33% of the patient was erroneously diagnosed as having usual ACS who later proved to have AAD(Wilcox,1988 ; European Myocardial Infarction Group, 1993).

2.2 Mechanisms

There are four possible mechanisms for coronary malperfusion in AAD(Ashida, 2000 ; Cambria, 1988; Massetti, 2003 ; Neri, 2001 ; Shapira, 1998,)

1. buldging of the dissected false lumen producing occlusion of the coronary artery orifice (Figure 1 A).
2. a retrograde extension of the dissection into the coronary arterial wall resulting in obstruction (Figure 1 B)
3. disruption or detachment of the coronary artery from the aortic root(Figure 1 C).
4. dynamic obstruction of the coronary orifice by flail intimal flap(Figure 1 D).

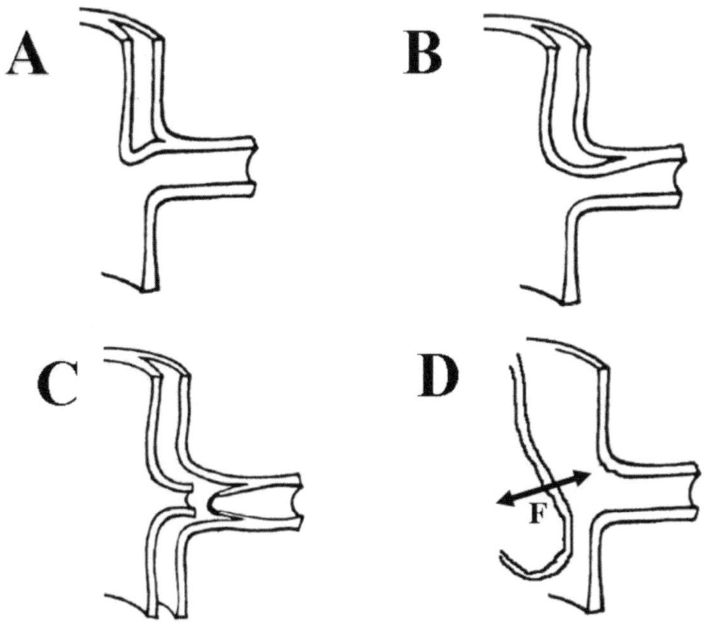

Fig. 1. Four possible mechanisms for coronary malperfusion in cases of acute type A aortic dissection. Mechanisms A to D correspond to mechanisms 1) to 4) in the text. See text in detail (modified from Neri E et al. Proximal aortic dissection with coronary artery malperfusion. J Thorac Cardiovasc Surg 2001 ; 121 : 552-560 with permission).

Distribution of the each mechanism has not been well defined. In our experience (Hirata,2010) , among 10 patients in whom actual mechanism of coronary malperfusion was identified during surgery, 5 patients had mechanism 1), 3 patients had mechanism 2) , and 2 patients had mechanism 3). Identification of the mechanism for coronary malperfusion is potentially important in relation to the therapeutic options described later.

2.3 Clinical pictures and electrocardiographic changes

Compared with patients of AAD without ACS, those with ACS had more severe clinical presentation as manifested with a higher incidence of cardiac tamponade and initial shock vital signs(Hirata K, 2010). The prognosis was also worse(Kawahito,2003; Metha 2002). If the right coronary artery is involved, ST segment elevation in the inferior leads is seen. Simultaneous ST elevation in leads V1-V3 may be seen as a result of obstruction of the conus branch or the right ventricular branch (Figure 2). If the left main trunk(LMT) is involved, elevation of the ST segment in leads aVR and aVL with diffusse ST depression in other leads(Figure 3), or ST elevation in V1-V6 and I, aVL are seen(Nikus,2007).

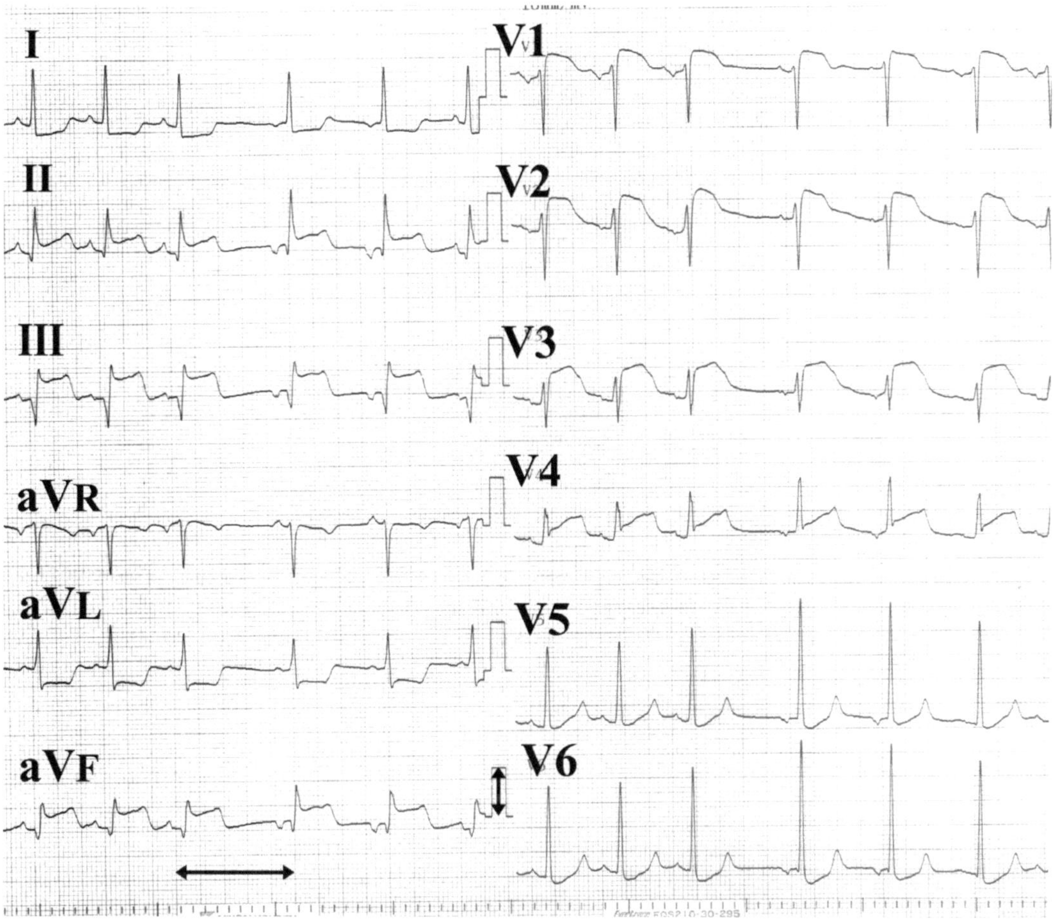

Fig. 2. Twelve-lead ECGs obtained from a 56-year-old male with type A AAD. This patient had shock (initial systolic blood pressure was 60mmHg), cardiac tamponade and mild aortic regurgitation. An ECG showed sinus pause with ectopic atrial escape rhythm, marked ST elevation in both inferior and precordial leads. This patient had disruption of the orifice of right coronary artery but the orifice of left main trunk was intact. Simultaneous ST elevation in inferior and anterior leads reflected involvement of the conus branch or right ventricular branch due to obstruction of the orifice of the right coronary artery. A horizontal arrow indicates 1 second and a vertical arrow indicates 1 mV (same in Figure 3). Reproduced with permission(Hirata K et al. Electrocardiographic changes in patients with type A acute aortic dissection. J Cardiol 2010;56:147-153).

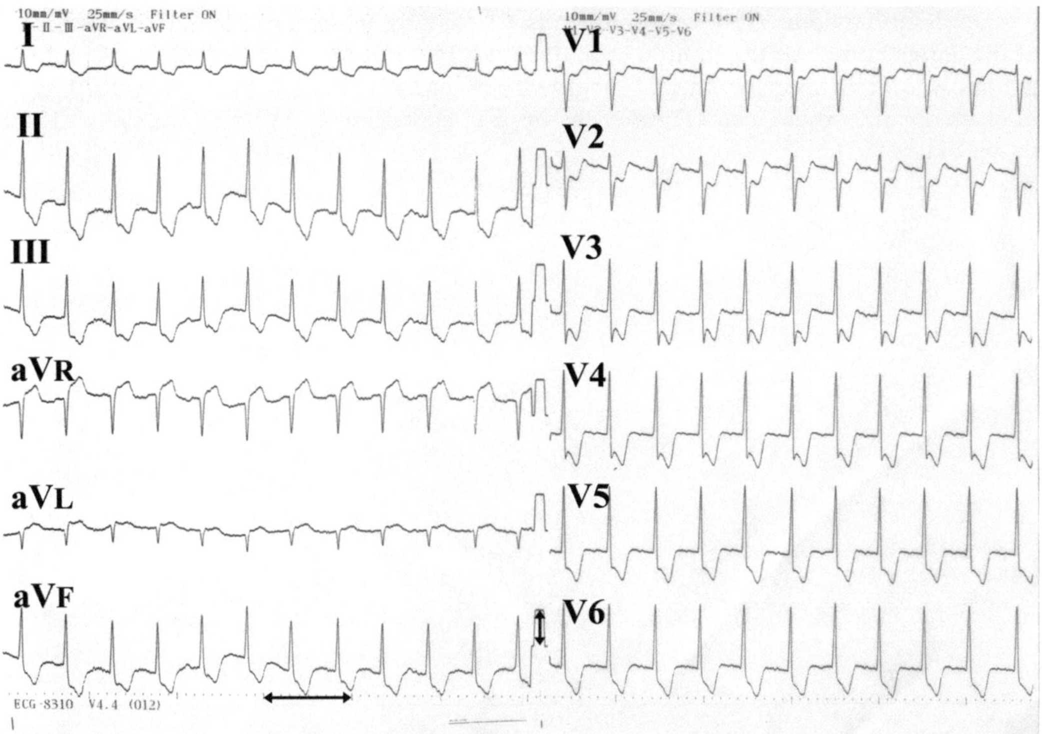

Fig. 3. Twelve-lead ECGs obtained from a 46-year-old female with type A AAD associated with Marfan syndrome. Note that ST segment was elevated in leads aVR and aVL, and diffuse severe ST depression was also seen. This patient had acute pulmonary edema due to severe acute aortic valvular regurgitation. Initial systolic blood pressure was preserved (120mmHg). A transesophageal echocardiogram showed flail intimal flap in the ascending aorta. The dissection was extended beyond the orifice of the left main trunk. Bentall surgery and coronary reconstruction were performed. Reproduced with permission(Hirata K et al. Electrocardiographic changes in patients with type A acute aortic dissection. J Cardiol 2010;56:147-153).

We recently reported that acute electrocardiographic changes(either ST depression and or T wave inversion) were rather common in patients with type A AAD even if there was no involvement of the coronary artery(Table 1, Hirata 2010). Only 27% of the patients with type A AAD had normal ECG. These observations were consistent with others(Hagan, 2000). Those acute ECG changes were closely associated with initial shock state(BP<90mmHg) and cardiac tamponade in our experience of 159 patients(Hirata K, 2010).

Pre-existing chronic coronary artery disease has been reported to coincide in some patients with type A AAD. In the international registry of AAD, Hagan et al reported that, among 464 patients, 4.3% had previous history of bypass surgery and 7.7% had evidence of old myocardial infarction(Hagan, 2000). Creswell et al. found that about one-third of the patients showed one or more coronary artery lesions greater than 50% with a coronary angiography (Creswell, 1995). At present, in type A AAD, the contribution of preexisting chronic coronary disease on clinical presentation, acute ECG change and needs for concomitant bypass surgery has not been well defined.

Chronic ECG abnormalities such as left ventricular hypertrophy with or without strain pattern, bundle branch block, etc. were also common in patients with type A AAD.

Acute change	79(49.7)
ST elevation (≧0.1mV)	13(8.2)
ST depression	54(34.0)
≧ 0.1 mV and < 0.2 mV	28(17.6)
≧ 0.2 mV and < 0.3 mV	18(11.3)
≧ 0.3 mV	8(5.0)
T inversion	34(21.4)
AVB	3(1.9)
New Af	1(0.6)
PAC/PVC	5(3.1)
Sinus bradycardia	18(11.3)
Chronic change	58(36.5)
LVH with strain	15(9.4)
LVH voltage	17(10.7)
Q waves	6(3.8)
BBB	8(5.0)
Chronic Af	8(5.0)
Both acute and chronic	21(13.2)
Normal	43(27.0)

AVB: Atrioventricular block (≧second degree), Af: Atrial fibrillation, PAC: Premature Atrial Contraction, PVC: Premature Ventricular Contraction, LVH: Left Ventricular Hypertrophy, BBB : Bundle Branch Block, Values are expressed as number(%). Reproduced with permission(Hirata K et al. Electrocardiographic changes in patients with type A acute aortic dissection. J Cardiol 2010;56:147-153)

Table 1. ECG changes in type A AAD(n=159)

2.4 Differentiation between acute coronary syndrome secondary to acute type A aortic dissection and usual form of acute coronary syndrome

Regardless of the difference of the mechanism, the results of coronary malperfusion is myocardial ischemia in both usual form of ACS and ACS secondary to AAD. So it is impossible to differentiate usual form of ACS from ACS secondary to AAD with electrocardiographic findings. At present, differential diagnosis is dependent on the clinical suspicion based on difference of clinical pictures, confirmed with imaging modalities such as a CT scan and an echocardiogram. Shirakabe et al. tried to differentiate AAD and ACS using scoring system utilizing clinical idexes obtainable in emergency room. Presence of back pain, mediastinal widening on chest X-ray, aortic regurgitation and aortic dilatation(>30mm) were closely associated with AAD (Shirakabe,2008) . They found that AAD can be differentiated from ACS at sensitivity of 93.1% and specificity of 77.6%, when more than 3 of the 4 features were positive. We found that ECG change in AAD is closely associated with initial shock vital sign(BP<90mmHg) and cardiac tamponade (Hirata, 2010) . To perform a trans-thoracic echocardiography at bedside in the emergency room appeared to be very important in ACS patients in whom underlying AAD is a possible cause of ACS. Those patients include abrupt onset with back pain, shock vital signs, mediastinal widening(ratio of greater than 30%), pericardial effusion, aortic regurgitation, and aortic root dilatation(>30mm). If there is a flail intimal flap, the diagnosis of AAD can be made at bedside

3. Treatment options for acute coronary syndrome secondary to acute type A aortic dissection

3.1 Surgery

If ACS secondary to AAD is erroneously diagnosed as usual form of ACS and received thrombolysis or catheter interventions, those patients may have an increased risk of developing harmful sequelae such as rupture of the aorta resulting in bleeding or cardiac tamponade (Blankenship, 1989; Butler 1990; Eriksen, 1992; Kamp,1994; Melchior,1993) . Surgical treatment to improve coronary malperfusion and underlying dissecting process at the same time is the most important and vital(Kawahito,2003; Neri,2001). Replacement of the dissected ascending aorta(sometimes beyond the arch) with artificial vessel prosthesis is necessary. If coronary involvement is seen, simultaneous bypass surgery or repair of the involved coronary artery may be required. Especially, if coronary malperfusion is due to mechanism 2) and 3), bypass surgery is mandatory(Figure 1 B and C). In mechanism 1), decompression of the false lumen may be sufficient enough to restore coronary perfusion(Figure 1A). In mechanism 4), removal of the flap with ascending aortic replacement may be effective and bypass may not be necessary(Figure1 D). Needless to say, aortic valve replacement is necessary, if the aortic valve regurgitation is severe.

3.2 Percutaneous catheter intervention

There have been several case reports of successful percutaneous catheter intervention (PCI) for ACS secondary to AAD. Barabas et al. reported a case of intermittent obstruction of the LMT in whom deployment of a stent in LMT was very effective to improve unstable hemodynamic (Barabas,2000). The patient was later sent to surgery as a definitive treatment. In their case, the diagnosis of ACS secondary to AAD was not made before the catheter intervention. The presence of AAD was diagnosed during the procedure and unplanned stenting was performed as an emergency bridge to surgery. Yunoki et al. reported a rare case of type A AAD in whom the right coronary orifice obstruction resulted in acute inferior and right ventricular myocardial infarction(Yunoki, 2010). Initially, the patient was sent for catheter intervention as having an usual form of ACS. During the procedure, AAD was diagnosed and the stent was deployed at the orifice of the right coronary artery. The patient was carefully followed medically and at one year, a false lumen in the ascending aorta had been resolved.

3.2.1 Report of a case

We recently experienced a case of ACS secondary to AAD in whom, emergency stenting in the LMT was intentionally necessary. The patient was a 56-year-old female who presented to the emergency room of Okinawa Hokubu Hospital complaining of chest pain. Initial systolic blood pressure was 60 mmHg and heart rate was 80 beats per minutes. A chest X ray showed mediastinal widening. A bedside echocardiography and a CT scan confirmed type A AAD(Figure 4). ECG showed ST elevation in aVR, aVL and V5-6. The patient developed repetitive episodes of ventricular fibrillation requiring multiple cardioversion and cardiopulmonary resuscitation. The patient was intubated and was taken to the catheterization laboratory. A percutaneous cardiopulmonary support equipment(PCPS) was inserted and emergency catheter intervention was performed as a last resort, because the hospital was not equipped for emergency cardiovascular surgery. A coronary angiography showed obstruction of the LMT with a dissecting hematoma(Figure 5). A bare metal stent was deployed at LMT. Shortly after, the patient's hemodynamic condition improved and the patient was transferred to Okinawa Chubu Hospital (with a support of PCPS). Emergency surgery (CABG on LAD and ascending aortic replacement) was performed. At the time of surgery, the surgeons noticed the ischemia of the small bowel and the part of the small bowel was also resected. The patient's condition improved temporarily, but unfortunately the patient died of pan-peritonitis secondary to intestinal ischemia and necrosis. In this particular patient, emergency left main stenting was the last resort in the situation of very unstable hemodynamic condition and inaccessibility of on-site cardiac surgery.

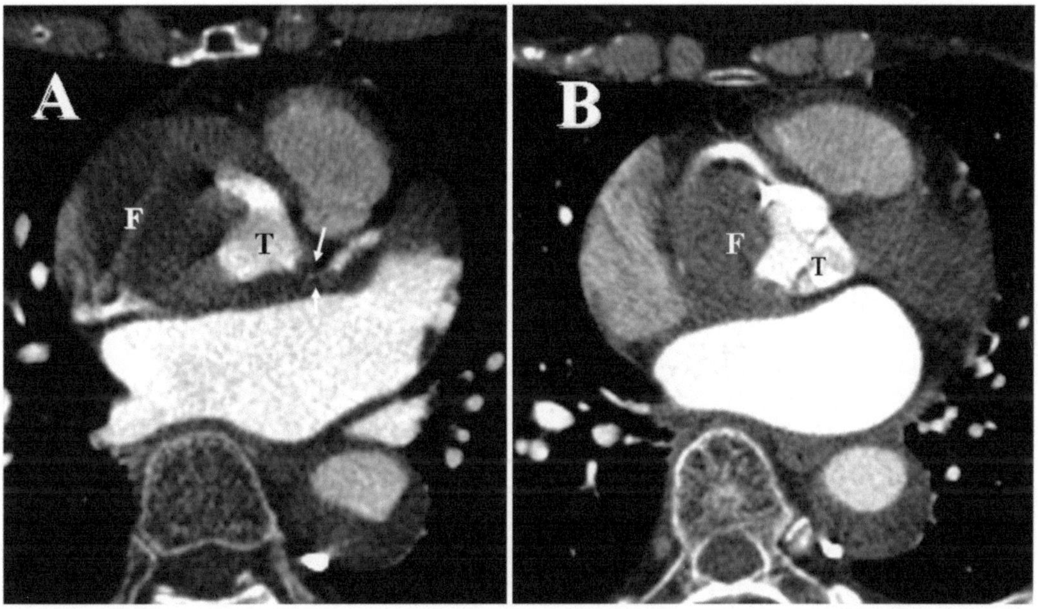

Fig. 4. A: A CT scan image showing severe narrowing of the left main coronary artey (between arrows)due to the extension of the dissecting hematoma. B: The ostium of the right coronary artery was not obstructed. T : True lumen, F: False lumen.

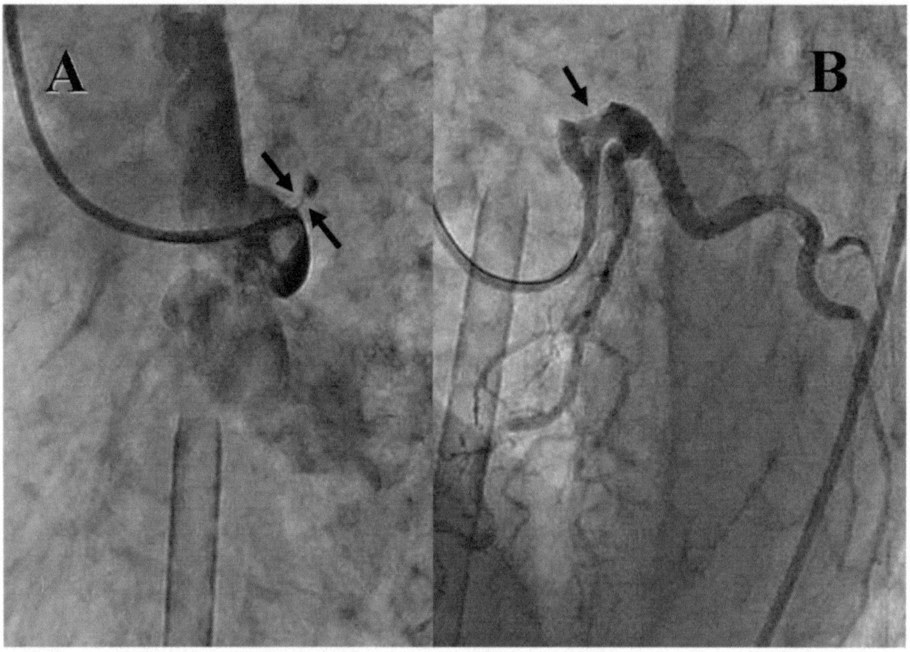

Fig. 5. Coronary angiograms before(A) and after(B) stenting the left main coronary artery. Note the severe narrowing of the orifice of the left main coronary artery resulting in poor visualization of both left anterior descending and circumflex artery. After stenting the left main tract became wide open and TIMI 3 flow was restored in both left anterior descending and circumflex arteries. A:Left anterior oblique view. B:Left anterior oblique and cranial view.

3.2.2 Current shortcomings of catheter intervention

Current shortcomings of PCI for ACS secondary to AAD include the followings:

1. Although PCI may be temporarily effective to improve coronary malperfusion, it has no effects on the ongoing dissection process itself. So the surgical approach to the dissecting process may be inevitably necessary
2. Medications used after PCI, such as antiplatelets or heparin, may result in increased risk of bleeding, rupture or cardiac tamponade.
3. To insert and to advance the guiding catheter in the injured aortic lumen may result in further injury of the aortic wall(sometimes, the true lumen is so shrunk and deformed). In addition, the guiding catheter may be erroneously inserted into the false lumen
4. Intra-aortic balloon pumping may be contraindicated and the safety of PCPS is not established.
5. If the mechanism of coronary malperfusion is due to mechanism 3), to pass the guidewire across the obstruction is impossible because there is no continuity of the wall of the coronary artery(Figure 1 C).
6. If the malperfusion is due to mechanism 4), deploying a stent in the orifice is not effective(Figure 1D).

So, at present, ACS secondary to AAD should be treated with surgery in most cases. PCI may be effective in selected cases as a bridge to definitive surgery.

4. Conclusion

Recognition and appropriate management of ASC secondary to AAD is very important. Because the mechanism of coronary malperfusion is totally different from usual ACS, the treatment of choice is also very different. Making a correct diagnosis regarding underlying dissection is very important.

5. Acknowledgment

We deeply express our thanks to Drs. Maeshiro, Henzan, Ie, Tengan, Yasumoto and Asato. We also appreciate the hard work of all the past and current fellow doctors in the division of cardiology, in Okinawa Hokubu and Chubu Hospital

6. References

Ashida K. (2000). A case of aortic dissection with transient ST-segment elevation due to functional left main coronary arterial obstruction. *Jpn Circ J* ,64,130-4

Barabas M.(2000). Left Main Stenting-as a Bridge to Surgery- for Acute Type A Aortic dissection and Anterior Myocardial Infarction. *Catheter Cardiovasc Intervnt,* 51, 74-77.

Blankenship J.(1989). Cardiovascular complications of thrombolytic therapy in patients with a mistaken diagnosis of acute myocardial infarction. *J Am Coll Cardiol,* 15 ,1579-82.

Butler J.(1990). Streptokinase in acute aortic dissection. *Br Med J* 1990, 300, 517-9.

Creswell LL. (1995). Coronary artery disease in patients with type A aortic dissection. *Ann Thorac Surg* , 59 ,585-90.

Eriksen UH(1992). Fatal haemostatic complications due to thrombolytic therapy in patients falsely diagnosed as acute myocardial infarction. *Eur Heart J* ,13 , 840-3.

Hagen PG.(2000). The international registry of acute aortic dissection(IRAD) : New insight into an old disease. *JAMA,* 283, 897-903.

Hirata K.(2010). Electrocardiographic changes in patients with type A acute aortic dissection-incidence, patterns and underlying mechanisms in 159 cases. *J Cardiol,* 56 , 147-153.

Kamp TJ.(1994) Myocardial infarction, aortic dissection, and thrombolytic therapy *Am Heart J* ,128, 1234-7.

Libby P.(2001). Current concept of the pathogenesis of acute coronary syndromes *Circulation* , 104, 365-372

Maseetti M.(2003). Flap suffocation : An uncommon mechanism ofcoronary malperfusion in acute type A dissection. *J Thrac Cardiovasc Surg,* 125, 6, 1548-1550.

Metha RH. (2002). Predicting death in patients with acute type A aortic dissection. *Circulation,* 105, 200-2006

Melchior T.(1993) Aortic dissection in the thrombolyitic era : early recognition and optimal management is a prerequisite for improved survival. *Int J Cardiol* 1993,42 , 1-6.

Neri E.(2001). Proximal aortic dissection with coronary malperfusion: presentation, management and outcome. *J Thrac Cardivasc Surg* ,121, 552-60 .

Nikus KC.(2007). Acute total occlusion of left main coronary artery with emphasis on electrocardiographic manifestations. *Timely Top Med Cardiovasc Dis* , 11 , E22.

Shapira OM.(1998). Functional left main coronary artery obstruction due to aortic dissection. *Circulation*,98,278-80.

Shirakabe A.(2008). Diagnostic score to differenciate acute aortic dissection in the emergency room. *Circ J*, 72, 986-990.

Spittel PC.(1993). Clinical features and differential diagnosis of aortic dissection :experience with 236 cases(1986 through 1990). *Mayo Clin Proc.* , 68 , 642-51.

The European Myocardial Infarction Project Group.(1993) Prehospital thrombolysis in patients with suspectedacute myocardial infarction. *N Engl J Med* , 329 ,383-9.

Wilcox RG.(1988) Trial of tissue plasminogen activator for mortality reduction in acute myocardial infarction. Anglo-Scandinavian Study of Early Thrombolysis(ASSET). *Lancet* , 2 , 525-30.

Yunoki K.(2010). Stenting of right coronary ostial occlusion due to thrombosed type A aortic dissection : One-year follow-up results. *J Cardiol case* , 1, e116-170.

Atypical Presentation in Patients with Acute Coronary Syndrome

Hyun Kuk Kim and Myung Ho Jeong
The Heart Center of Chonnam National University Hospital, Gwangju, Korea

1. Introduction

Chest pain has been reported as a cardinal clinical feature among the patients with acute coronary syndrome (ACS). However, several patients exhibit the atypical or no symptom on initial evaluation. Atypical symptom was defined as the absence of chest pain before or during admission, and may have included gastrointestinal or respiratory symptoms such as dyspnea, nausea, vomiting, and abdominal discomfort.

Patients who present without chest pain are frequently misdiagnosed, and less likely to receive optimal treatment for ACS. Consequently, greater in-hospital morbidity, and mortality are noted. Therefore, understanding the factor associated with atypical presentations may help in the earlier detection and treatments in patients with ACS.

Prior to discussing the risk factor, clarifying the concept of symptom in patients with ACS is needed to figure out this theme. In this manuscript, atypical presentation is used interchangeably 1 or 1+2 in figure 1 according to each reference (Fig.1).

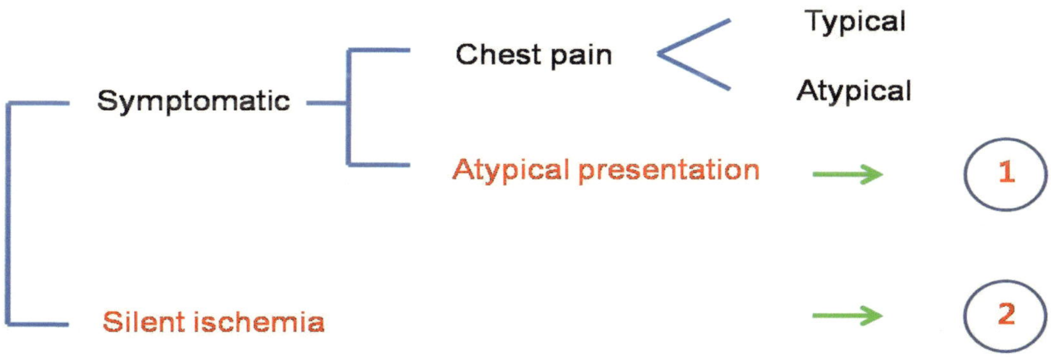

Fig. 1. Definition of atypical presentation; 1 or 1+2

2. Definition of clinical presentation

2.1 Ischemic chest pain

There are several features that tend to distinguish ischemic chest pain from non-cardiac pain.

- **Quality** - patients with ischemic pain often describe more as a discomfort than pain. Typical pain is expressed by terms include squeezing, tightness, pressure, constriction, strangling, burning, heavy weight on chest. It is not generally described as sharp, knife-like, stabbing, and pins.
- **Site** - ischemic pain is a diffuse discomfort that may be difficult to localize. The sensation is often located in the retro-sternal area but may be felt in the epigastrium, back, arms, or jaw. Pain radiating to the upper extremities is highly suggestive of ischemic pain.
- **Onset** - ischemic pain is described as having a crescendo pattern (wax and wane), and is typically gradual in onset.
- **Provocation and relieving factors** - ischemic pain is usually developed by situations such as exercise, emotional stress which increases cardiac oxygen demands. Chest pain that is reproduced on respiration, coughing, position change, palpation is often associated with not-ACS disease. Relief of pain after administration of nitroglycerin or gastro-intestinal cocktails (GI cocktails; viscous lidocaine and antacid) could not guarantee the cardiac or gastric origin pain.

2.2 Atypical chest pain and presentation

The following characteristics were considered as more non-ischemic chest discomfort.

- Sharp or knife like pain related to respiration, coughing
- Reproduced pain by movement or palpation
- Localized pain with one finger
- Radiating pain into the lower extremities or above the mandible
- Pain lasting for days or a few seconds

Atypical presentation was defined as the absence of chest pain before or during admission, and may have included gastrointestinal or respiratory symptoms such as dyspnea, nausea, vomiting, and abdominal discomfort. The prevalence of this presentation was 8.4% in the Global Registry of Acute Coronary Events (GRACE), 33% in the National Registry of Myocardial Infarction 2 (NRMI-2) and the dominant symptoms in these patients were dyspnea, nausea, syncope (Fig.2).

3. Clinical characteristics and prognosis with atypical symptom

In NRMI-2 report, patients with atypical presentation had a longer delay before hospital seek (mean, 7.9 vs. 5.3 hours), were less likely to be diagnosed with a myocardial infarction on admission (22% vs. 50%), and were less likely to be treated with optimal medical therapy [aspirin (60% vs. 85%), β-blocker (28% vs. 48%), heparin (53% vs. 83%)] and to receive thrombolytic therapy or primary percutaneous coronary intervention (25% vs. 74%).[6] Its results were similar with GRACE report. Not surprisingly, in-hospital mortality rates were much higher in patients with atypical presentation in both registry data (NRMI-2, 23% vs. 9%; GRACE 13% vs. 4%). Moreover, in-hospital complications were developed more in atypical presentation group.

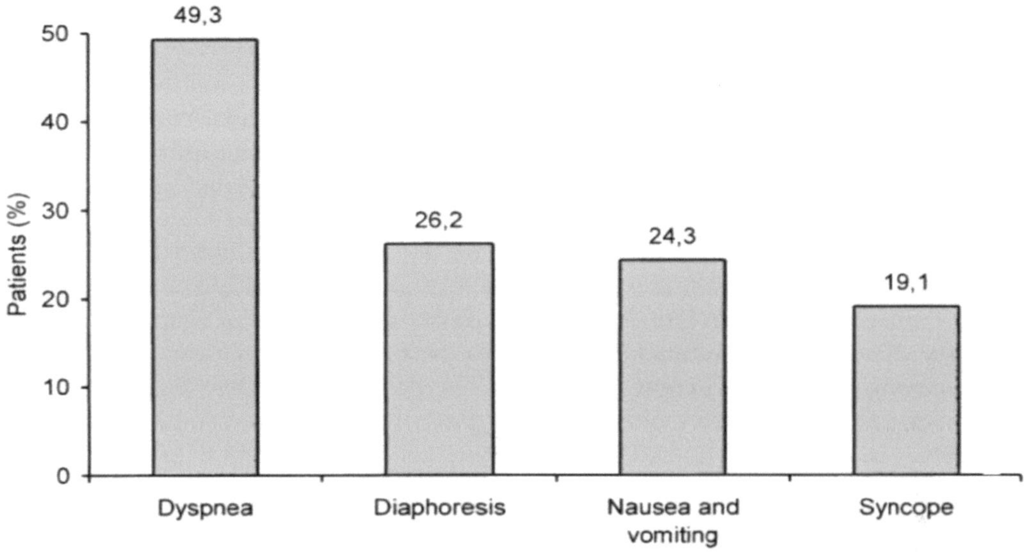

Fig. 2. Dominant symptom among patients with atypical presentation (Adopted from Brieger D, et al. Chest. 2004;126: 461-9)

4. Risk factors of atypical presentation

In NRMI-2 registry, Variables such as older age, gender, race, and co-morbidities (diabetes, stroke, heart failure) were considered as a risk factor for atypical symptom (Table.1), and many studies have described the association of aging, gender, and diabetes mellitus.

Variables	Odds Ratio (95% confidential interval)
Nonwhite	1.05 (1.03-1.07)
Women	1.06 (1.04-1.08)
Diabetes mellitus	1.21 (1.19-1.23)
Age (10-year interval)	1.28 (1.26-1.28)
Prior stroke	1.43 (1.40-1.47)
Prior heart failure	1.77 (1.74-1.81)

Table 1. Independent risk factor for atypical presentation (Adopted from Canto J.G, et al. JAMA. 2000;283:3223-9)

4.1 Women

Atypical presentation in ACS was observed more commonly in women than men in large cohort studies (Table 2). Women with coronary heart disease are older by 10 years and have more risk factors than men. It might be due to lack of early recognition and management.

There are several differences between men and women in presentation. Women were less likely to have typical angina, rated their pain as more intense, used different words to describe it (more burning, sharp), and reported more non-pain-related symptoms than men. They experienced pain and other sensations in the neck area more frequently. Another feature of chest pain in women is that angina being induced by rest, sleep, mental stress instead of or addition to physical exertion. Psychosocial factors might also affect symptom presentation and diagnostic approach in women. For example, a history of anxiety disorders is associated with a lower probability of significant angiographic disease among women with chest pain symptoms. As women underestimate their own risk of coronary artery disease, diagnostic approach by physician could be altered less aggressively than men. Compared with men, women are less likely to perform cardiac monitoring, cardiac enzyme measurement, electrocardiogram, cardiac consultation, admission to a coronary care unit, undergo less coronary angiography, angioplasty, and bypass surgery.

Study name	Study years	Sample size	Atypical symptom (%)	
			Men	Women
GRACE	1999-2002	20881	7.3	10.6
NRMI-2	1994-1998	434877	28.6	38.6
Alabama UA registry	1993-1999	4167	50.2	53.0
United kingdom	1995	2096	17.6	24.6
Worcester MI study	1986-1988	1360	18.0	23.0
Worcester MI study	1997-1999	2073	30.9	45.8
26 hospitals, CCU Israel	2000	2113	18.7	29.7
Croatia	1990-1995	1996	12.4	20.3
Olmsted County	1985-1992	2271	25.0	19.0
Cumulative			**27.4**	**37.5**

Table 2. Prevalence of atypical presentation in large cohort

4.2 Diabetes mellitus

Some patients with diabetes mellitus (DM) have a blunted perception of ischemic chest pain, which could result in atypical presentation. The suggested mechanisms of this phenomenon are as follows; 1) autonomic neuropathy, 2) prolongation of the anginal perceptual threshold.

Sympathetic denervation diabetic patients have evidence of a significant reduction in MIBG uptake, most likely on the basis of autonomic dysfunction. Furthermore, diabetic patients with silent myocardial ischemia have evidence of a diffuse abnormality in metaiodobenzylguanidine (MIBG) uptake, suggesting that abnormalities in pain perception may be linked to sympathetic denervation. Similar finding has also been observed with positron emission tomography. Moreover, regional heterogeneity in sympathetic denervation could result in potentially life-threatening myocardial electrical instability that may lead to life-threatening arrhythmias.

Another mechanism of abnormal perception is prolongation of the angina perceptual threshold during exercise. Anginal perceptual threshold (the time from onset of 0.1 mV of ST segment depression to onset of angina during treadmill exercise) is prolonged in diabetic patients with coronary artery disease. The permissive effect of a prolonged anginal perceptual threshold on exercise capacity is undesirable as reflected by its correlation with ischemia at peak exercise ($r = 0.6$, p less than 0.001): the longer the threshold, the greater the exercise capacity and the more severe the ischemia.

4.3 Age and atypical presentation

Advanced age is an important predictor of atypical presentation and poor prognosis. Recent study in Korea examined and compared the risk factor associated with atypical presentation according to the age parameter. In this study, diabetes and hyperlipidemia significantly predicted atypical symptom in relatively young (<70 years) age group. Otherwise, co-morbid conditions such as stroke or chronic obstructive pulmonary disease were the positive predictors in relatively old age group (>70 years) (Table 3).

	Younger (n=49) Adjust OR (95% CI)	P	Older (n=41) Adjust OR (95% CI)	P
Female gender	0.861 (0.576-1.769)	0.069	0.721 (0.780-2.599)	0.385
Hypertension	0.740 (0.712-1.875)	0.352	0.628 (0.780-2.599)	0.208
Diabetes	2.494 (1.108-4.014)	0.023	0.841 (0.416-1.515)	0.719
Hyperlipidemia	0.486 (0.285-0.828)	0.006	0.840 (0.438-1.611)	0.465
Co-morbidity	2.029 (0.889-4.633)	0.093	3.315 (1.357-8.729)	0.001
Smoking	0.595 (0.345-1.025)	0.061	0.575 (0.255-1.297)	0.157
ACS type	1.243 (0.675-1.235)	0.883	1.041 (0.744-1.417)	0.877
Constant	0.162	<0.001	0.258	0.001

Table 3. Predicting factors on atypical presentation in younger and older patients (Adopted from Hwang S.Y, et al. J Korean Med Sci. 2009;24:789-94)

5. Conclusions

ACS patients with atypical presentation are under-diagnosed and under-treated high risk group. Several clinical risk factors could be helpful in prediction of ACS in this group.

Health care providers should have more concerns about the presence of ACS in patients who have these risk factors.

6. References

Panju A.A., Hemmelgarn B.R., Guyatt G.H., Simel D.L. (1998). The rational clinical examination. Is this patient having a myocardial infarction? JAMA, 280, 1256-1263.

Swap C.J., Nagurney J.T. (2005). Value and limitations of chest pain history in the evaluation of patients with suspected acute coronary syndromes. JAMA, 294, 2623-2629.

Servi R.J., Skiendzielewski J.J. (1985). Relief of myocardial ischemia pain with a gastrointestinal cocktail. Am J Emerg Med, 3, 208-209.

Henrikson C.A., Howell E.E., Bush D.E., et al. (2003). Chest pain relief by nitroglycerin does not predict active coronary artery disease. Ann Intern Med, 139, 979-986.

Brieger D., Eagle K.A., Goodman S.G., et al. GRACE Investigators. (2004). Acute coronary syndromes without chest pain, an underdiagnosed and undertreated high-risk group: insights from the Global Registry of Acute Coronary Events. Chest, 126, 461-469.

Canto J.G., Shlipak M.G., Rogers W.J., et al. (2000). Prevalence, clinical characteristics, and mortality among patients with myocardial infarction presenting without chest pain. JAMA, 283, 3223-3229.

Gregoratos G. (2001). Clinical manifestations of acute myocardial infarction in older patients. Am J Geriatr Cardiol, 10, 345-347.

Patel H., Rosengren A., Ekman I. (2004). Symptoms in acute coronary syndromes: does sex make a difference? Am Heart J, 148, 27-33.

Arslanian-Engoren C., Patel A., Fang J., Armstrong D., et al. (2006). Symptoms of men and women presenting with acute coronary syndromes. Am J Cardiol. 2006, 98, 1177-1181.

DeVon H.A., Ryan C.J., Ochs A.L., Shapiro M. (2008). Symptoms across the continuum of acute coronary syndromes: differences between women and men. Am J Crit Care, 17, 14-24; quiz 25.

Canto J.G., Goldberg R.J., Hand M.M., Bonow R.O., Sopko G., Pepine C.J., Long T. (2007). Symptom presentation of women with acute coronary syndromes: myth vs reality. Arch Intern Med,167, 2405-2413.

Lerner D.J., Kannel W.B. (1986). Patterns of coronary heart disease morbidity and mortality in the sexes: a 26-year follow-up of the Framingham population. Am Heart J, 111, 383-390.

Kannel W.B., Vokonas P.S. (1992). Demographics of the prevalence, incidence, and management of coronary heart disease in the elderly and in women. Ann Epidemiol, 2, 5-14.

Stangl V., Witzel V., Baumann G., Stangl K. (2008). Current diagnostic concepts to detect coronary artery disease in women. Eur Heart J, 29, 707-717.

Alexander K.P., Shaw L.J., Shaw L.K., Delong E.R., Mark D.B., Peterson E.D. (1998). Value of exercise treadmill testing in women. J Am Coll Cardiol, 32, 1657-1664.

D'Antono B., Dupuis G., Fortin C., Arsenault A., Burelle D. (2006). Angina symptoms in men and women with stable coronary artery disease and evidence of exercise-induced myocardial perfusion defects. Am Heart J, 151, 813-819.

Pepine C.J., Abrams J., Marks R.G., Morris J.J., Scheidt S.S., Handberg E. (1994). Characteristics of a contemporary population with angina pectoris. TIDES Investigators. Am J Cardiol, 74, 226-231.

Rutledge T., Reis S.E., Olson M., et al. Women's Ischemia Syndrome Evaluation (WISE). (2001). History of anxiety disorders is associated with a decreased likelihood of angiographic coronary artery disease in women with chest pain: the WISE study. J Am Coll Cardiol, 37, 780-785.

Birdwell B.G., Herbers J.E., Kroenke K. (1993). Evaluating chest pain. The patient's presentation style alters the physician's diagnostic approach. Arch Intern Med, 153, 1991-1995.

Lehmann J.B., Wehner P.S., Lehmann C.U., Savory L.M. (1996). Gender bias in the evaluation of chest pain in the emergency department. Am J Cardiol, 77, 641-644.

Anand S.S., Xie C.C., Mehta S., et al. CURE Investigators. (2005). Differences in the management and prognosis of women and men who suffer from acute coronary syndromes. J Am Coll Cardiol, 46, 1845-1851.

Yu H.T., Kim K.J., Bang W.D., et al. (2011). Gender-based differences in the management and prognosis of acute coronary syndrome in Korea. Yonsei Med J, 52, 562-568.

Langer A., Freeman M.R., Josse R.G., Armstrong P.W. (1995). Metaiodobenzyl-benzolguanidine imaging in diabetes mellitus: assessment of cardiac sympathetic denervation and its relation to autonomic dysfunction and silent myocardial ischemia. J Am Coll Cardiol, 25, 610-618.

Di Carli M.F., Bianco-Batlles D., Landa M.E., et al. (1999). Effects of autonomic neuropathy on coronary blood flow in patients with diabetes mellitus. Circulation, 100, 813-819.

Stevens M.J., Raffel D.M., Allman K.C., et al. (1998). Cardiac sympathetic dysinnervation in diabetes: implications for enhanced cardiovascular risk. Circulation, 98, 961-968.

Ranjadayalan K., Umachandran V., Ambepityia G., Kopelman P.G., Mills P.G., Timmis A.D. (1990). Prolonged anginal perceptual threshold in diabetes: effects on exercise capacity and myocardial ischemia. J Am Coll Cardiol, 16, 1120-1124.

Stern S., Behar S., Leor J., Harpaz D., Boyko V., Gottlieb S. Israeli Working Group on Intensive Cardiac Care, Israel Heart Society. (2004). Presenting symptoms, admission electrocardiogram, management, and prognosis in acute coronary syndromes: differences by age. Am J Geriatr Cardiol, 13, 188-96.

Calle P., Jordaens L., De Buyzere M., Rubbens L., Lambrecht B., Clement D.L. (1994). Age-related differences in presentation, treatment and outcome of acute myocardial infarction. Cardiology, 85, 111-20.

Hwang S.Y., Park E.H., Shin E.S., Jeong M.H. (2009). Comparison of factors associated with atypical symptoms in younger and older patients with acute coronary syndromes. J Korean Med Sci, 24, 789-94. .

Hwang S.Y., Jeong M.H. (2010). Cognitive factors that influence delayed decision to seek treatment among older patients with acute myocardial infarction in Korea. Eur J Cardiovasc Nurs, in-press.

Hwang S.Y., Zerwic J.J., Jeong M.H. (2011). Impact of prodromal symptoms on prehospital delay in patients with first-time acute myocardial infarction in Korea. J Cardiovasc Nurs, 26, 194-201.

9

Exercise Training for Patients After Coronary Artery Bypass Grafting Surgery

Ching Lan, Ssu-Yuan Chen and Jin-Shin Lai
Department of Physical Medicine and Rehabilitation, National Taiwan University Hospital, and National Taiwan University, College of Medicine, Taipei, Taiwan

1. Introduction

Patients with coronary artery disease (CAD) who suffer persistent symptoms and reduced quality of life while receiving medical therapy are considered for revascularization.[1] Coronary artery bypass grafting (CABG) and percutaneous coronary intervention (PCI) are the most common methods of revascularization for symptomatic CAD. These two interventions can reduce ischemic symptoms such as angina or dyspnea,[2] thus improving the ability to undertake physical training. Shorter length of hospitalization,[3] earlier return to work,[4] and better life adaptation[5] were reported in patients undergoing PCI. However, the incidence rate of restenosis following PCI is higher than CABG,[6] and PCI patients who required further interventions outnumbered the patients who underwent CABG.[7-8] A recent meta-analysis study found that the mortality rate and the rate of revascularization were significantly lower in the CABG group than the PCI group (9.9% vs 24.5%).[9] In a subgroup analysis, the 5-year mortality rate of DM patients was also lower in the CABG group.
In the era of drug-eluting stent (DES), the Synergy between PCI with Taxus and Cardiac Surgery (SYNTAX) trial[10] found that major adverse cardiovascular events rates at 12 months were significantly higher in the PCI group (17.8% vs 12.4%), and the rate of revascularization was lower in the CABG group (5.9% vs 13.5%), but stroke was significantly higher in the CABG group (2.2% vs 0.6%). However, the application of new surgical technique, such as off-pump CABG (OPCAB) may reduce the rate of stroke after surgery. In general, CABG remains the method of choice in patients with left main disease, multivessel disease, especially in diabetic patients, or patients with left ventricular dysfunction, in the event of failure of PCI, and in-stent restenosis.[11] Although the procedure risk is higher for patients receiving CABG, the extent of revascularization is more complete,[12] and hence the potential of training is higher than patients with PCI. The objective of this study is to review the effect of exercise training program in patients with CABG.

2. Principle of exercise training

Exercise is a major component for patients with CAD. Cardiac rehabilitation (CR) usually beginning during hospitalization (phase I, inpatient), followed by a supervised outpatient program lasting 3-6 months (phase II), and continuing in a lifetime maintenance stage in minimally supervised or unsupervised setting (phase III). According to the recommendations of American College of Sports Medicine,[13] patients with CABG should perform aerobic exercise 3-5 times per week and 20-60 minutes for each session, at the intensity of 40-80% of $\dot{v}O_{2peak}$. Strength training is suggested to perform 2-3 times per week at the intensity of 40-50 % of maximal voluntary contraction with 10-15 repetitions.

For the coronary patients, exercises with moderate intensity have been shown to improve functional capacity, and it may provide greater safety during unsupervised training. Lower intensity exercise training also increases the acceptance of exercise program, particularly unfit and elderly patients. Therefore, some oriental conditioning exercises deserve more attention because they are less intense, easily accessible, low cost and therefore suitable for implementation in the community.

3. Benefits of exercise training

3.1 Cardiorespiratory fitness

Cardiac rehabilitation exercise training improves exercise capacity, without significant complications or other adverse effects. Peak oxygen uptake is the best indicator for cardiorespiratory fitness, and attaining a high $\dot{v}O_{2peak}$ requires integration of high levels of pulmonary, cardiovascular and neuromuscular function. In patient with CAD, the level of $\dot{v}O_{2peak}$ is also a good predictor for mortality rate. Kavanagh et al.[14] reported exercise test data for 12,169 male rehabilitation candidates, and found the most powerful predictor of cardiac and all-cause mortality was $\dot{v}O_{2peak}$. Values of <15, 15 to 22, and >22 $mL \cdot kg^{-1} \cdot min^{-1}$ yielded respective hazard ratios of 1.00, 0.62, and 0.39 for cardiac deaths and 1.00, 0.66, and 0.45 for all-cause deaths. Additionally, the mortality rate might decrease 9% for each 1 $mL \cdot kg^{-1} \cdot min^{-1}$ increase of $\dot{v}O_{2peak}$.[14] For patients with CABG, previous studies reported 10.5%-48.2% increase of $\dot{v}O_{2peak}$ in outpatient CR, and the increase of absolute value was 1.9-6.6 $mL \cdot kg^{-1} \cdot min^{-1}$ (Table 1),[15-32] depended on different exercise protocol and the initial level of fitness.

Study	Patients	Intervention	Outcomes
Haennel et al[15] (1991)	24 men 9-10 wk after CABG	Cycle training (n=8): cycling 24 min, 3 times/wk for 8 wk Hydraulic circuit training (HCT, n=8): 24 min circuit training 3 times/wk for 8 wk Control (n=8)	$\dot{V}O_{2peak}$ between baseline and 8 wk: Cycling: 21.4 vs 25.7 $mL \cdot kg^{-1} \cdot min^{-1}$ (20.1%) HCT: 21.2 vs 23.6 $mL \cdot kg^{-1} \cdot min^{-1}$ (11.3%) Cardiac output between baseline and 8 wk: Cycling:14.3 vs 16.8 $L \cdot min^{-1}$ (17.5%) HCT: 13.1 vs 15.1 $L \cdot min^{-1}$ (15.3%)
Engblom et al[16] (1992)	171 men 2 mon after CABG	Rehabilitation group (n=93) 3- wk exercise followed by 2-day refresher for 8 m Reference group (n=78)	Maximal work load increased in both groups, but the increase is greater in rehabilitation group than in reference group 12 months post-operatively.

Study	Patients	Intervention	Outcomes
Dubach et al[17] (1995)	42 men 1 mon after CABG	Exercise group (n=22): walking 1 h twice daily for 1 m, followed by 1 m of usual care Control group (n=20): usual care for 1 m, followed by walking 1 h twice daily for 1 m	$\dot{V}O_{2peak}$ between baseline and 1 mon: Ex: 22.6 vs 24.5 mL·kg^{-1}·min^{-1} (8.4%) Control: 21.0 vs 23.7 mL·kg^{-1}·min^{-1} (12.9%) $\dot{V}O_{2peak}$ between 1 mon and 2 mon: Ex: 24.5 vs 26.4 mL·kg^{-1}·min^{-1} (7.8%) Control: 23.7 vs 25.0 mL·kg^{-1}·min^{-1} (5.5%)
Daida et al[18] (1996)	15 M, 2 F 53±3 y/o, 3 m after CABG	6-8 wk aerobic training, 3 times/wk, 40 min each time, at RPE 12-13	$\dot{V}O_{2peak}$ between baseline and 9 mon: 21.9 vs 27.4 mL·kg^{-1}·min^{-1} (25.1%) ↑Exercise time, O2 pulse, peak HR
Mariorana et al [19] (1997)	26 Men 60±8.5 y/o, 18 mon after CABG	Circuit weight training group, (CWT, n=12):10 wks CWT at 40-60% max. contraction Control group (n=14)	Strength increased by 18% in five out of seven exercise in the CWT group, but unchanged in the control group $\dot{V}O_{2peak}$: no increase in both groups
Lan et al[20] (1999)	20 men 56.5±7.4 y/o 5 mon after CABG	Tai Chi group (n=9): 1-yr TC training, 3.8 times/wk, 1 h each time, at 48-57% of HR reserve Control group (n=11)	$\dot{V}O_{2peak}$ between baseline and 1 yr: TC : 26.2 vs 28.9 mL·kg^{-1}·min^{-1} (10.3%) Control: 26.0 vs 25.6 mL·kg^{-1}·min^{-1} (-1.5%)
Goodman et al[21] (1999)	31 subjects 53±1 y/o 8-10 wk after CABG	12-wk of walking program Initial intensity at 50-60% of $\dot{V}O_{2peak}$, then increase to 75-80% of $\dot{V}O_{2peak}$, 5 times/wk, 45-60 min each session for 3 m	$\dot{V}O_{2peak}$ between baseline and 3 mon: CABG: 19.0 vs 21.0 mL·kg^{-1}·min^{-1} (10.5%) Ejection Fraction (EF): At 40% of $\dot{V}O_{2peak}$: 60 vs 63% At 70% of $\dot{V}O_{2peak}$: 61 vs 64% ↑18% ischemic exercise calf blood flow
Takeyama[22] (2000)	28 patients (26M/2F) 1 wk after CABG	Exercise group (n=13): 30 min bicycle exercise, twice daily for 2 wk, intensity at ventilatory threshold (VeT) Control group (n=15): walking 200-500 meters for 2 wk	$\dot{V}O_{2peak}$ between 1 wk and 3 wk: Ex: 13.1 vs 16.1 mL·kg^{-1}·min^{-1} (22.9%) Control:13.7 vs 14.8 mL·kg^{-1}·min^{-1} (8.0%) Peak CO between 1wk and 3 wk: Ex: 10.6 vs 13.4 L/min (26.4%) Control:11.9 vs 12.0 L/min (0.1%)

Study	Patients	Intervention	Outcomes
Adachi et al[23] (2001)	57 patients (46 M/ 11F) 1 wk after CABG	Exercise group (n=34): 30 min exercise, twice daily for 2 wk, intensity at VeT Control group (n=23)	$\dot{V}O_{2peak}$ between 1 wk and 3 wk: Ex: 13.7 vs 20.3 mL·kg^{-1}·min^{-1} (48.2%) Control:13.7 vs 14.3 mL·kg^{-1}·min^{-1} (4.4%) ↑Ventilatory efficiency and cardiac output in exercise group
Kodis et al[24] (2001)	1,042 patients 6-8 wk after CABG	Supervised Ex (n=713): 2 times per wk, at 40-70% of functional capacity for 6 m Home Ex (n=329)	Supervised Ex group: ↑23.7% in $\dot{V}O_{2peak}$, ↑HDL-C, ↓LDL-C Home Ex group: ↑17.2% in $\dot{V}O_{2peak}$, ↑HDL-C
Lan et al[25] (2002)	20 men 56.5±7.4 y/o 2 mon after CABG	Aerobic exercise for 3 m, 3 time/ wk, 30 min each session, at 51-59 % of functional capacity	$\dot{V}O_{2peak}$ between baseline and 3 m: Ex: 19.8 vs 26.3 mL·kg^{-1}·min^{-1} (32.8%) $\dot{V}O_2$ at VeT between baseline and 3 m: Ex: 11.9 vs 14.7 mL·kg^{-1}·min^{-1} (23.5%)
Chuang et al[26] (2005)	32 patients 2-3 mon after CABG	Virtual reality (VR, n=17) group: simulated exercise 2 times per wk, 30 min for 3 m Non-VR (n=15) group: exercise without simulation	$\dot{V}O_{2peak}$ between baseline and 3 m: VR: 17.7 vs 22.5 mL·kg^{-1}·min^{-1} (27.1%) Non-VR: 15.1 vs 16.8 mL·kg^{-1}·min^{-1} (11.3%) ↑ $\dot{V}O_2$ at VeT in both groups
Sumide et al[27] (2009)	42 patients (40 M/ 2F) 61±8 y/o	Aerobic and resistance exercise for 6 m, 1-2 time/wk, 60 min each session	$\dot{V}O_{2peak}$ between baseline and 6 m: Ex: 15.1 vs 21.7 mL·kg^{-1}·min^{-1} (43.7%) ↑Peak torque in knee extensor/ flexor, and calf circumference
Moholdt[28] (2009)	59 patients AIT: 24M/ 4F MCT:24M/7F	Aerobic interval training (AIT) Moderate continuous training (MCT) 4 wk in rehab center, then 6- m home-based exercise	$\dot{V}O_{2peak}$ between baseline and 4 wk: AIT: 27.1 vs 30.4 mL·kg^{-1}·min^{-1} (12.2%) MCT:26.2 vs 28.5 mL·kg^{-1}·min^{-1} (8.8%) $\dot{V}O_{2peak}$ between 4wk and 6 m: AIT: 30.4 vs 32.2 mL·kg^{-1}·min^{-1} (5.9%) MCT:28.5 vs 29.5 mL·kg^{-1}·min^{-1} (3.5%)
Onishi et al[29] (2009)	32 patients with metabolic syndrome 5-14 days after CABG	Supervised CR program for 6 months, including aerobic exercise (60 min) and resistance training, at VeT	$\dot{V}O_{2peak}$ between baseline and 6 m: Ex: 14.2 vs 19.2 mL·kg^{-1}·min^{-1} (35.2%) ↑peak torques of knee extensor (13.4%) and knee flexors (15.3%) ↓Triglyceride, LDL-C and CRP

Study	Patients	Intervention	Outcomes
Bilinska et al[30] (2010)	120 Men 55±6 y/o 3 mon after CABG	Ex group (n= 60), 6 wk aerobic training, 3 times/wk, at 70-80% HRmax Control group (n=60)	Handgrip-induced increases in HR, BP, and TPR were lower, whereas SV and CO were higher (by 13% and 15%, respectively) in Ex group. A higher increase in NO level and a lower increase in noradrenaline in Ex group.
Shabani et al[31] (2010)	60 women	Ex group (n=30): 12 wk aerobic exercise Control group (n=30): usual care	Estimated exercise capacity and 6 min walking test increased in Ex group Exercise duration time↑49.2% and rate pressure product↑10.3% in Ex group
Smith et al[32] (2011)	196 patients	Hospital Ex group: aerobic Ex 30-50 min per session, 3 times/wk, at 60-80% HR reserve for 6 m Home Ex group: walking in home 5 times per wk	MET between baseline and 6 m: Hospital Ex: 4.5 vs 6.2 MET (37.8%) Home Ex: 5.1 vs 6.4 MET (25.5%) Home-based exercise maintained higher physical capacity during 6 yrs follow up than hospital-based exercise

Table 1. Effect of Exercise Training to Functional Capacity in Patients with CABG

3.2 Muscular strength

Traditionally, CR program involving aerobic exercise training such as walking and cycling is emphasized. However, muscular strength is important in vocational activities and activities of daily living. Previous studies showed that moderate intensity resistance exercise might significantly increase muscular strength for cardiac patients.[33-34] It is recommended that cardiac patient should start a low weight and perform one set of 10-15 repetitions using 8-10 different exercises. Some studies reported that resistance training might increase aerobic power,[15,33-34] but other study found that resistance training can only improve muscular strength.[19] Therefore, resistance training should be integrated into an aerobic exercise program. Sumide et al[27] reported a 6-month aerobic exercise and resistance training program was beneficial to patients with CABG. After training, the $\dot{v}O_{2peak}$ and peak lower limb torques significantly increased, and the circumferences of thigh and calf were also increased. In a recent study, Onishi et al.[29] reported a 6-month aerobic and resistance training program also improved $\dot{v}O_{2peak}$ and isokinetic peak torques of knee extensor and flexor in patients after CABG. It appears that a combined aerobic and resistance training program significantly increased exercise tolerance and lower limb muscle strength.

3.3 Cardiac function

Exercise training in healthy individuals may enhance physical capacity by both an increase in cardiac output, a central mechanism, and a widening of the arteriovenous oxygen difference, a peripheral mechanism. In patients with heart disease, previous studies suggested the enhancement of $\dot{v}O_{2peak}$ only relied on peripheral adaptations,[35-37] however, recent studies found the increase of $\dot{v}O_{2peak}$ might be partially attributed to an elevation in cardiac output.

Nakai et al.[38] reported the effects of exercise training on recovery of cardiac function in 115 patients after CABG. After training, stroke index increased significantly in the exercise group, but not in the usual care group. Takeyama et al[22] applied a 2-week bicycle program to 13 patients with CABG, and they exercised 30-minute twice daily. The peak cardiac output increased 22.9% from 10.6 L/min to 13.4 L/min, while the control group showed no significant improvement. Adachi et al.[23] assigned 34 patients with CABG to a 2-week exercise program, and cardiac output during exercise at 20 watt and at peak exercise significantly increased in the exercise group. In a recent study, Bilinska et al[30] reported that after 6 weeks of aerobic training at 70–80% of HR_{peak}, the stroke volume and cardiac output were higher (by 13% and 15%, respectively) in trained patients compared with controls.
Goodman et al.[21] has explored central and peripheral adaptations after exercise training in 31 patients with CABG. Patients underwent 12 weeks of exercise training consisting of walking and jogging, at 75% to 80% $\dot{V}O_{2peak}$. The results showed a significant improvement in $\dot{V}O_{2peak}$ and an increase of the ejection fraction during submaximal exercise (60 ± 3% vs 63 ± 2% at 40% $\dot{V}O_{2peak}$; 61 ± 3% vs 64 ± 3% at 70% $\dot{V}O_{2peak}$). Peak ischemic exercise calf blood flow and vascular conductance were also increased. The result indicated that exercise training in patients after CABG can elicit significant improvements in functional capacity that, for the most part, are secondary to peripheral adaptations, with lesser contribution of central adaptation.

3.4 Ventilatory efficiency

Shortness of breath is a major complaint when ventilation is accelerated during exercise. Although exercise training may attenuate exertional dyspnea during exercise, whether exercise training improves ventilatory efficiency in patients after CABG was not clear. Adachi et al.[23] reported the effects of exercise training on ventilatory response and cardiac output during exercise in patients following CABG. The minute ventilation–carbon dioxide output ($\dot{V}E$–$\dot{V}CO2$) slope decreased from 38.9±8.1 to 35.1±6.7 in the exercise group, and there was a correlation between improvement of the $\dot{V}E$–$\dot{V}CO2$ slope and peak cardiac output in the exercise group. The results showed that short-term physical training after CABG might improve ventilatory efficiency to exercise.

3.5 Lipid profile

Exercise training is not recommended as a sole intervention for lipid modification because the inconsistent effect on lipid and lipoprotein levels. Optimal lipid management requires dietary and pharmacologic management, in addition to CR exercise training.
Wosornu et al. [39] compared the effects of 6-month aerobic or strength exercise training after CABG. Both groups showed a significant increase in physical capacity, but there were no changes in lipoprotein levels. Brügemann et al.[40] randomized 137 men who underwent an coronary procedure (111 received CABG) to two types of CR, and blood lipid profile was unaffected by exercise training. However, Kodis et al.[24] conducted a retrospective review of 1,042 patients with CABG and found that exercise might induce beneficial changes to lipid profile. Following 6 months of exercise training, the supervised exercise group had significant lower cholesterol and LDL-cholesterol than the home-based group. Patients in the supervised exercise group had significant improvements in triglyceride, LDL-cholesterol and HDL-cholesterol, whereas the home-based group showed improvement in HDL-cholesterol only. In a recent study, Onishi et al.[29] also reported CR exercise training might

improve LDL-cholesterol and total cholesterol in CABG patients with metabolic syndrome. Additionally, metabolic scoring defined by the number of the modified Adult Treatment Panel criteria of the US National Cholesterol Education Program was significantly improved.

3.6 Hemodynamic and neurohormonal response

In order to measure hemodynamic and neurohormonal response to static exercise, Bilinska et al[30] randomized 120 male patients to either 6 weeks of aerobic training at a 70–80% of the HR_{peak} or to a control group. After 3 months of training, handgrip-induced increases in HR, BP, and total peripheral resistance were lower, whereas stroke volume and cardiac output were higher (by 13% and 15%, respectively) in trained patients compared with controls. Moreover, a higher increase in nitric oxide level (46% vs 14%) and a lower increase in noradrenaline (11% vs 20%) were observed in trained patients compared with controls. The result showed that short-term dynamic training caused significant improvement of hemodynamic and neurohormonal responses to static exercise.

3.7 Quality of life

Heather et al.[40] recruited 249 patients on a waiting list for elective CABG and randomized them into an intervention group and a control group. During the waiting period, the training group exercised twice per week, with education and reinforcement. After surgery, both groups participated in a CR program. Quality of life was measured by short-form 36 (SF-36) questionnaire during the waiting period, and patients in the intervention group showed a significant increase in the scores of physical role, physical functioning, bodily pain and composite physical summary score. The intervention group displayed better quality of life than the control group, but mainly in physical component, and the improvement continued up to 6 months after surgery.

In a recent study, Brügemann et al.[41] randomized 137 men to one of two types of CR: physical training plus information ('Fit' program) during 6 weeks or comprehensive CR which, on top of the Fit-program, included weekly psycho-education sessions and relaxation therapy ('Fit-Plus' program) for 8 weeks. The results showed that quality of life improved in both treatment groups in the course of time up to 9 months after training, and there was no difference between the two types of CR.

3.8 Graft patency, cardiac events and readmission

Nakai et al.[38] reported the effects of exercise training on recovery of cardiac function and graft patency in 115 patients after CABG. The patients were divided into Group I (n = 60) with and Group II (n = 55) without a CR program. The rate of graft patency was 98% in Group I and 80% in Group II. After training, the exercise stroke index increased significantly in Group I, but not in Group II. The result suggested that physical exercise training should be started as early as possible after CABG to improve graft patency and recovery of cardiac function.

Perk J et al.[42] reported in a study including 49 CABG patients participating in a comprehensive CR program and 98 matched patients receiving standard care. During the first year after CABG, fewer study group patients were readmitted to hospital (14% vs 32%) and on fewer occasions (1.1 vs 2.9). There were no differences in the rates of returning to work (59% vs 64%). In a long-term follow-up, the study group patients rated their physical work capacity higher, and more patients had continued with regular physical training (66% vs 46%). Hedbäck et al.[43] reported in a study included 49 patients who underwent CABG and were offered a CR program consisting of education in risk-factor control and a physical training program. After 10 years of follow up, the study group had lower cardiac events than in the control group (18.4% versus 34.7%). The number of readmissions to hospital (2.1 versus 3.5 per patient) and length of admissions (11 versus 26 days per patient) were significantly lower in the study group. The result proved that a comprehensive CR program after CABG will improve long-term prognosis and reduce the need for hospital care.

In a recent study, Plüss et al.[44] randomized 224 patients with acute myocardial infarction or undergoing CABG to expanded CR (a one-year stress management program, increased physical training, staying at a 'patient hotel' for five days after the event, and cooking sessions), or to standard CR. The number of cardiovascular events was reduced in the expanded CR group compared with the standard CR (47.7% versus 60.2%). This was mainly because of a reduction of myocardial infarctions in the expanded CR group. Days at hospital for cardiovascular reasons were significantly reduced in patients who received expanded CR (median 6 days) compared with standard CR (median 10 days). The result showed that expanded CR reduces cardiovascular morbidity and days at hospital.

4. Tai Chi Chuan training

Tai Chi Chuan (TCC) is a popular Chinese conditioning exercise. The exercise intensity of TCC was low to moderate, depends on its training style, posture and duration. Participants can choose to perform a complete set of TC or selected movements according to their needs. Previous research substantiates that TC enhances aerobic capacity, muscular strength, endothelial function and psychological well-being. In addition, TC benefits to some cardiovascular risk factors, such as hypertension and dyslipidemia. Recent studies also prove that TC is safe and effective for patients with myocardial infarction, bypass surgery and heart failure. Channer et al. [45] reported that the application of TCC for patients with acute myocardial infarction was safe and showed benefits to blood pressure. There are several reasons to recommend TCC as an exercise program for patients with CABG. First, TCC did not need special facility or expensive equipment. Second, TCC is effective for enhancing health fitness and improving cardiovascular risk factors. Third, TCC is low cost and low technology, and can be easily implemented in the community. We have applied a 12-month TCC program to patients with CABG as a phase III cardiac rehabilitation program.[25] After training, the TCC group showed an increase of 10.3% in $\dot{V}O_{2peak}$ and 11.9% in peak work rate. Therefore, TC may be prescribed as an alternative exercise program for selected patients with CABG.

5. Off-pump and minimally invasive CABG

Off-pump coronary artery bypass grafting (OPCAB) uses fewer resources than conventional CABG with cardiopulmonary bypass (CABG-CPB). It was estimated that 20% of CABG operations using OPCAB in western countries, but over 60% of isolated CABG have been performed in Japan using the OPCAB technique. OPCAB grafting reduces the risk of postoperative morbidity, length of hospital stay than conventional surgery with cardiopulmonary bypass.

In a recent study, Angelini et al.[46] reported the graft patency 6-8 years after CABG was similar between OPCAB and CABG-CPB, and the major adverse cardiovascular events or death showed no difference between the two groups. The health-related quality of life was similar between the OPCAB and CABG-CPB groups. In addition, with increasing expertise and technology, minimally invasive and robotic techniques have been developed to enhance post-operative recovery and patient satisfaction.[47] However, there is no study compare the effect of exercise training on conventional CABG and those new techniques, further study is needed to evaluate the difference between conventional and new surgical techniques to the outcomes in patients with CABG.

6. Conclusion

Short-term exercise training for patients with CABG showed benefits to cardiorespiratory function, muscular strength, metabolic profile, cardiac function, ventilatory efficiency, hemodynamic function and quality of life. Additionally, exercise training may improve graft patency, reduce cardiac events and readmission rate. Thus, CR exercise training is an important intervention and should be recommended to most of the patients after CABG.

7. References

[1] Hamm CW, Reimers J, Ischinger T, et al. A randomized study of coronary angioplasty compared with bypass surgery in patients with symptomatic multivessel coronary disease. N Engl J Med 1994;331:1037-43.
[2] Bourassa MG, Knatterud GL, Pepine CJ, et al. Asymptomatic Cardiac Ischemia Pilot (ACIP) Study. Improvement of cardiac ischemia at 1 year after PTCA and CABG. Circulation 1995;92:II1-II7.
[3] Holmes DR, Vlietstra RE, Mock MB. Employment and recreation patterns in patients treated by percutaneous transluminal coronary angioplasty: a multicenter study. Am J Cardiol 2000;52:710-3.
[4] Holmes DR, Jr., Van Raden MJ, Reeder GS, et al. Return to work after coronary angioplasty: a report from the National Heart, Lung, and Blood Institute Percutaneous Transluminal Coronary Angioplasty Registry. Am J Cardiol 1984;53:48C-51C.
[5] Raft D, McKee DC, Popio KA, et al. Life adaptation after percutaneous transluminal coronary angioplasty and coronary artery bypass grafting. Am J Cardiol 1985;56:395-8.
[6] Popma JJ, Califf RM, Topol EJ. Clinical trials of restenosis after coronary angioplasty. Circulation 1991;84:1426-36.
[7] Five-year clinical and functional outcome comparing bypass surgery and angioplasty in patients with multivessel coronary disease. A multicenter randomized trial. Writing Group for the Bypass Angioplasty Revascularization Investigation (BARI) Investigators. JAMA 1997;277:715-21.
[8] King SB, III, Lembo NJ, Weintraub WS, et al. A randomized trial comparing coronary angioplasty with coronary bypass surgery. Emory Angioplasty versus Surgery Trial (EAST) N Engl J Med 1994;331:1044-50.
[9] Hlatky MA, Boothroyd DB, Bravata DM, et al. Coronary artery bypass surgery compared with percutaneous coronary interventions for multivessel disease: a

collaborative analysis of individual patient data from ten randomised trials. Lancet 2009; 373: 1190–97
[10] Serruys PW, Morice, MC, Kappetein AP, et al. Percutaneous coronary intervention versus coronary artery bypass grafting for severe coronary artery disease. N Engl J Med 2009; 360: 961-72.
[11] Hannan EL, Racz, MJ, Gary Walford G, et al. Long-term outcomes of coronary artery bypass grafting versus stent implantation. N Engl J Med 2005;352:2174-83.
[12] Whitlow PL, Dimas AP, Bashore TM, et al. Relationship of extent of revascularization with angina at one year in the Bypass Angioplasty Revascularization Investigation (BARI). J Am Coll Cardiol 1999;34:1750-9.
[13] American College of Sports Medicine: Guidelines for Exercise Testing and Exercise Prescription. 8th ed. Philadelphia: Lea & Febiger, 2010.
[14] Kavanagh T, Mertens DJ, Hamm LF, et al. Prediction of long-term prognosis in 12,169 men referred for cardiac rehabilitation. Circulation 2002;106:666-71.
[15] Haennel RG, Quinney AH, Kappagoda CT. Effects of hydraulic circuit training following coronary artery bypass surgery. Med Sci Sports Exerc 1991;23:158-65.
[16] Engblom E, Hietanen EK, Hämäläinen H, et al. Exercise habits and physical performance during comprehensive rehabilitation after coronary artery bypass surgery. Eur Heart J 1992;13:1053-9.
[17] Dubach P, Myers J, Dziekan G, et al. Effect of residential cardiac rehabilitation following bypass surgery. Chest 1995;108:134-9.
[18] Daida H, Squires RW, Allison TG, et al. Sequential assessment of exercise tolerance in heart transplantation compared with coronary artery bypass surgery after phase II cardiac rehabilitation. Am J Cardiol 1996; 77:696-700.
[19] Mariorana AJ, Briffa TG, Goodman C, et al. A controlled trial of circuit weight training on aerobic capacity and myocardial oxygen demand in men after coronary artery bypass surgery. J cardiopulm Rehabil 1997;17:239-47.
[20] Lan C, Chen SY, Lai JS, et al. The effect of Tai Chi on cardiorespiratory function in patients with coronary artery bypass surgery. Med Sci Sports Exerc 1999;31:634-8.
[21] Goodman JM, Pallandi DV, Reading JR, et al. Central and peripheral adaptations after 12 weeks of exercise training in post-coronary artery bypass surgery patients. J Cardiopulm Rehabil 1999;19:144-50.
[22] Takeyama J, Itoh H, Kato M, et al. Effect of physical training on the recovery of the autonomic nervous activity during exercise after coronary artery bypass grafting. Jpn Circ J 2000; 64:809-13.
[23] Adachi H, Itoh H, Sakurai S, et al. Short-term physical training improves ventilatory response to exercise after coronary arterial bypass surgery. Jpn Circ J 2001; 65: 419–23.
[24] Kodis J, Smith KM, Arthur HM, et al. Changes in exercise capacity and lipid after clinic versus home-based aerobic training in coronary artery bypass graft surgery patients. J Cardiopulm Rehabil 2001;21:31-6.
[25] Lan C, Chen SY, Hsu CJ, et al. Improvement of cardiorespiratory function in patients with percutaneous transluminal coronary angioplasty or coronary artery bypass grafting during outpatient rehabilitation. Am J Phys Med Rehabil 2002;81:336-41.
[26] Chuang TY, Sung WH, Lin CY. Application of a virtual reality-enhanced exercise protocol in patients after coronary bypass. Arch Phys Med Rehabil 2005;86:1929-32.

[27] Sumide T, Shimada K, Ohmura H, et al. Relationship between exercise tolerance and muscle strength following cardiac rehabilitation: comparison of patients after cardiac surgery and patients with myocardial infarction. J Cardiol 2009; 54: 273-81.
[28] Moholdt TT, Amundsen BH, Rustad LA, et al. Aerobic interval training versus continuous moderate exercise after coronary artery bypass surgery: a randomized study of cardiovascular effects and quality of life. Am Heart J 2009;158:1031-7
[29] Onishi T, Shimada K, Sunayama S, et al. Effects of cardiac rehabilitation in patients with metabolic syndrome after coronary artery bypass grafting. J Cardiol 2009;53:381-7.
[30] Bilinska M, Kosydar-Piechna M, Gasiorowska A, et al. Influence of dynamic training on hemodynamic, neurohormonal responses to static exercise and on inflammatory markers in patients after coronary artery bypass grafting. Circ J 2010;74:2598-604.
[31] Shabani R, Gaeini AA, Nikoo MR, et al. Effect of cardiac rehabilitation program on exercise capacity in women undergoing coronary artery bypass graft in hamadan-iran. Int J Prev Med 2010;1:247-51.
[32] Smith KM, McKelvie RS, Thorpe KE, et al. Six-year follow-up of a randomized controlled trial examining hospital versus home-based exercise training after coronary artery bypass graft surgery. Heart 2011;97:1169-74.
[33] Kelemen MH, Stewart KJ, Gillilan RE, et al. Circuit weight training in cardiac patients. J Am Coll Cardiol 1986;7:38-42.
[34] McCartney N, McKelvie RS, Haslam DR, et al. Usefulness of weightlifting training in improving strength and maximal power output in coronary artery disease. Am J Cardiol 1991;67:939-45.
[35] Hagberg JM, Eshani AA, Holloszy JO. Effect of 12 months of intense exercise training on stroke volume in patients with coronary artery disease. Circulation 1983; 1194-9.
[36] Ehsani AA, Biello DR, Schultz J, et al. Improvement of left ventricular contractile function by exercise training in patients with coronary artery disease. Circulation 1986; 64: 1116-24.
[37] Laslett LJ, Paumer L, Ammsterdam EA. Increases in myocardial oxygen consumption indexes by exercise training at onset of ischemia in patients with coronary artery disease. Circulation 1985; 72: 958-62.
[38] Nakai Y, Kataoka Y, Bando M, et al. Effects of physical exercise training on cardiac function and graft patency after coronary artery bypass grafting. J Thorac Cardiovasc Surg 1987;93:65-72.
[39] Wosornu D, Bedford D, Ballantyne D. A comparison of the effects of strength and aerobic exercise training on exercise capacity and lipids after coronary artery bypass surgery. Eur Heart J 1996;17:854-63.
[40] Heather AM, Daniels C, Mckelvie R, et al. Effect of a preoperative intervention on preoperative and postoperative outcomes in low-risk patients awaiting elective coronary artery bypass graft surgery. Ann Intern Med 2000;133:253-62.
[41] Brügemann J, Poels BJ, Oosterwijk MH et al. A randomized controlled trial of cardiac rehabilitation after revascularisation. Int J Cardiol. 2007;119:59-64.
[42] Perk J, Hedbäck B, Engvall J. Effects of cardiac rehabilitation after coronary artery bypass grafting on readmissions, return to work, and physical fitness. A case-control study. Scand J Soc Med 1990;18:45-51.

[43] Hedbäck B, Perk J, Hörnblad M, et al. Cardiac rehabilitation after coronary artery bypass surgery: 10-year results on mortality, morbidity and readmissions to hospital. J Cardiovasc Risk 2001;8:153-8.
[44] Plüss CE, Billing E, Held C, et al. Long-term effects of an expanded cardiac rehabilitation programme after myocardial infarction or coronary artery bypass surgery: a five-year follow-up of a randomized controlled study. Clin Rehabil 2011;25:79-87.
[45] Channer KS, Barrow D, Barrow R, et al. Changes in hemodynamic parameters following Tai Chi Chuan and aerobic exercise in patients recovering from acute myocardial infarction. Postgrad Med J 1996;72:349-51.
[46] Angelini GD, Culliford L, Smith DK, et el. Effects of on- and off-pump coronary artery surgery on graft patency, survival, and health-related quality of life: long-term follow-up of 2 randomized controlled trials. J Thorac Cardiovasc Surg 2009;137:295-303.
[47] Atluri P, Kozin ED, Hiesinger W, et al. Off-pump, minimally invasive and robotic coronary revascularization yield improved outcomes over traditional on-pump CABG. Int J Med Robot 2009;5:1-12.

10

Risk Evaluation of Perioperative Acute Coronary Syndromes and Other Cardiovascular Complications During Emergency High Risky Noncardiac Surgery

Maria Milanova and Mikhail Matveev
University Hospital of Emergency Medicine,
Institute of Biophysics and Biomedical Engineering, BAS
Bulgaria

1. Introduction

The cardiac risk (CR) in noncardiac surgery represents the probability of acute cardiovascular conditions appearance, assessed as perioperative complications.
The most frequent perioperative complications are the acute manifestations of coronary or noncoronary ischemia; acute or exacerbated chronic heart failure (CHF); acute rhythm and conductive disorders; acute cardiac inflammatory processes; increased arterial blood pressure or hypertensive crisis; cardiogenic shock and sudden cardiac death. These conditions are either early signs, or represent a manifestation of progress or decompensation of present cardiac diseases. Specific indication may be found in their origin, if it is explicitly or implicitly associated with the present surgical disease or with a completed surgical intervention, giving weight to the special features of the perioperative period [1].
The major surgical interventions, e.g. in the thoracic cavity and the upper abdominal cavity, as well as the neurosurgical and the major orthopedic operations, are related to increased CR. Previous myocardial infarction, unstable stenocardia and decompressed chronic cardiac insufficiency are powerful predictors for the emergence of acute perioperative cardiovascular complications (CVC) and mortality. The patients with such specified pathologies need additional evaluation before major surgical intervention.
The cardiac postoperative morbidity and mortality are closely related to the basic surgical disease and the corresponding intervention. Many scientific publications report on the high number of complications, accompanying the major surgical abdominal and intrathoracic interventions, emergency surgical interventions, surgery of malignant neoplasm, major peripheral vascular manipulations [1, 2, 3].
The CR evaluation will not change the course and the result of the intervention in emergency conditions, e.g. rupture of abdominal aortic aneurism, heavy trauma, perforations etc., but may have influence upon the care during the early postoperative period. In emergency but noncritical states (e.g. biliary obstruction), the evaluation may contribute to risk reduction without influence upon the decision about the necessity of the intervention. In some cases, the CR evaluation may influence the surgical intervention planning and the choice of less invasive

intervention, e.g. the preference for peripheral arterial angioplasty before infrainguinal bypass, even though the long-term result of the surgery may be altered. In other cases, the CR assessment must support the decision for a given intervention, e.g. for removal of small aneurisms from asymptomatic patients with carotidal stenosis, when the compromise is between the expected life duration and the risk of the intervention.
Below are presented some practices for cardiac risk assessment in emergency noncardiac surgery, including high risk one. Part of them are discussed on the basis of own studies over the applicability of models for CP evaluation in groups of subjects, differentiated upon the urgency, the severity of the surgical disease and intervention, with or without cardiovascular and other concomitant nonsurgical diseases [4, 5, 6, 7].

2. Short review of preoperative cardiac risk assessment schemes in major noncardiac surgery

2.1 General preoperative clinical assessment

The tentative general assessment of the cardiac perioperative risk may be completed on the basis of factors with known contribution.

2.1.1 Risk in patients with ischemic heart disease (IHD)

The perioperative mortality reaches 9.6% in case of IHD, otherwise it is just about 2.8% [8, 9]. Besides the hemodynamically induced complication, other manifestations like thrombosis, coronary spasm, serious rhythm disorder, spontaneous psychogenic nocturnal or preoperative complications, are also possible. The patients with IHD, subjected to major noncardiac surgery, can be divided into 3 groups:

a. Patients with angina pectoris (AP).

The preoperative assessment of patients with angina, who will be subjected to major noncardiac surgery (MNCS), has to clarify the following questions: stable or unstable angina; functional class (FC); is the medicamentous treatment adequate; necessity of specific diagnostic tests.
Except for the surgery of abdominal aortic aneurism, the patients with I-II FC stable stenocardia have the resources to bear the stress of MNCS, while this intervention presents serious threats to patients with III-IV FC.
The patients with I-II FC stable AP are with increased risk of cardiac complications after MNCS [10] (about 10 times higher relative risk compared to patients without IHD). However, this tenfold increase corresponds to a relatively low risk of myocardial infarction (MI), approximately of 4%, and of cardiac death, about 1-2% [8, 9]. FC is decisive in predicting the risk level of patients with stenocardia. Those of them that succeed to reach 85% of the maximum cardiac frequency (even with appearance of ST-depression) have no complications during surgery [11, 12]. Just the opposite, *the presence of ST-depression and the bad tolerance of physical stress identify the high-risk patients.*

b. Patients with MI

The number of perioperative reinfarctions decreases with the improvement of the anesthesiologic methods from 30% to 6% after survived MI during the last 3 months, and from 15% to 2% after preceding MI during the preoperative 3-6 months.
The MI manifestation during intra- or early postoperative periods is often preceded by prolonged or recidivistic ischemia. There are two important mechanisms in the context of the perioperative MI:

1. Chronic imbalance between the need and the providing of blood stream that is clinically manifested as stable IHD (due to coronary arteries' stenosis, limiting the blood stream);
2. Rupture of coronary plaque with clinical manifestation of acute coronary syndrome (ACS).

c. Patients with high risk of asymptomatic IHD.

Such are the patients with diabetes mellitus (DM) or peripheral vascular disease, when either the ECG stress-test cannot be carried out, or the results obtained are not reliable.

2.1.2 Risk in patients with heart failure (HF)

The congestive heart failure (CHF) increases the risk of postoperative complications. Here, it is important to clarify as far as possible, the HF etiology. For example, HF due to hypertension runs a different risk, compared to HF due to IHD [13, 14].

Many general anesthetics cause direct myocardial depression. Very often, a large quantity of liquids is infused during the perioperative period in MNCS and overburden the patients with left ventricular dysfunction or HF. The risk of perioperative cardiogenic pulmonary edema among subjects aged over 40 years, who have been subjected to MNCS, vary from about 2%, if CHF anamnesis is absent, through about 6% for patients with preceding HF, which is not present during physical and X-ray examinations, and reaches up to 16% with persisting physical and X-ray data about pulmonary stagnation [8].

Large abdominal or thoracic surgery, which is followed by CHF that has not been identified before the intervention, is usually associated with elderly patients with ECG abnormalities or other cardiac symptoms [15].

The presence of CHF represents another risk factor for perioperative MI [16, 17, 18, 19].

2.1.3 Risk in patients with heart valvular disease

The patients with heart valvular disease, who have been subjected to MNCS, are subject to an increased risk of cardiac complications, mostly because of their susceptibility for development of CHF, hypo- and hypervolemia and cardiac arrhythmias in the perioperative period [13]. About 20% of the patients with severe heart disease (II or higher FC) either evolve new or complicate the present cardiac decompensation during the MNCS [15]. It is accepted, that the subjects with aortic stenosis are the higher risk patients among these with valvular cardiac disease, as they bear with difficulty hypo- and hypervolemia [20].

The patients with combined rheumatic mitral and aortic heart disease represent a considerable group. Their risk during noncardiac intervention is high, because of their limited resources and capabilities to support changes in pre- and afterloads.

2.1.4 Risk in patients with cardiac arrhythmias

The arrhythmias, either atrial or ventricular, are often related to IHD or CHF and specify increased risk during MNCS. Although both arrhythmias are pointed out as independent risk factors in the perioperative period [20, 21, 22], they probably have significance only as a manifestation of serious heart disease, which itself increases the risk of CVC. In similar cases, the arrhythmias correlate as a marker of cardiac suffering with ischemic and HF complications and do not contribute additional risk during noncardiac surgery. According to Detsky *et al* and Goldman *et al,* the prognosis in patients with arrhythmias, but without supporting cardiac pathology, is usually good and the risk of intervention is very unlikely to be increased, although the same authors determine the atrial fibrillation as an independent risk factor [20, 23].

High risk of the supraventricular tachiarrhythmias progress subsists among elderly patients subjected to pulmonary surgery, patients with subcrucial valvular stenosis and patients with primary anamnesis of similar tachyarrhythmias [24].
Patients with anomalies in the conductive system as AV block, fascicular or bundle branch block often have cardiac diseases. Many anesthetics suppress the cardiac contractility and/or provoke peripheral vasodilatation. The anesthesia may give rise to further depression of the automatism and, consequently, of the ventricular frequency in patients with heart block. The complication of biphascicular block after MI may progress to a third degree AV block, often accompanied by serious hemodynamic disorders [24, 25].
Patients with bundle branch blocks are not subject to increased risk of third degree AV block progress in the perioperative period, although they may acquire it in a long-term context. The presence of bundle branch block does not represent an independent predictor of heavy postoperative cardiac complications if there is no evidence of other severe disease [15, 20].
According to the recommendations of the ACC/AHA the arrhythmias with high risk are as followed [2]:

- high-degree AV block;
- symptomatic ventricular arrhythmias, combined with presence of cardiovascular diseases (CVD);
- supraventricular arrhythmias at high and out-off-control heart rate (HR).

2.1.5 Arterial hypertension

Despite contemporary achievements in arterial hypertension (AH) diagnosis and monitoring, a large percent of the subjects with AH remain without diagnosis or have been inadequately treated. The patient arterial blood pressure (BP) may increase in a hospital environment as a result of a stress. Prys Roberts *et al,* report higher perioperative BP instability among subjects with high preoperative BP [26]. According to Goldman and Caldera [8], the mean intraoperative BP, the necessity of infusion and adrenergic agents for supporting the pressure during the intervention, as well as the progress of considerable postoperative hypertension, practically are not influenced by the fact whether the hypertension was not treated, inadequately treated or well monitored.
Several communications [15, 20, 23, 27] point out that patients with mild through moderate hypertension can be subjected to anesthesia and intervention without high risk of CVC [8]. Other studies cite as evidence that patients with AH are subjected to higher risks of cardiac complications during, or immediately after, MNCS, compared to normotensive subjects. The reasons of the increased risk are due to IHD, left ventricular dysfunction, renal failure, or other disorders commonly encountered among patients with AH [26]. The subjects with AH have increased IHD and CHF risk and tendency towards most frequent manifestations of silent myocardial ischemia during surgery [28].

2.1.6 Cardiomyopathies

The hypertrophic cardiomyopathy raises some specific problems. The reduction of the blood volume, the decreased vascular system resistance and the increased venous volume can reduce the left ventricular volume and increase the tendency towards obstruction of the left ventricular output tract. In addition, the decreased pressure of the ventricular filling may lead to considerable reduction of stroke volume, due to reduced compliance of the hypertrophic ventricle.

2.1.7 Peripheral vascular diseases

They add certain perioperative risks, since they are often associated with accelerated atherosclerosis and IHD [2].

2.1.8 Other risk factors

2.1.8.1 Age

Advanced age is an independent risk factor for perioperative complications [2, 17, 18, 25], not only because of the increased probability of coronary disease, but also because of the senescent effect on the myocardium - decrease of the myocytes number. The mortality caused by acute MI considerably increases with the age. The perioperative MI have higher mortality among the elderly patients [29].

2.1.8.2 Sex

The women have lower cardiac risk except for present early climax or DM [2]. They have lower frequency of IHD, and coronary disease is observed 10 years later, compared to men. In the case of early climax and DM, the risk is equal to that of men at the same age. Mortality, due to acute MI, is greater among women than men, and this difference is even more evident with advancement of age and presence of DM.

2.1.8.3 Diabetes mellitus

DM increases the probability of IHD appearance, but the myocardial ischemia is often silent. DM frequently is considered as a risk factor for cardiac complications in the MNCS perioperative period [17, 30, 31].

2.1.8.4 The chronic pulmopathies

The chronic pulmopathies present a high perioperative risk [32], which is dependent on the severity of the pulmonary disease and the intervention duration.

2.1.9 Type of surgical intervention

The surgical risk represents a complex assessment, which includes the severity of the basic surgical disease, the treatment method and the patient condition. In addition to the present data about cardiovascular pathology that influences the prognosis, other basic surgical factors can provoke exacerbation of present chronic cardiac diseases or appearance of perioperative CVC. Their number is twice higher with infectious inflammation (sepsis) or neoplastic disease [33].

The basic surgical disease is a leading factor for localization, size and duration of the intervention, as well as for the conditions necessary for its performance [34]. The surgery of the thoracic and abdominal aorta contributes the highest risk among the noncardiac interventions, because of the accompanying problems with the water balance, bleeding and oxygenation. The abdominal interventions take the second place in frequency of concomitant CVC, following the thoracic ones [35]. The interventions of carotidal and peripheral vessels are also associated with increased risk of cardiac complications. It is known, that up to 50% of patients undergoing interventions of the peripheral arteries suffer MI in the next 2-3 years [36].

2.1.9.1 Surgical factors

Surgical factors, which influence the cardiac risk, are associated with the emergency, the complication, the type and the duration of the intervention, as well as with the change of the body temperature, the loss of blood and the body liquids exchange. The intervention emergency represents an issue of special importance. The survival rate increases twofold with preoperative intensive cardiac care that is related to eventual delayed emergency intervention, whenever that is possible [37]. Each surgery provokes a stress reaction, due to tissue damages and is mediated by neuroendocrine factors that may lead to tachycardia and hypertension. The perioperative stress reaction includes effusion of catecholamine, provoked by the hemodynamic stress, vasospasm, reduced fibrinolitic activity, activated trombocytes and extracoagulation. Coronary plaque rupture leads to thromboses and subsequent vessel occlusion, which are important factors for the occurrence perioperative ACS. The MI among patients with significant IHD may be a result of a continuous imbalance between the available and the necessary myocardial blood steam (in cases of tachycardia and increased myocardial contractility). Studies on performed autopsies, demonstrate that half of the fatal MI have directly destroyed plaque fissure, rupture or plaque bleeding. Although the specific patient factors are more important for cardiac risk prediction than the surgical ones, the type of the surgical intervention cannot be ignored.

2.1.9.2 Type of the anesthesia

Recent studies indicate, that the operative period is more reliable than it was in the past, mostly because of the careful monitoring of hemodynamics and respiration during the anesthesia [20]. No data are available for determining some significant differences in the severity of the cardiac complications due to the different anesthesia techniques. However, the assessment of the type and the conditions of the anesthesia may have important implications for the cardiac risk prognosis.

2.2 Indices and scales for cardiac risk evaluation and their applicability on cardiac risk assessment in patients with emergency high risky noncardiac surgery

The preoperative assessment of cardiac risk during noncardiac surgery (specifically for emergency surgery) is based on quantitative indices and rated scales. They were proposed and introduced initially for assessment of the anesthesiology risk and consequently, for the cardiac one [20, 23, 38, 39].

The synthesis of methods for preoperative cardiac risk assessment began intensively at the end of the seventies, as a result of the communication by Goldman *et al* [17, 19, 20, 23, 40, 41, 42, 43, 44, 45, 46]. The methods and indices for the cardiac risk assessment can be characterized as:

- common for CR [20, 25, 27, 42];
- specifically related to the risk of ischemic complications – underestimated by Goldman *et al*, although it is the most dynamic and dangerous risk factor (RF) [17,19, 40, 41, 43, 44, 45, 46].

From another point of view, the methods and indices for cardiac risk assessment are:

- quantitative [20, 23, 27];
- qualitative [17, 19, 40, 41, 42, 43, 44, 45, 46, 47].

2.2.1 Quantitative (point) indices

The CR index in noncardiac surgeries that was introduced by Goldman et al [20] represents a point assessment and is still largely applied in practice. This index is derived over data of patients with MNCS, such as aortic, pleural, intraoperational and intrathoracic interventions. It includes 9 preoperative assessable indices with own quantitative contribution to the amount, which determines the perioperative CVC risk. The risk is distributed in 4 classes: I-st class (0 to 5 points) with live-threatening complications and cardiac death of 0.9%; II-nd class (6 to 12 points) with 7% rate of such complications; III-rd class (13 to 25 points) with 14% rate; IV-th class (26 and over points) with expected rate of live-threatening complications and cardiac death of 77%. The indicator "Poor general condition" includes the criteria: $PO2 < 60$; $PCO2 > 50$; $K < 3$; $HCO3 < 20$; $BUN > 50$; Creat > 3; elevated SGOT; chronic liver disease; bedridden.

Detsky *et al* [23] modified Goldman's index on the basis of clinical evaluation and monitoring of non-selected patients over 40 years old with MNCS. Within that index, the timing of the previous MI is divided into less or more than 6 mounts ago, while the influence of the stenocardia is specified according the adopted division as stable (with differentiated classes) and unstable; the anamnesis of the pulmonary edema is also included. It is accepted, that Goldman's index is equally informative as the extended index of Detsky *et al* [23], but the first does not include III and IV class stenocardia, while Detsky *et al* introduced such corrections. The atrial fibrillation is included as RF too. Subsequent studies establish its significance, whenever this cardiac disorder is currently manifested [53]. AH was also evaluated at a later stage, but from the heart defects, only aortic stenosis is included.

The pivotal points of Goldman's index are the presence of MI and HF. The index of Larsen *et al* [27] includes metabolic deviations in parallel with CVD. Here the volume, the nature and, especially, the surgical conditions (emergency or planned) are assessed in greater detail. On the basis of that, Larsen *et al* managed to integrate the CR index with the type of surgical intervention. The index of Larsen *et al* can reach a maximum value of 54 points - divided by the level and actuality of HF and IHD, as well as other conditions.

In 1999, Lee *et al* [48] reevaluated the significance of some clinic risk factors, associated with patients undergoing noncardiac surgery. The revised index sets 6 predictors of major cardiac complications: high risk surgery, IHD, HF, cerebrovascular disease, type 1 DM and renal insufficiency. The presence of 0, 1, 2 or 3 of the predictors sets the risk level of major cardiac complications at 0.4%, 0.9%, 7% and 11%, respectively. The index of Lee *et al* has better prognostic value than those of Goldman *et al* and Detsky *et al,* due to the smaller number of variable risk factors. For the time being, the clinicians and the researchers accept Lee's index as the most applicable for prediction of the perioperative cardiac risk in noncardiac surgery. However, the patients examined by Lee *et al* do not constitute a representative population of patients undergoing noncardiac surgeries, since the thoracic, the vessel and the orthopedic cases are over-represented.

2.2.2 Non-point scales for cardiac risk assessment

The scale of Kleinman [42] includes remoteness of MI, angina pectoris, valvular disease, rhythm disorders, arterial hypertension, abnormal ECG, peripheral vascular diseases.

The scale of Eagle *et al* [47] includes age over 70 years, DM, angina pectoris, presence of pathological Q-wave in ECG and ventricular extrasystoles. The presence of one RF determines low risk, the presence of 2 to 3 - moderate risk, while more than 3 risk factors leads to high risk assessment.

Later on, *diagrams and tables for risk assessment of ischemic complications* [19, 41, 43], life-threatening ischemic complications [17, 36, 44, 45], tachyarrhythmias [24], and ventricular arrhythmias [49] were proposed. The scales and the statements about the probability of ischemic complications comprise of several symptoms, derived from clinical, laboratory, imaging, and electrophysiological examinations. Hopf and Tarnow [41] propose intraoperative ECG monitoring, transesophageal echocardiography, which is a semi-invasive and expensive method, cardio-kymography, radio-marked erythrocytes and small gamma camera, as well as metabolic parameters. Lette *et al* [43] reach the conclusion that the clinical parameters can not predict incoming ischemic incidents. They accentuate on dipyridamole-thallium scintigraphy. Leppo [19] includes ECG examinations, treadmill, stress-echocardiography with dobutamine or exercise, thallium scintigraphy with test burden in the preoperative assessment. Symptomatic angina, CHF, survived MI, ventricular extrasystoles, and age over 70 years, are also taken into consideration.

Mangano *et al* [50] evaluate the significance of the following clinic symptoms, related to the appearance of post-operative ischemic complications: 1) presence of left ventricular hypertrophy in ECG; 2) remoteness of the arterial hypertension; 3) diabetes mellitus; 4) manifested IHD; 5) HF needing the use of digoxine. According to the presence of the five preoperative symptoms for postoperative ischemia, the probability of its perioperative appearance is divided into 5 levels: without any symptom presence - 22%; presence of one symptom - 31%; 46% with two symptoms; 70% with three; 77% with four symptoms.

Other studies of the same authors emphasize the significance of the following conditions, contributing to unfavorable outcomes from ischemic complications [44, 45]:

1. intraoperative hypotension and tachycardia (the assessment of hypertension is contradictory);
2. appearance of acute ischemic events in the postoperative period (acute MI), unstable stenocarida or ECG ischemia. Note that CHF and ventricular tachycardia are not associated with unfavorable outcomes;
3. instrumentally determined intra- and postoperative changes: appearance of ECG ischemia (doubles the MI risk); increases of the endmost left camera diastolic pressure that are accepted as evidence of ischemia - note that the mean pulmo-capillary pressure and the diastolic pulmonary arterial pressure do not correlate with the incidents; segmental disorder of the left camera wall assessed by transesophageal echocardiography - that is accepted as the most sensitive predictor [51], although the same authors specify later on, that transesophageal echocardiography weakly correlates with postoperative complications;
4. the presence of AH, heavy limiting lung disease, creatinine clearance lower than 0.8 ml/s - factors independently associated with high risk of cardiac death [45]. The death probability is 80% when two or more factors are present.

If the total rate of complications with all monitored patients is 12%, then 24% of those with old MI or cardiomegaly have postoperative complications - cardiac death, acute MI, ischemia. The rate of patients without the mentioned consequences is only 7% [52].

A standard for CR assessment during noncardiac surgeries [22, 53, 54] was adopted, on the basis of the debates, concerning the applicability of the schemes and indices for CR assessment and the ACC/AHA proposals [22, 53, 54]. According to it, CR is further divided into three groups - high, moderate, and low, depending on the severity of the perioperative

CVC and the probability of a fatal outcome; the significance of the clinical predictors is determined, as well as the volume and type of the surgery.

1. Risk, related to CVD:

a. high:
   the unstable coronary syndromes - new MI and unstable stenocardia;
   the decompensated HF;
   the significant arrhythmias - high-degree AV block, symptomatic ventricular arrhythmias accompanying cardiac disease, as well as supraventricular arrhythmias with uncontrolled HR;
   critical valvular cardiac lesion.

b. moderate:
   stable stenocardia - I-II FC;
   old MI or present pathological Q wave in ECG ;
   compensated HF;
   diabetes mellitus.

c. lower:
   advanced in years;
   ECG abnormalities;
   non-sinus rhythm;
   bad functional capacity;
   past apoplexy;
   uncontrolled arterial hypertension.

2. Risk, related to surgical intervention:

a. high:
   emergency major interventions, specifically with elderly patients;
   aortic and other major vessel interventions;
   peripherally vessel surgeries;
   extended surgeries, accompanied by loss of many liquids and blood .

b. moderate:
   carotid endarteriectomy;
   cranial and vertebral surgeries;
   intraperitoneal and intrathoracic surgeries;
   orthopedic surgeries;
   prostate surgery.

c. lower:
   endoscope procedures;
   procedures on the body surface;
   cataract and breast surgeries.

The ACC/AHA classification merits consist of classification of the risk categories, as well as the consideration of the cardiac state and type of surgery. Are specified the rhythm disorders, the low risk predictors and the pathological ECG findings.

There are several investigations and analyses on the applicability of the CR indices evaluation [1, 11], including such on large number of patients [23]. Basic disadvantages of indices are the high percent of false-positive conclusions [38] and the impossibility of obtaining accurate diagnosis and assessment of the most serious and dynamic RF - the ischemia, with pain or silent [9, 31, 45, 56]. The CR indices do not determine the appearance

probability of acute ischemic incidents [9, 31, 57] and that is what significantly affects the reliability of the cardiac death prognosis.
The point indices of Goldman *et al* and Larsen *et al* include the emergency and the operation volume in the criteria set for the index calculation, but with the lowest possible weights: 4 and 3 with Goldman *et al* (in the assessment range from 3 through 11) and 3 and 3 with Larsen *et al* (in the range from 3 through 12). The detailed analysis of the two schemes gives a satisfactory answer to both the low discrimination coefficients (used for calculation of the emergency and severity of the surgery with both models), and their unavoidable presence among the criteria. Table 1.1 details systematically the required data.

Data for investigation of :	**Goldman et al**	**Larsen et al**
Total number of surgeries (TNS)	1001	2609
Total number of heavy cardiac complications including cardiac death (HCC)	58	68
Emergency surgeries (ES)	197	605
Heavy cardiac complications (including cardiac death) in emergency surgeries (HCC_{ES})	31	38
Emergency surgeries /Total number of surgeries (ES/TNS)	19.7%	23.2%
Heavy cardiac complications in ES/Total number of heavy cardiac complications (HCC_{ES}/HCC)	35.4%	56%
Exceeding index (EI_{ES})	**271%**	**241%**
Major surgeries * (MNCS)	437	857
Heavy cardiac complications (including cardiac death) in major noncardiac surgeries (HCC_{MS})	43	40
Major surgeries/Total number of surgeries (MS/TNS)	43.7%	32.8%
Heavy cardiac complications in major surgeries/ Total number of heavy cardiac complications (HCC_{MS}/HCC)	74.1%	58.8%
Exceeding index (EI_{MS})	**170%**	**179%**

* Major surgeries: aortic, pleural, intraperitoneal, intrathoracic.

Table 1.1. Exceeding indices for emergency and major noncardiac surgery

The proportion between the cardiac complication rates, accompanying the emergency and major surgeries on the one hand, and the total cardiac complication rates for all patients on the other, considerably exceeds the corresponding proportion between the emergency and major intervention rates to the total number of interventions. We devoted special attention to that fact, in our targeted study [5, 6] introducing the so called **"Exceeding Indices."** The Exceeding Index, applied to the emergency surgeries (EI_{ES}) expresses the quotient (in percent) between the relative rate of the heavy cardiac complications (including cardiac death) accompanying the emergency surgeries (HCC_{ES}), towards the total number of heavy cardiac complications (HCC), and the relative rate of the emergency surgeries (ES) towards the total number of surgeries (TNS):

$$EI_{ES}\ (\%) = (HCC_{ES}/HCC)/(ES/TNS).$$

Respectively, the Exceeding Index of the major surgeries (EI_{MS}) expresses the quotient (in percent) between the relative rate of the heavy cardiac complications (including cardiac death) accompanying the major surgeries (HCC_{MS}) towards the total number of heavy cardiac complications (HCC), and the relative rate of the major surgeries (MS) towards the total number of surgeries (TNS):

$$EI_{MS}\ (\%) = (HCC_{MS}/HCC)/(MS/TNS).$$

The emergency surgeries, representing about 1/5 of a relatively small group used with both studies [5, 6], demonstrated a specific rate of cardiac complications that is 2.5-3 times higher than the one, observed for the entire group. The same parameter for MNCS indicates an increase of 1.5-2 times.

It is worth noting that the "Exceeding Indices" makes evident the practically total coincidence between the results obtained by Goldman et al and Larsen et al about the "weights" of the emergency and the intervention volume, despite some differences within the constellations of the other criteria used by both point systems. The reason for the mentioned emergency and major surgery "classification", completed by both systems becomes clear - on the one hand, they do not predominate over the total number of interventions, i.e. they do not determine the nature of the used samples; on the other hand, they bring considerable CVC risk in the perioperative period that can not be ignored by the used statistical analysis.

The analysis of the results obtained, when applying both indices of CR assessment towards the three specific patient groups, generally indicates a significant discrepancy between the formally calculated assessments and the concretely recorded cardiac complications in the perioperative period. There are certain possible hypotheses, offering reasons for the limited applicability of the index models for CR evaluation under the emergency MNCS conditions:

1. The criteria with considerable contribution to the total risk assessment (point assessment above the mean for a given criterion of the corresponding model) have a relatively low rate and/or are weakly informative in emergency surgeries, while the criteria with lower contribution (point assessment below the mean for a given criterion) have a relatively high rate or are highly informative in emergency surgeries.
2. More important contribution to the cardiac risk evaluation in cases of emergency MNCS have other criteria, which are not included in both models.

In our opinion, both hypotheses are realistically supported by the analysis performed. We reiterate, that the emergency and the surgery severity (markedly demonstrated with the first group of patients) dominate as cardiac risk predictors. *However, these criteria are not direct detectors of the heart status; they specify the surgical heart burdening, which is the reason for their predominance in patients with cardiac diseases.* The constellation parameters of both models are deficient in direct criteria for cardiac status evaluation; this fact is relevant to a greater extent for Goldman's model.

The relative advantages of Larsen's model may be well explained by the adequately introduced cardiac status criteria. The IHD assessment criterion includes: 1) MI presence during the 3 last months (Goldberger *et al* specify 6 months); 2) older infarction or angina pectoris (missing in Goldberger's model). The data analysis shows that the second index, even appreciated by 3 points only, is significantly more frequent, about 15% of the cases with critical patient complications. At the same time, MI presence during the last 3 or 6 months (indices with high value, 10 and 11 in both models, respectively) is recorded with one patient, who did not demonstrate perioperative complications. Our interpretation is that the recent (and generally severe) cardiovascular incidents have no explicit contribution to the risk evaluation, since they are subject to therapeutic monitoring. This is not the case with patients with chronic and mild incidents and generally more distant in time CVD and their complications. In emergency cases, the possibilities for correction are missing, that are inherent to planed surgery, even when the complications are under- or decompensated.

Considerable contribution to the cardiac risk assessment in the model of Larsen *et al,* have indices characterizing in aggregate the "heart failure" criterion. Within the investigated by us patient group, with present or preceding pulmonary stagnation, heart failure is a considerably more frequent postoperative CVC. The conclusion is highly valid among patients with stagnations, confirmed by X-ray examination. In such cases, the corresponding cardiac risk assessment increases by 12 points (at persistent pulmonary stagnation) or by 8 points (without stagnation but with preceding pulmonary edema).

Important for the correct cardiac risk evaluation are the cases, offering indices for combined criteria, that are assessed by low point amounts from 2 to 4, such as preceding HF without stagnation or edema; preceding IHD with or without old MI; diabetes; increased serum creatinine. The combination of three of the mentioned indications, accompanying the emergency abdominal surgeries (very common case in practice), leads to a risk increase in the range of 12 through 50%.

Special comment is needed on diabetes, included as a indicator in Larsen's model. In addition to the specific complication, diabetes is associated with the IHD. Introduction of diabetes in cardiac risk evaluation is appropriate, bearing in mind its frequency. It was encountered in 22.4% of the patients, examined by us. The percent of the heavy CVC in patients with diabetes is 14.5. In comparison, it is 8 with patients with mild CVC complications.

The discussion on the applicability of the index models does not cover the problems related to the adequate evaluation of the used criteria constellations for CR assessment in emergency noncardiac surgery. Evidently, there are other criteria, which reliably predict (directly or indirectly) the probability of cardiovascular incidents during the perioperative period.

3. Real and relative myocardial ischemia as a risk factor for appearance of acute cardiac complications in emergency noncardiac surgery – Index for cardiac risk assessment, through ST-depression in the preoperative ECG

Most well known studies indicate the manifested myocardial ischemia as a proven predictor of perioperative cardiac incidents. Different investigations report preoperative ischemia found in 28% through 32% [50, 58] of the examined cases; other refer to a value of up to 60% [59]. The preoperative ischemia, established by Holter monitors, is a predictor of the perioperative one [60]. When the preoperative ischemia is determined by two-days of ECG monitoring, the perioperative complications are specified as 18%, 21% of them being cardiac death, AMI, and unstable stenocardia; 35% are HF; 44% - ventricular tachycardia [9]. The influence of the real and relative myocardial ischemia on perioperative CVC appearance is evident. Therefore, it is useful to associate the CR evaluation with the ECG determined ST-depression. The introduction of an index for CR assessment provides an understandable and objective method for CVC risk determination in cases of preoperative ECG manifested myocardial ischemia (MMI) during emergency noncardiac surgeries. This paragraph presents a synthesis of the cardiac risk assessment index (CRI) for CVC prediction in the postoperative period, based on ST-depression in preoperative ECG, as an expression of real/relative myocardial ischemia.

Data obtained by monitoring the disease process within a group of 466 patients is used for CRI synthesis. The patients have been emergency treated against acute abdominal surgical diseases or abdominal traumas. The patient distribution within the investigated surgical nosological groups (ING) is presented in increasing order of surgical disease (SD) severity in Table 2.1.

The CRI synthesis is related to assessment and comparison of the CVC rate of patients with and without MMI in the ING. CVC appeared in 169 (36.3%) of ING patients: 51 (64.5%) of them with MMI and the remaining 118 (30.9%) - without MMI. The statistically significant difference ($p<0.001$) shows that MMI is an important RF. This general evaluation of the MMI influence on the patients in the postoperative period has to be specified for ING in increasing order of their severity. Table 2.2 presents the CVC rate (in percent) found in ING patients with and without MMI.

The frequency of CVC in patients without MMI marks the anticipated increasing trend in accordance with the increased SD severity - from the low 5.5% among patients with acute appendicitis, through the significant 33, 34, and 35% for patients with hernia, abdominal and biliary-pancreatic diseases, to the high 54% related to acute states, provoked by pathologies of the lower part of the gastrointestinal tract.

The CVC rates in patients with MMI are obviously higher, but as a trend, they do not repeat the monotonic CVC rate increase with SD deterioration of patients without MMI. A characteristic peak may be observed in group B (77%); high rate in group E (71%); limited increase in C (62%) and D (65%) groups. Group A remains with the most rare CVC cases (40%).

The statistically significant difference between the CVC rates in ING, among patients with and without MMI, underlines the specificity of the two trends. Significant, even at different levels, are the differences in groups A, B, C and D. The high level ($p<0.005$) in group B corresponds to the highest recorded increase of the CVC rate, when comparing the results of patients with and without MMI (from 33% to 77%). The differences in groups A and D ($p<0.005$) are also derived with high significance, due to the considerable CVC percentage among the MMI patients. At the same time, the difference in group E between the CVC rate among patients with and without MMI is not significant.

The analysis of the trends in the CVC rates demonstrates the necessity of a detailed discussion on the MMI influence as an ING risk factor.

The CVC are separated as lethal and nonlethal, depending on the recorded disease outcome. Nonlethal CVC appeared in 136 (29.2%) patients of the investigated group: 38 (48.1%) of them with and 98 (25.3%) without MMI. Lethal CVC were observed in 33 (7.1%) patients, 13 (16.5%) with and 20 (5.2%) without MMI.

Surgical disease	Code	Number
Acute appendicitis	**A**	**102**
acute phlegmonous appendicitis		
acute gangrenous and perforated appendicitis		
Complicated hernia	**B**	**92**
Incarceration inguinal and ventral hernia without complications		
Incarceration inguinal and ventral hernia with intestinal necrosis or intestinal phlegmon		
Gastro-duodenal	**C**	**84**
Gastro-duodenal ulcer with perforation		
Gastro-duodenal ulcer with hemorrhage		
Gastro-duodenal ulcer with stenosis		
Gastric neoplasia with perforation or hemorrhage		
Hepatopancreatobiliary	**D**	**108**
Acute or chronic exacerbated cholecystitis		
Complicated cysts, tumors and abscess of liver		
Mechanical icterus		
Acute pancreatitis-with edema, necrotic pancreatitis or absceding necrotizing pancreatitis		
Intestinal	**E**	**80**
Benignant ileus		
Malignant ileus		
Spontaneous intestinal perforation (including intestinal diverticulum, ulcerative or necrotic colitis)		
Colo-rectal neoplasia with perforation or hemorrhage		
Mesenteric thrombosis		
Inflammatory and neoplastic tumors of abdominal wall		

Table 2.1. The patient distribution of the surgical nosological groups in increasing order of severity.

Group of surgical diseases	Total number of CVC to the number of patients (in %) in the group accordingly		Number of lethal CVC to the total number of CVC (in %) in patients		Number of nonlethal CVC to the total number of CVC (in %) in patients		Number of lethal CVC to the number of patients (in %) in the group accordingly		Number of lethal to the number of non-lethal CVC (in %) in patients		Mean age of the patients in the surgical groups	
	Without MMI	With MMI	Without MMI	With MMI	Without MMI	With MMI	Without MMI	With MMI	Without MMI	With MMI	Without MMI	With MMI
A	5,5	40	0	0	5,5	40	0	0	0	0	37	58
B	33	77	4	10	32	69	1	8	3	12	69	75
C	34	62	8	25	31	46	3	15	10	33	61	68
D	35	73	21	24	28	50	7	23	25	46	55	63
E	54	71	32	50	37	35	17	35	50	100	62	72

Table 2.2. CVC and age profiles in surgical groups

Lethal CVC were not recorded among patients in group A, either with or without MMI. These complications among patients without MMI increase gradually, even weakly in groups B (1%), C (3%) and D (7%), but considerably in group E (17%). The trend of the lethal CVC rates among MMI patients is also increased, but highly expressed in the range of severity groups: 8%, 15%, 23% and 35% in B, C, D and E, respectively. Except for group A, there are significantly higher CVC rates among MMI patients, compared to these without MMI ($p<0.05$). The nonlethal CVC rate in patients without MMI increases from 5.5% in group A to approximately equal levels in groups B (32%), C (31%) and D (28%), but more expressively in group E (37%). This rate reaches the peak among MMI patients in group B (69%), compared to the almost equal and lower rates in A (40%), C (46%) and D (50%). The low rate (35%) of nonlethal CVC patients with MMI in group E is impressive, and practically equal to the rate of patients without MMI. This is true also for the many times higher CVC rate in group A among MMI patients, comparing to patients without MMI ($p<0.001$). These data determine the high significance of the rate differences in group A and the lack of such difference in group E. Nonlethal CVC were observed in groups B and D as statistically significant more often with MMI patients than among those without MMI, although the calculated significant level is lower ($p<0.05$). The difference in group C is not significant.

The consequence of the differentiated analysis on the CVC rates with and without lethal outcomes is that the above mentioned specificity of the rate trends of all CVC in patients with MMI is totally determined by the rate trend of the low (nonlethal) complications. The lethal complications rate in the MMI group follows the increasing trend from group A with the low surgical severity to group E with the considerable severity of SD, but this trend is to some extent higher in patients without MMI. Among the nonlethal CVC, the most significant differences are in the groups A and B with low severity SD, while group A shows the highest relative increase in complications (7.3 times). The increased value of 2.2 times in group B is obtained with highest absolute percent of 69% of nonlethal complications among MMI patients.

The differentiated MMI evaluation as a risk factor, reveals its different contribution to the critical complications structure (lethal and nonlethal) of ING patients with and without MMI. Both ratios equal zero due to lack of lethal CVC in group A. In this group, with low severity SD, MMI is a risk factor only in cases of mild complications.

In group B, despite the lesser level of significant difference ($p<0.1$), MMI stands out as a factor emphasizing the CVC and their prognoses. In groups with increased severity SD (C and D) this difference is $p<0.05$,which is convincing proof of the MMI importance for the CVC structuring. The significance of the MMI contribution has its logical maximum ($p<0.001$) with the CVC appearances and outcomes in group E, the group with considerable surgical severity.

The results obtained, outlining the role of MMI as a risk factor of increased severity of CVC rate in SD with increased severity, need specification of the factor, which underlines the specifics of the nonlethal CVC rate trend among MMI patients, reflected also in the structure of the total number of CVC.

The role of age as risk factor in CVC appearance and their complicated duration is known. We will limit our scope to clarification of its specific contribution to the CVC structure in the ING, thus evaluating the CVC risk among patients with and without MMI. The highest mean age of such patients is recoded with the lowest level of significance in group B - 69 and 75 years, respectively, with the lowest level of significance of $p<0,05$. This expressed high and near mean age in both types of patients in group B, may be well interpreted by the SD nature - the complicated abdominal hernias. The age discrimination among patients with and without MMI (37 and 58 years) is most expressed in group A, where the significance level of difference is high: $p<0.005$. Practically the patients of this group are clustered in two sets - young without MMI and elderly with MMI. Such clusters have considerably nearer values in groups C, D and E (61 and 68 years, 55 and 63 years, 62 and 72 years, respectively) that determines the lower significance levels of difference. The mean age of MMI patients in the very serious SD (group E) is relatively high (72 years) and come close to that in group B.

The low surgical severity group A of MMI patients often contains nonlethal CVC; it is characterized by a relatively high mean age. Such age, combined with MMI, determines the frequency peak of the nonlethal CVC in group B, which also consists of relatively low surgical severity SD. The lethal CVC are more frequent in group E, because of the considerable surgical severity SD and the high mean age of the MMI group; the nonlethal CVC rates among patients with and without MMI are equaled. In comparison to MMI, the age has prevalent importance towards the appearance of nonlethal CVC, in the cases discussed above.

The performed analysis and the results obtained allow quantitative assessment of the increasing risk of CVC in patients with MMI in ING, taking into consideration the age profile, expressed by indices synthesis: **general** – for prognosis of all CVC, and **specific** – for the lethal CVC prognosis only. Based on the related to the SD groups content of Table 2.2:

1. relation between rates of all CVC in patients with and without MMI

$$(FAC^{+MMI}/FAC^{-MMI})_{SD};$$

2. mean ages of patients with and without MMI

$$(MA^{+MMI}/MA^{-MMI})_{SD},$$

we can constitute a relation between the rates of all CVC in patients with and without MMI, adjusted to the corresponding mean ages:

$$TCRI_{SD} = (FAC^{+MMI}/FAC^{-MMI})_{SD}/(MA^{+MMI}/MA^{-MMI})_{SD}$$

The last equation is the total, age-corrected CRI, which gives assessment of the MMI "net contribution" to the increased risk of CVC appearance individually in each SD group, and is relevant for a "conditional" patient whose age is equal to the mean age within the group. The MMI assessment of a given patient is corrected by the ratio between his own age (PA) and the mean age within the MMI group of SD:

$$P(TCRI_{SD}) = TCRI_{SD}*(PA/MA^{+MMI})$$

This formula can be used for interval assessments of the general CRI in ING, according to the recommended by the WHO age intervals for patient grouping - Table 2.3.
Analogously, one may assess the specific CRI, related to lethal CVC prediction by the equation

$$LCRI_{SD} = (FLC^{+MMI}/FLC^{-MMI})_{SD}/(MA^{+MMI}/MA^{-MMI})_{SD}$$

and its personalized value

$$P(LCRI_{SD}) = LCRI_{SD}*(PA/MA^{+MMI}),$$

where FLC^{+MMI} and FLC^{-MMI} are the presented in Table 2.3 lethal CVC rates of patients with and without MMI.
Table 2.4 contains the age interval assessments (compliant with WHO recommendations) of the specific CRI in the SD groups. The trend towards increasing the value of the index can be clearly followed as a function of the severity of the SD.
The research conducted, leads to the following conclusions. The CVC prediction during emergency surgeries is very important, due to the exceptionally high CVC rate - 45% in the investigated patient groups. In its turn, the significantly higher CVC rate among patients with MMI proves that it is an independent, important and leading risk factor. In this context, MMI determines not only the probability of occurrence, but also the CVC severity: fully nonlethal (group A); predominantly nonlethal (groups B, C, D); predominantly lethal (group E).
The rate trends of the nonlethal (low severity) and lethal (considerable severity) complications among patients in the SD groups with and without MMI take into consideration the age influence, since it can not be disregarded in risk factor evaluation. Therefore, the MMI presence qualitatively determines the following, influenced by the age CVC risks:

- group A (low surgical severity): rare and mild CVC in young patients, who dominate in the group; relatively frequent, but mild CVC among the more elderly;
- group B (relatively low surgical severity): high rate of mild CVC due to the specific high mean age;
- groups C and D (increased surgical severity): increased probability of mild CVC with the age increase; increased probability of high severity CVC with the SD severity increase;
- group E (considerable surgical severity): high probability of high severity CVC, due to the specific high mean age; the risk of mild CVC is identical in patients with and without MMI.

Age >	18 - 40	41 -55	56 - 65	66 - 75	76 - 90	> 90
A	1,4 - 3,2	3,2 - 4,3	4,3 - 5,1	5,1 - 5,9	5,9 - 7,1	> 7,1
B	0,5 - 1,1	1,1 - 1,5	1,5 - 1,8	1,8 - 2,1	2,1 - 2,5	> 2,5
C	0,4 - 0,95	0,95 - 1,3	1,3 - 1,5	1,5 - 1,8	1,8 - 2,2	> 2,2
D	0,5 - 1,2	1,2 - 1,7	1,7 - 2,0	2,0 - 2,3	2,3 - 2,7	> 2,7
E	0,3 - 0,6	0,6 - 0,8	0,8 - 1,0	1,0 - 1,1	1,1 - 1,4	> 1,4

Table 2.3. Values of TCRI according to surgery groups and age intervals

Age >	18 - 40	41 -55	56 - 65	66 - 75	76 - 90	> 90
A	0	0	0	0	0	0
B	0,06 - 0,13	0,13 - 0,18	0,18 - 0,22	0,22 - 0,25	0,25 - 0,30	> 0,30
C	0,13 - 0,31	0,31 - 0,43	0,43 - 0,50	0,50 - 0,59	0,59 - 0,73	> 0,73
D	0,22 - 0,53	0,53 - 0,75	0,75 - 0,88	0,88 - 1,01	1,01 - 1,19	> 1,19
E	0,30 - 0,60	0,60 - 0,80	0,80 - 1,00	1,00 - 1,10	1,10 - 1,40	> 1,40

Table 2.4. Values of LCRI according to surgery groups and age intervals

4. Extended quantitative schemes for risk evaluation of perioperative acute coronary syndromes and other cardiovascular complications during emergency high risky noncardiac surgery

The proposed, in the preceding paragraph, index for cardiac risk assessment based on the ST-depression has to be interpreted as an express method, applied under the specific conditions of emergency noncardiac surgery for prediction of acute CVC during the postoperative period. The mentioned index is powerful, as it pays attention to manifested myocardial ischemia, which is among the proven factors, determining the high cardiac risk in patients with MNCS. This concept, combined with the conclusion about the limited applicability of the known schemes for CR assessment under emergency MNCS conditions, raises the actual problem related to the synthesis of extended schemes for risk evaluation that offer a compromise between the requirement of highly significant assessment and its achievement, based on available patient data. Below, we propose such schemes, synthesized on the basis of real patient data undergoing emergency abdominal surgery.

The study uses data obtained by the same 466 patients with emergency treated acute surgical abdominal diseases or traumas (see Table 2.1). The data from large sets of indicators have been collected. The pilot investigation on the potential contributions of indicators that may reliably characterize the CVC, resulted in the constellation shown in Table 3.1. The data cover the three periods of the disease process: preoperative, intraoperative and postoperative. Each indicator has its own structure of category-related or quantitative values, appropriately coded to be processed through a multidimensional statistical approach. We used discriminant analysis (DA) for the synthesis of rules, allowing quantitative evaluation of the CVC risk appearance probability, during the intra- and postoperative periods. The categorisation of individual patients to the CVC group with a given CR level, or to the group without CVC, is performed by substituting the patient's indicators values in the linear discriminator. The patient belongs to the control group if the discriminator value is below the limit. Such are the operated patients without perioperative CVC, even only with transient CVD or abnormal values of some indicators related to the cardiovascular system. Discriminator value above the limit classified the patient to the corresponding risk level group. The hypothesis about CVC appearance with higher risk level is verified by the next discrimination rule, which assesses the probability of higher risk of CVC.

Age	Diabetes mellitus
Surgical conditions	Lung breathing
Volume of surgery	Lung auscultatory
Duration of anesthesia	Systolic blood pressure
Total duration of intubation	Diastolic blood pressure
Intraoperative surgery complications	Central venous pressure
Intraoperative CVC with low risk	Heart rate
Intraoperative CVC with moderate risk	Heart rhythm
Intraoperative CVC with high risk	Heart auscultatory
Postoperative surgery complications	Hemoglobin
Postoperative CVC with low risk	Glucose
Postoperative CVC with moderate risk	Urea
Postoperative CVC with high risk	Creatinine
Cause of death, noncardiac	Potassium
Cause of death, cardiac	Enzymes - SGOT
Arterial hypertension, class	Enzymes - SGPT
Ischemic heart disease	X-ray lung
Myocardial infarction	Exercise ECG
Arrhythmias	Myocardial ischemia - preoperative
Heart failure	Myocardial ischemia - intraoperative
Chronic pulmonary disease	

Table 3.1. Used indicators

The level of discrimination significance depends on the patient numbers, correctly or incorrectly assigned to the training groups. In our case, training groups are the control patient group and the groups with specified CR level. The 446 operated persons are distributed in training groups, which correspond almost totally to the ACC/AHA classification of intra- and postoperative CVC [2, 20]. Two corrections are introduced, since the analysis of the false positive and false negative errors in previous own research, following strictly the ACC/AHA classification, showed the expedience of these corrections in the specific practice with emergency noncardiac surgeries:

- the transient hypotension of the intraoperative CVC scheme is re-classified from low risk to moderate risk;
- the compensated HF of the postoperative CVC scheme is re-classified from high risk to moderate risk; the decompensate HF is determined as a high risk complication.

According to these corrections, the patients are distributed in CVC groups with different CR level, as it is shown in Table 3.2 and Table 3.3. The control group consists of 97 patients. The intraoperative CVC groups are with: low risk - 42; moderate risk - 206; high risk - 41. The postoperative CVC groups are: 1 with low risk; 201 with moderate risk; 40 with high risk (21 of them with, and 19 without cardiac death).

Further on, the procedure for optimum discriminator synthesis was applied on the already differentiated patient groups. Tables 3.4, 3.5, and 3.6 present the weighting discrimination coefficients of the corresponding groups, within the models that determine the appearance of the risk of: postoperative CVC, based on data from the preoperative period; postoperative CVC based on the pre- and intraoperative data period; intraoperative CVC based on data from the preoperative period. The lack of a weighting coefficient for a given index in some columns means that the step procedure of the discriminant analysis has rejected this index as non-contributing to the correct patient distribution in the corresponding groups.

Level of risk	**Type of complication**	**Number of patients**
Low	Short transient hypertension Supraventricular extrasystoles Ventricular extrasystoles	42
Moderate	Transient hypotension Unprovoced prolonged hypotension (> 1 hour) Prolonged hypertension (> 1 hour) Supraventricular arrhythmias (atrial fibrillation, supraventricular tachycardia) Increased heart rate (> 120 bpm) Sinus bradycardia ECG manifestations of myocardial ischemia Frequent ventricular extrasystoles	206
High	Hypotension during sudden heart failure Ventricular extrasystoles class IV Ventricular tachycardia Acute myocardial infarction Acute cardiogenic pulmonary edema Cardiac arrest	41

Table 3.2. Intraoperative cardiovascular complications

Level of risk	Type of complication	Number of patients
Low	Hypotension Supraventricular extrasystoles Ventricular extrasystoles	1
Moderate	Hypertension Supraventricular arrhythmias (atrial fibrillation, supraventricular tachycardia) Angina attack Increased heart rate (> 120 bpm) Sinus bradycardia Ventricular extrasystoles class III ECG manifestations of myocardial ischemia Compensated heart failure NYHA-FC I - II	201
High	Decompensated heart failure, high NYHA-FC Acute cardiogenic pulmonary edema Acute myocardial infarction Cardiac arrest	40

Table 3.3. Postoperative cardiovascular complications

Indicators	Discrimination				
	CVC with moderate risk vs. control group	CVC with high risk vs. control group	Cardiac death vs. control group	CVC with high risk vs. cardiac death	CVC with moderate risk vs. CVC with high risk
Age				8.0	
Arterial hypertension	10.5				
Ischemic heart disease	2.5	15.0		14.0	6.5
Myocardial infarction			18.5	55.5	
Arrhythmias		4.5			
Heart failure	12.0	17.5	57.0	3.5	
Chronic pulmonary disease	8.5				
Diabetes mellitus			3.0	2.0	4.5
Lung breathing, preoperative		10.0			
Lung auscultatory, preoperative					
Systolic blood pressure, preoperative			0.5		
Diastolic blood pressure, preoperative					
Central venous pressure, preoperative					19.5
Heart rate, preoperative	19.5	6.5	6.0		
Heart rhythm, preoperative					
Heart auscultatory, preoperative		1.0	4.0		3.0
Hemoglobin, preoperative	3.0	18.0	11.0		7.0
Glucose, preoperative	3.5				
Urea, preoperative					
Creatinine, preoperative				13.5	43.5
Potassium, preoperative					
Enzymes - SGOT, preoperative					
Enzymes - SGPT, preoperative					
X-ray lung, preoperative		27.5		3.5	16.0
Exercise ECG, preoperative					
Myocardial ischemia - preoperative	40.5				
Limit value for positive test:	**40**	**30**	**60**	**35**	**30**

Table 3.4. Quantitative models for postoperative CVC risk assessment according to preoperative data

Indicators	Discrimination				
	CVC with moderate risk vs. control group	CVC with high risk vs. control group	Cardiac death vs. control group	CVC with high risk vs. cardiac death	CVC with moderate risk vs. CVC with high risk
Age					
Surgical conditions					
Volume of surgery	1.0			8.0	
Duration of anesthesia			2.0		
Intraoperative surgery complications	0.5			5.0	
Intraoperative CVC with low risk	4.5	5.0	3.5		
Intraoperative CVC with moderate risk	81.0	69.0	41.0		
Intraoperative CVC with high risk	8.5	21.5	43.0	8.5	
Arterial hypertension, class	2.0				
Ischemic heart disease				3.5	5.5
Myocardial infarction				7.0	
Arrhythmias					
Heart failure				15.5	
Chronic pulmonary disease			1.5		
Diabetes mellitus				7.5	3.5
Lung breathing, preoperative					
Lung breathing, intraoperative					
Lung auscultatory, preoperative	1.5		1.5		
Lung auscultatory, intraoperative				6.5	
Systolic blood pressure, preoperative			0.5		
Diastolic blood pressure, preoperative	0.5				
Systolic blood pressure, intraoperative					
Diastolic blood pressure, preoperative					
Central venous pressure , preoperative				3.5	11.5
Central venous pressure, intraoperative				17.0	15.0
Heart rate, preoperative			1.0		
Heart rate, intraoperative				9.0	
Heart rhythm, preoperative					
Heart rhythm, intraoperative			5.0		
Heart auscultatory, preoperative					2.5
Hemoglobin					4.5
Glucose					
Urea					
Creatinine				3.5	30.0
Potassium					
Enzymes - SGOT					
Enzymes - SGPT					
X-ray lung				2.5	12.5
ECG LVH		0.5	0.5		
Myocardial ischemia - preoperative					
Limit value for positive test:	**20**	**20**	**55**	**65**	**25**

Table 3.5. Quantitative models for postoperative CVC risk assessment according to pre- and intraoperative data

Indicators	Discrimination				
	CVC with low risk vs. control group	CVC with moderat e risk vs. control group	CVC with high risk vs. control group	CVC with moderat e risk vs. CVC with low risk	CVC with high risk vs. CVC with moderate risk
Age	24.0	18.5	7.0	6.0	
Arterial hypertension	22.0	6.5	2.5	9.5	
Ischemic heart disease		5.5	3.0		
Myocardial infarction	11.0		8.0		20.5
Arrhythmias	42.0			19.5	
Heart failure		12.0	13.0		11.0
Chronic pulmonary disease		9.0		4.5	
Diabetes mellitus					
Lung breathing, preoperative		8.0	19.0		17.0
Lung auscultatory, preoperative			8.5		
Systolic blood pressure, preoperative					
Diastolic blood pressure, preoperative					7.5
Central venous pressure, preoperative					10.0
Heart rate, preoperative		23.5		15.5	
Heart rhythm, preoperative					
Heart auscultatory, preoperative					8.5
Hemoglobin, preoperative		2.5	20.5		25.5
Glucose, preoperative			6.0		
Urea, preoperative					
Creatinine, preoperative					
Potassium, preoperative					
Enzymes - SGOT, preoperative					
Enzymes - SGPT, preoperative					
X-ray lung, preoperative	1.0				
Exercise ECG, preoperative			2.0		
Myocardial ischemia - preoperative		12.5	14.5	45.0	
Limit value for positive test:	90	80	40	60	30

Table 3.6. Quantitative models for intraoperative CVC risk assessment according to preoperative data

Tables 3.7 and 3.8 show the results of correct and incorrect classification of patients, on the basis of the used training groups, ranged according to the CVC risk. The greater informative value of the combination of pre- and intreoperative data for prognosis of postoperative CVC becomes obvious, and the more distinct significance for prognosis of each higher-risk level of the post- and intraoperative CVC.

Cadiovascular complications	Data from period	Number of patients with complications	Number of patients without complications	True classified patients with complications (%)	False classified patients with complications (%)	True classified patients without complications (%)	False classified patients without complications (%)	Weighted average % of true classified patients
Postoperative with high risk	Preoperative	19	97	63,2	36,8	95,4	4,6	91,4
	Pre- and intraoperative	19	97	94,7	5,3	100	0	99,1
Postoperative with moderate risk	Preoperative	201	97	69,1	30,9	94,5	5,5	86,2
	Pre- and intraoperative	201	97	92	8	100	0	94,6
Postoperative with low risk	Preoperative	1	97					
	Pre- and intraoperative	1	97					
Intraoperative with high risk	Preoperative	41	97	65	35	97,9	2,1	88,3
Intraoperative with moderate risk	Preoperative	206	97	95,1	4,9	59,8	40,2	83,8
Intraoperative with low risk	Preoperative	42	97	66,7	32,3	92,8	7,2	84,9
Cardiac death	Preoperative	21	97	71,4	28,6	96,9	3,1	92,4
	Pre- and intraoperative	21	97	95,2	4,8	100	0	99,2

Table 3.7. Predictive value of models for evaluation of cardiovascular complications

Cadiovascular complications	Data from period	Number of patients with high risk	Number of patients with cardiac death	True classified patients with high risk (%)	False classified patients with high risk (%)	True classified patients with cardiac death (%)	False classified patients with cardiac death (%)	Weighted average % of true classified patients
Postoperative with high risk vs. cardiac death	Preoperative	19	21	89,5	10,5	95,2	4,8	92,5
	Pre- and intraoperative	19	21	100	0	100	0	100

Cadiovascular complications	Data from period	Number of patients with high risk	Number of patients with moderate risk	True classified patients with high risk (%)	False classified patients with high risk (%)	True classified patients with moderate risk (%)	False classified patients with moderate risk (%)	Weighted average % of true classified patients
Postoperative with high risk vs. moderate risk	Preoperative	19	206	52,6	47,4	96,5	3,5	89,5
	Pre- and intraoperative	19	206	52,6	47,4	96	4	92,3

Cadiovascular complications	Data from period	Number of patients with high risk	Number of patients with moderate risk	True classified patients with high risk (%)	False classified patients with high risk (%)	True classified patients with moderate risk (%)	False classified patients with moderate risk (%)	Weighted average % of true classified patients
Intraoperative with high risk vs. moderate risk	Preoperative	19	206	57,5	42,5	97,6	2,4	91,1

Cadiovascular complications	Data from period	Number of patients with moderate risk	Number of patients with low risk	True classified patients with moderate risk (%)	False classified patients with moderate risk (%)	True classified patients with low risk (%)	False classified patients with low risk (%)	Weighted average % of true classified patients
Intraoperative with moderate risk vs. low risk	Preoperative	206	42	97,6	2,4	42,3	57,7	88,2

Table 3.8. Predictive value of models for evaluation of cardiovascular complications (in patient groups with adjacent levels of cardiac risk)

Generally, the proposed models for risk assessment of acute CVC appearances, and of incidents with patients undergoing emergency noncardiac interventions, manifest not only high significance, but also point out:

- the importance of the intraoperative CVC (especially that with moderate risk) for prognosis of all risk level postoperative CVC, based on preoperative and intraoperative data;
- the obtained discrimination between the groups with cardiac death and high risk complications, which is impossible when directly using the ACC/AHA classification of intra- and postoperative CVC;
- certain decrease of the discrimination importance of the preoperatively ECG detected myocardial ischemia together with keeping its role in prognosticating the intraoperative CVC with moderate and high risk, which are among the factors that determine the rate and the severity of the postoperative CVC.

5. Cardiac risk reduction strategies

The topical risk assessment of perioperative cardiac incidents during noncardiac surgery, attracts the attention of the specialists, and is the reason for permanent updating of the practices leading to significant evaluation. It is sufficient to list the handbooks published by competent professional societies, including the ESC Guidelines, issued in 2009, on preoperative cardiac risk assessment and perioperative cardiac management in non-cardiac surgery [61, 62, 63]. *The final goal of these strategies for evaluating the cardiac risk and the optimization of heart management during noncardiac surgery, based on this evaluation, is the reduction of perioperative acute cardiac incidents.* The strategies can be summarized, without reiteration of the available algorithms, in following three directions.

5.1 Pharmacological strategy

Surgeries of patients with moderate and low FC and moderate CR can be performed by inclusion of statins and low dose beta-blockers. ACE inhibitors are recommended to be introduced before intervention on patients with LV dysfunction (EF less than 40%).

Continued use of **beta-blockers** is advised with patients having positive preoperative stress-tests. The latest cardioprotection concepts recommend the use of cardio-selective beta-1-blockers without internal simpatico-mimetic activity and long half-life time, e.g. bisopropol.

The **statins** induce coronary plaque stabilization. Multiple clinical investigations show the positive effect of the perioperative use of statins.

The **inhibition of ACE** may prevent myocardial ischemia and LV dysfunction, therefore the perioperative treatment with ACE inhibitors is expedient.

Aspirin is widely taken by patients with IHD, especially after intracoronary stent implantation. The apprehension of perioperative hemorrhaging complications often leads to suspension of the aspirin in the perioperative period. However, this is related to triplicate the risk of heavy cardiac incidents. The aspirin admission has to be interrupted only if the bleeding risk exceeds the cardiac benefit.

5.2 Noninvasive stress-tests

Patients with one or more cardiac risk factors are advised to be ECG monitored for changes in the postoperative period. Noninvasive testing is recommended for patients with 3 or

more risk factors. The last can be accomplished during each surgery, depending on the change in the perioperative strategy – the intervention type and the anesthetic technique.
Patients without stress-induced moderate or heavy ischemia (orienting towards single- or two-branch coronary disease) can continue with the planned intervention by inclusion of statins and low dose beta-blockers. Individual approach is recommended for patients with heavy stress-induced ischemia, after discussing the potential benefit of the advised surgery in comparison with the bad prognosis. It is necessary to specify the effect of the medicamentous therapy and/or coronary revascularization not only in the postoperative plan, but also in a long-term plan.

5.3 Revascularization

When a life-threatening state, requiring surgical intervention, is combined with ACS, it is advisable to give advantage to the surgery. However, a second stage necessities aggressive medicamentous therapy and revascularization, according to the NSTEMI and STEMI-ACS recommendations.
ACS without ST-elevations is interpreted as a high risk clinical state, requiring accurate diagnosis, risk stratification and revascularization. That means that if no life-threatening surgical state is present, advantage has to be given to the diagnosis and the appropriate treatment of the unstable angina. The corner-stones of the treatment are the double antiaggregating therapy, the beta-blocker and the revascularization.
The antiaggregation and the anticoagulations have to be carefully appreciated before applying to patients with unstable AP and forthcoming surgery state, in order to avoid the risk of subsequent enhanced bleeding. Most of the patients with unstable AP need interventional revascularization and advantage must be given to metal stents, in order not to delay the surgery more than three months.
The main goal of the prophylactic myocardial revascularization is the prevention of lethal perioperative MI. As far as the revascularization may be only partially effective in treatment of high risk stenosis, it cannot prevent the rupture of vulnerable plaque during the surgery stress. This one is found at least in the half of the perioperative MI cases, and can explain the lack of specificity in the stress-imaging methods for infarct-related coronary lesions discovery. Patients with previous PCI can be with higher risk during or after noncardiac surgery, especially in the cases of unplanned or emergency surgery that follow coronary stent setting. The intervention duration and the specificity of the process (malignant tumor, vascular aneurism, etc.) have to be adequately balanced against the risk of stent-provoked thrombosis during the first year after the implantation of drug emitting stent. Careful discussion is recommended in every individual case by a team, including a surgeon, an anesthesiologist and a cardiologist.
Despite the specific strategies for risk reduction, the perioperative CR assessment gives an opportunity for optimized control of all cardiovascular risk factors.

6. Index

7. References

[1] Wong CB, Porter TR. Cardiac management of patients undergoing major noncardiac surgery. Nebr Med J 1995; 80: 350-353.

[2] Eagle KA, Brundage BH, Chaitnam BR, *et al.* Guidelines for Perioperative Cardiovascular Evaluation for noncardiac surgery. Report of ACC/AHA Task Force on Practice Guidlines. Circulation 1996; 93: 1286–1317.

[3] Fleisher L, Pasternak L, Herbert R, Anderson G. Inpatient hospital admission and death after outpatient surgery in elderly patients: imoprtance of patient and system characteristics and location of care. Arch Surg 2004; 139:67-72.

[4] Milanova M, Matveev M. Cardiac risk evaluation in noncardiac surgical procedures. Journal of Emergency Medicine 1998; vol. 6, 2:27-32.

[5] Milanova M, Matveev M. Heart risk assessment indicators in emergency noncardiac surgery. I. Practicability in patients presenting periopertative cardiovascular accodents. Journal of Emergency Medicine 1999; 7(2):45-52.

[6] Milanova M, Matveev M. Heart risk assessment indicators in emergency noncardiac surgery. I. Practicability in patients free periopertative cardiovascular accodents. Journal of Emergency Medicine 2001; 9(2):60-63.

[7] Milanova M, Matveev M. Index for myocardial ischemia assessment as a risk factor of nonsurgical postoperative complications in emergency abdominal surgery. Journal of Emergency Medicine 1999; vol. 7, 4:43-49.

[8] Goldman L, Caldera D. Risks of general anasthesia and elective operative in the hypertensive patient. Anesthesiology 1979; 50: 285-293.

[9] Mangano DT, Browner WS, Hollenberg M *et al.* Association of perioperative myocardial ischemia with cardiac morbidity and mortality in men undergoing noncardiac surgery. New Engl J Med 1990; 323: 1781-1788.
[10] Foster ED, Davis KB, Carpenter JA *et al.* Risk of noncardiac operation in patients with defined coronary disease: The Coronary Artery Surgery Study (CASS) registry experience. Ann Thorac Surg 1986; 41: 42-50.
[11] Massie BM, Mangano DT. Risk stratification for noncardiac surgery. How (and why)? Circulation 1993; 87: 1752 -1755.
[12] Gerson MC. Cardiac risk evaluation and management in noncardiac surgery. Clin Chest Med 1993;14: 263-281.
[13] Kloner RA, Goldman L, Lee TH. Noncardiac surgery in the cardiac patient; Cardiovasc Rev Rep1992; 13: 24-47.
[14] Jollis J. Outcomes in heart failure patients after major noncardiac surgery. J Am Coll Cardiol 2004; 44:1446-53.
[15] Goldman L, D. Caldera, F. Southwick *et al.* Cardiac risk factors and complications in noncardiac surgery, Medicine 1978; 57: 357-370.
[16] Ashton CM, Petersen NJ, Wray NP *et al.* The incidence of perioperative myocardial infarction in men undergoing noncardiac surgery. Ann Intern Med 1993; 118: 504-510.
[17] Hollenberg M, Mangano DT, Browner WS. Predictors of postoperative myocardial ischemia in patients undergoing noncardiac surgery. The study of Perioperative Ischemia Reserch Group. JAMA 1992; 268 (2): 205-209.
[18] Joyce WP, Ameli FM, Mc Ewan P *et al.* Failure of bicycle exercise electrocardiogram to predict major post-operative cardiac complications in patients undergoing abdominal aortic surgery. Ir Med J 1990; 83: 65-66.
[19] Leppo JA. Preoperative cardiac risk assessment for noncardiac surgery. Am J Cardiol 1995; 75: 42D-51D.
[20] Goldman L, Caldera D, Hussbaum S *et al.* Multifactorial index of cardiac risk in noncardiac surgical procedures. N Engl J Med 1977; 297: 845-850.
[21] Amar D, Roistacher N, Burt M, Reinsel RA, Ginsberg-RJ, Wilson-RS. Clinical and echocardiographic correlates of symptomatic tachydysrhythmias after noncardiac thoracic surgery. Chest 1995; 108: 349-354.
[22] Eagle KA. Surgical patients with heart disease: summary of the ACC/AHA guidelines. American College of Cardiology/American Heart Association. Am Fam Physician 1997; 56(3): 811-818.
[23] Detsky AL, Abrams HB, Mc Laughlin JR *et al.* Predicting cardiac complications in patients undergoing noncardiac surery. J Gen Intern Md 1986; 1: 211-219.
[24] Lin M, Yang YF, Lin SL *et al.* Supraventricular tachiarrhythmias after noncardiac surgery. Acta Cardiol Sin 1994; 10: 128-136.
[25] Goldman L, Braunwald E. General anaesthesia and noncardiac surgery in patients with heart disease In: Braunwald E, ed. Heart disease, 4-th ed., Philadelphia: Sounders, 1992, 1708-1720.
[26] Prys Roberts C, Meloche R, Foex P. Studies of anesthesia in relation to hypertension. I. Cardiovascular responses of treated and untreated patients. J Anaesthesiol 1971; 43: 122-

[27] Larsen SF, Olesen KH, Jacobsen E et at. Prediction of cardiac risk in noncardiac surgery. Eur Heart J 1987; 8: 179-87.
[28] Fleisher LA, Barash PG. Preoperative cardiac evaluation for noncardiac surgery: a functional approach. Anesth Analg 1992, 74: 586-598.
[29] Khoja H, Gard D, Gupa M, *et al.* Evaluation of risk factors and outcome of Surgery in Elderly patients. Journal of the Indian Acad. of Geriatrics 2008; 1:14-17.
[30] Carliner NH, Fisher ML, Plotnik GD *et al.* The preoperative electrocardiogram as an indicator of risk in major noncardiac surgery. Can J Cardiol 1986; 2: 134-137.
[31] Cohen JR, Cooper B, Sardari F *et al.* Risk factors for myocardial infarction after distal arterial reconstructive procedures. Am Surg 1992; 58: 478-483.
[32] Kroenke K, Lawrence VA, Theroux JF *et al.* Operative risk in patients with severe obstructive pulmonary disease; Arch Intern Med 1992; 152/5: 967-971.
[33] Goldman L. Medical care of the surgical patient. JB Lippincott Co, Phyladelphia 1983: 41-47.
[34] Schouten O, Bax J, Poldermans D. Assessment of cardiac risk before non-cardiac general surgery. Heart 2006; 92:1866-72.
[35] Bunker JP, Wennberg RD. Operation rates, mortality statistic and the quality of life. N Engl J Med 1973; 289: 1249–1254.
[36] Eisenberg MJ, London MJ, Leung JM *et al.* Monitoring for myocardial ischemia during noncardiac surgery. A technology assessment of transesophageal echocardiography and 12-lead ECG. SPI Research Group. JAMA 1992; 268: 210-216.
[37] American College of Surgeons Committee on pre- and postoperative care: Manual of preoperative and postoperative care. ed 3, WB Saunders Co, Phyladelphia 1983: 87-111.
[38] Goldman L. Cardiac risk in noncardiac surgery: An Update. Anesth. Analg 1995; 80: 810 – 820.
[39] Lawrence VA, Hilsenbeck SC, Mulrow CD, Dhanda R, Sapp J, Page CP. Incidence and hospital stay for cardiac and pulmonary complications after abdominal surgery. J Gen Intern Med 1995; 10: 671-678.
[40] Hollenberg M, Mangano DT. Therapeutic approaches to postoperative ischemia. Am J Cardiol 1994; 73: 30B - 33B.
[41] Hopf HB, Tarnow J. Perioperative diagnosis of acute myocardial ischemia. Anaesthesist 1992; 41: 509-519
[42] Kleinman B. Assessment and preparation of a cardiac patient scheduled for noncardiac surgery: A cardiologist and anesthesiologist's viewpoint. Probl Crit Care 1991; 5: 493-512.
[43] Lette J, Colleti BW, Cerino M *et al.* Artificial intelligence versus logistic regression statistical modelling to predict cardiac complications after noncardiac surgery. Clin Cardiol 1994; 17: 609-614.
[44] Mangano DT. Dynamic predictors of perioperative risk. Study of Perioperative Ischemia (SPI) Research Group. J Card Surg 1990; 5 (3 Suppl): 231-236.
[45] Mangano DT, Browner WS, Hollenberg M *et al.* Long-term cardiac prognosis following noncardiac surgery. J Am Med Assoc 1992; 268: 233 – 239.
[46] Mangano DT. Perioperative cardiac morbidity. Can J Anaesth 1994; 41/5 II (R13 - R16).

[47] Eagle K, Coley C, Newell J *et al.* Combining clinical and thallium data optimizes preoperative assessment of cardiac risk before major vascular surgery. Ann Intern Med 1989; 110: 859-866.
[48] Lee T, Marcantonio D, Mangione C *et al.* Derivation and Prospective Validation of a Simple Index for Prediction of Cardiac Risk of Major Noncardiac Surgery. Circulation 1999; 100:1043-49.
[49] O'Kelly B, Browner WS, Massie B *et al.* Ventricular arrhythmias in patients undergoing noncardiac surgery. J Am Med Assoc 1992; 268: 217-221.
[50] Mangano DT, Hollenberg M, Fegert G *et al.* Perioperative myocardial ischemia in patients undergoing noncardiac surgery - I: Incidence and severity during the 4 day perioperative period. J Am Coll Cardiol 1991; 17: 843 - 850 .
[51] Greim CA, Roewer N, Schulte am Esch J. Assessment of changes in left ventricular wall stress from the end-systolic pressure-area product. Br J Anaesth 1995; 75: 583-587.
[52] Charlson ME, MacKenzie CR, Gold JP *et al.* The preoperative and intraoperative hemodynamic predictors of postoperative ischemia in patients undergoing noncardiac surgery. Ann Surg 1989; 210: 637-643.
[53] Eagle KA, Berger PB, Calkins H, Chaitman BR, Ewy GA, Fleischmann KE *et al.* ACC/AHA guideline update for perioperative cardiovascular evaluation for noncardiac surgery: executive summary: a report of the American College of Cardiology/ American Heart Association Task Force on practice guidelines (Committee to update the 1996 guidelines for perioperative cardiovascular evaluation for noncardiac surgery). Circulation 2002; 105: 1257-1267.
[54] Eagle KA, Rihal CS, Mickel MC, Holmes DR, Foster ED, Gersh BJ. Cardiac risk of noncardiac surgery: influence of coronary disease and type of surgery in 3368 operations. CASS Investigators and University of Michigan Heart Care Program. Coronary Artery Study. Circulation 1997; 96: 1882-1887.
[55] Goldman L. When the cardiac patient has noncardiac surgery. Prim Cardiol 1985; 11: 72-80.
[56] Abraham SA, Eagle KA. Preoperative cardiac risk assessment for noncardiac surgery. J Nucl Cardiol 1994; 1: 389-398.
[57] Mangano DT, London MJ, Hollenberg M *et al.* Predicting cardiac morbidity in surgical patients. Prim Cardiol 1992; 18: 27-36.
[58] Marsch SC, Schaefer HG, Skarvan K *et al.* Perioperative myocardial ischemia in patients undergoing elective hip arthroplasty during lumbar regional anesthesia. Anesthesiology 1992; 76: 518-527.
[59] Mangano DT. Characteristics of electrocardiographic ischemia in high-risk patients undergoing surgery SPI Research Group. J Electrocardiol 1990; 23 Suppl : 20-27.
[60] Dodds TM, Stone JG, Coromilas J *et al.* Prophylactic nitroglycerin infusion during noncardiac surgery does not reduce perioperative ischemia. Anesth Analg 1993; 76: 705-713.
[61] Bassand J, Hamm C, Ardissino D *et al.* Guidelines for the diagnosis and treatment of non-ST-segment elevation acute coronary syndromes. European Heart Journal 2007; 28(13): 1598-660.

[62] Van de Werf F, Bax J, Betriu A *et al.* Management of acute myocardial infarction in patients presenting with persistent ST-segment elevation: Task Force on the Management of ST-Segment Elevation Acute Myocardial Infarction of the European Society of Cardiology. European Heart Journal 2008; 29(23): 2909-45.
[63] ESC Guidelines on Perioperative Cardiac Risk Assessment and Perioperative Cardiac Management in Non-Cardiac Surgery. European Heart Journal 2009; 30: 2769-812.

11

Early Evaluation of Cardiac Chest Pain – Beyond History and Electrocardiograph

Ghulam Naroo and Aysha Nazir
Rashid Hospital, Dubai
United Arab Emirates

1. Overview

Acute Coronary Syndrome (ACS) represents a continuous spectrum of disease including Unstable Angina (UA), acute non-ST elevation myocardial infarction (NSTEMI), and acute ST elevation myocardial infarction (STEMI). In spite of major advances in prevention and treatment, Acute Coronary Syndrome remains a leading cause of death as well as a major cause of hospital admissions both within Europe and worldwide.[1-3]

Recent advances have allowed for early detection and disposition of patients with Acute Coronary Syndrome. The first step in the management of patients with ACS is prompt recognition. The diagnosis of ACS is largely based on the history, the electrocardiogram (ECG) and changes in cardiac biomarkers. It is a universally acknowledged fact that history remains the most essential tool in directing the need for further workup which includes serial ECGs and measurement of cardiac biomarkers.

2. Diagnostic challenges

The ECG is an important diagnostic and risk stratification tool. Most patients who have UA/NSTEMI have some ECG changes, although the ECG may be normal in 1% to 6% of patients who have NSTEMI and in approximately 4% of patients who have UA.[4]ST elevation myocardial infarction (STEMI) is diagnosed by the symptoms and the characteristic ST elevation on the ECG. The other two variants of ACS, non-ST elevation myocardial infarction and unstable angina are differentiated from each other by the presence of positive cardiac biomarker in the former and the treatment varies accordingly.[5-7]

Of the number of available markers and assays that detect myocardial necrosis, the cardiac troponins T and I and the creatinine kinase–MB (CK-MB) isoform are the most commonly used, with troponins gaining acceptance as the markers of choice in ACS. These have achieved an important role in diagnostic, prognostic, and treatment pathways by virtue of their high degree of sensitivity and specificity and their relative ease of use and interpretation. However, troponins are detectable only 6 hours after myocardial injury and are measurable for up to 2 weeks.

For a patient presenting with a suspected acute MI, the characteristics of the chest pain and the ECG findings permit initial risk stratification. The gold standard in the care of a patient with cardiac chest pain is that an ECG and an abbreviated history and physical examination be obtained within 10 minutes of patient arrival.[8]

The early diagnosis of acute myocardial infarction (AMI) is however sometimes difficult due to: [9]

1. Equivocal electrocardiogram (ECG) changes and other conditions with ECG changes that mimic acute myocardial infarction. Atypical chest pains with many differentials confuse to make a diagnosis.
2. Acute myocardial infarction patients without ST-segment elevation.
3. Delayed liberation and detection of cardiac markers of myocardial necrosis such as troponin and creatine kinase (CK).

Cardiac troponin is frequently not detected until after 4-6 hours and in many cases, repeated measurement is needed 8-12 hours after admission. The importance of early risk stratification in the management of acute myocardial infarction is emphasized in the American Heart Association task force guidelines.[10]Risk stratification is an important objective in the evaluation of patients with ACS. The presence of positive biomarkers indicates higher risk and worse prognosis.[11]

When initiating reperfusion therapy, door-to-needle time of less than or equal to 30 minutes for initiation of fibrinolytic therapy and a door-to-balloon time of less than or equal to 90 minutes for percutaneous coronary perfusion is the standard of care.[12-14]Although, more and more hospitals are meeting this benchmark, diagnosing and excluding ACS often poses a diagnostic challenge to the clinicians.[15]A misdiagnosis may lead to considerable increase in morbidity and mortality. An ideal marker which can predict the onset of the disease, could aid in reducing the deaths due to ACS.

3. Cardiac biomarkers

Acute myocardial infarction refers to irreversible myocardial necrosis caused by an imbalance between oxygen supply and demand. In 75% cases, plaque rupture or erosion leading to thrombus formation are the causes of acute coronary syndromes. Early diagnosis and subsequent reperfusion therapies within 4 to 6 hours of onset of symptoms can salvage myocardium at risk. Therefore, optimal markers of myocardial necrosis need to be rapidly detectable in blood.

Myocardial injury causes release into the extracellular space of intracellular constituents including detectable levels of a variety of biologically active cytosolic and structural proteins such as troponin, creatine kinase, myoglobin, lactate dehydrogenase, etc.

Cardiac biomarkers have characteristic release and clearance kinetics. However, the time to presentation and comorbidities that affect clearance may confound the interpretation of biomarkers. Myoglobin is the earliest biochemical marker of myocardial cell damage, and it is detectable in blood within 1 to 2 hours of myocyte damage. Blood levels of CK-MB may be detectable in blood after 4 to 6 hours of myocardial ischemia. [16] Cardiac troponins are elevated within 4 to 12 hours of symptom onset and remain elevated for 4 to 10 days. [17]

Based on these patterns of release and clearance, a diagnostic algorithm of serial biomarker measurements has been developed. Serial sampling of multiple cardiac markers beginning at the time of presentation is recommended currently. The sensitivity of serial measurements of multiple markers nears 100%, whereas the sensitivity of a single measurement of any biomarker at the time of presentation is poor. The recommended time between the first and second blood draw is 6 to 7 hours. [18] If cardiac marker levels are not elevated but clinical suspicion remains high, a third set of markers should be drawn at 12 to 24 hours after presentation. [19] The markers currently used in this multimarker approach are myoglobin, CKMB, and troponin.

3.1 Myoglobin

Myoglobin is a heme protein found in the cytoplasm of cardiac and skeletal muscle cells that rises most rapidly after myocardial injury but is not cardiac-specific. [16] Myoglobin levels are frequently elevated in patients who have renal failure, skeletal muscle injury, trauma, and other diseases. Myoglobin is not used in most hospital laboratories.

3.2 Creatine kinase-MB isoform

CK-MB is an enzyme present primarily in cardiac muscle and active in energy generation. CK-MB is released rapidly after myocardial injury and is more cardiac-specific than myoglobin. However, CK-MB also comprises up to 5% of skeletal muscle and can be elevated in noncardiac disease states. Before the use of troponin, CK-MB was the gold standard for the biochemical diagnosis of AMI. CK-MB is released early during AMI, and it plays an important role in defining infarct size, infarct expansion, and reinfarction.[20]

3.3 Cardiac troponins

Cardiac troponins and tropomyosin form the thin filament component of the contractile structure in striated muscle. Troponins are released into the blood stream following irreversible ischemic myocardial cell injury and remain elevated for a prolonged time. There is no clinical difference between TnT and TnI for diagnosing cardiac necrosis. There are separate cardiac and skeletal isoforms of both TnI and TnT, allowing for the development of highly cardiac-specific assays. [17, 21] Troponin assays can detect as little as 1 g of myocardial tissue necrosis, and even minute elevations in cardiac troponins have been associated with myocardial necrosis and increased rate of short- and long-term mortality. [19,22-24]

Cardiac troponins have been studied in symptomatic and asymptomatic patients who have renal dysfunction. It is important that emergency physicians include the patient's history and physical examination when considering an elevated troponin level in patients who have renal dysfunction. In patients in whom acute coronary syndrome is not suspected, renal failure may be associated with chronic elevations of TnI and TnT, without evidence of acute myocardial necrosis. However, an acute increase from baseline troponin levels may be associated with increased mortality[25, 26]

Therefore, baseline troponin levels are helpful when differentiating between acute and chronic elevations in cardiac troponins. Elevated levels of cardiac troponins in patients who have renal dysfunction may be attributable to decreased renal clearance and increased release from cytoplasm because of the loss of membrane integrity. TnT is of higher molecular weight and is more commonly present in the free, unbound form in the cytoplasm, potentially explaining why TnT is more frequently elevated than TnI. [25] A study of asymptomatic patients who had renal failure did not show TnI levels to be elevated in this population. The previously noted false-positive TnI results in patients who have renal failure were measured during acute disease states, including sepsis or pulmonary embolism, which may independently cause elevated troponin levels. [27]

In symptomatic patients who have chest pain and renal dysfunction, elevated levels of cardiac troponin predict patients at an increased risk for adverse cardiovascular outcomes. In a study of 7033 patients who had suspected acute coronary syndromes, the elevated levels of TnT were predictive of death or myocardial infarction across the spectrum of creatinine clearance. [28]

Despite the value of cardiac troponin as a very sensitive marker for myocardial damage, elevated troponin levels do not reflect the mechanism of damage and should not be used alone to diagnose myocardial infarction. Troponin levels may be elevated in patients who have myocarditis, pericarditis, decompensated heart failure, and septic shock. The use of troponin measurements as a screening tool in patients whose conditions have a low suspicion for ACS lowers the sensitivity and positive predictive value to 47% and 19%, respectively. A high sensitive troponin could be available in future to turn out an ideal biomarker for ACS. [29]

4. Heart-type fatty acid-binding protein

Heart-type fatty acid-binding protein (h-FABP) has been researched since 1988, due to its high potential as an early marker for myocardial infarction. It bears considerable resemblance to myoglobin in terms of size, location within the cell, release and clearance kinetics. It is a relatively low molecular mass cytoplasmic protein (15 kDa) available in abundance in myocardial tissue. [30-32]It is important for myocardial homeostasis since 50 – 80% of the heart's energy is provided by lipid oxidation and h-FABP ensures intracellular transport of insoluble fatty acids. It is released from the heart during cell necrosis, it diffuses much more rapidly than troponins through the interstitial space and appears in the circulation as early as 90 minutes after the onset of symptoms, reaching its peak within 6 hours and clearing within 24 hours.

This combination of early h-FABP release after symptom onset, rapid kidney clearance from the circulation and high cardiac specificity suggests great potential for its clinical use.[30-32]Therefore,it can be derived that h-FABP may not only be of value in detecting myocardial injury in the early hours of the insult but may also be ideal for the diagnosis of reinfarctions. H-FABP has been found to be superior to troponins due to its higher sensitivity.[33, 34]A recent study showed h-FABP had a sensitivity of 75.76% and a specificity of 96.97% compared with 58.59% and 98.94% for cTnT and 68.69% and 97.54% for CK-MB in the initial 6 hours after the onset of chest pain. [35]Recent data also suggests h-FABP may provide some prognostic information which appears superior to that of troponins. [36].

4.1 h-FABP in the pre-hospital setting

There is some evidence to suggest the utility of h-FABP in the pre-hospital setting.[37]According to the literature, early assessment of H-FABP in patients presenting with chest pain improves the diagnosis of an ongoing myocardial infarction. An h-FABP self-testing kit can be helpful in the pre-hospital setting. Though an h-FABP testing kit (h-

FABP Quanta) is used for the quantitative measurement, especially in next one hour of the initial testing to see if there is a rise of titre. This kit is more useful in emergency department/CCU and ICU setting. ConformitéEuropéenne (CE) certification approving it for sale in the European Union member countries.

5. References

[1] World Health Organization Department of Health Statistics and Informatics in the Information, Evidence and Research Cluster (2004).The global burden of disease 2004 update. Geneva: WHO. ISBN 9241563710.

[2] Thom T, Haase N, Rosamond W, et al. Heart disease and stroke statistics - 2006 update: a report from the American Heart Association Statistics Committee and Stroke Statistics Subcommittee. Circulation.2006; 113:85-151.

[3] World Health Organization. Estimated deaths per 100,000 population by cause and Member State. http://www.oint/research/en (14 November 2008)

[4] Slater DK, Hlatky MA, Mark DB, et al. Outcome in suspected acute myocardial infarction with normal or minimally abnormal admission electrocardiographic findings. Am J Cardiol 1987;60:766–70.

[5] Alpert JS, Thygesen K, Antman E, Bassand JP. Myocardial infarction redefined-a consensus document of the Joint European Society of Cardiology/American College of Cardiology Committee for the redefinition of myocardial infarction. J Am CollCardiol 2000;36 (3):959-69.

[6] Antman EM, Anbe DT, Armstrong PW, Bates ER, Green LA, Hand M, et al. ACC/AHA guidelines for the management of patients with ST-elevation myocardial infarction-executive summary. A report of the American College of Cardiology/American Heart Association Task Force on Practice Guidelines (Writing Committee to revise the 1999 guidelines for the management of patients with acute myocardial infarction). J Am CollCardiol 2004;44 (3):671-719.

[7] Braunwald E, Antman EM, Beasley JW, Califf RM, Cheitlin MD, Hochman JS, et al. ACC/AHA guideline update for the management of patients with unstable angina and non-ST-segment elevation myocardial infarction-2002: summary article: a report of the American College of Cardiology/American Heart Association Task Force on Practice Guidelines (Committee on the Management of Patients With Unstable Angina). Circulation 2002;106(14):1893-900.

[8] Antman EM, Anbe DT, Armstrong PW, et al. ACC/AHA guidelines for the management of patients with ST-elevation myocardial infarction: a report of the American College of Cardiology/American Heart Association Task Force on Practice Guidelines (Committee to Revise the 1999 Guidelines for the Management of Patients with Acute Myocardial Infarction). Circulation 2004; 110:e82.

[9] Okamoto F, Sohmiya K, Ohkaru Y, Kawamura K, Asayama K, Kimura H, et al. Human heart-type cytoplasmic fatty acid-binding protein (H-FABP) for the diagnosis of acute myocardial infarction. Clinical evaluation of H-FABP in

comparison with myoglobin and creatine kinase isoenzyme MB.ClinChem Lab Med 2000;38(3):231-8.

[10] Ryan TJ, Antman EM, Brooks NH, Califf RM, Hillis LD, Hiratzka LF, et al. 1999 update: ACC/AHA guidelines for the management of patients with acute myocardial infarction: executive summary and recommendations: a report of the American College of Cardiology/American Heart Association Task Force on Practice Guidelines (Committee on Management of Acute Myocardial Infarction). Circulation 1999;100(9):1016-30.

[11] Antman EM, Tanasijevic MJ, Thompson B, Schactman M, McCabe CH, Cannon CP, et al. Cardiac-specific troponin I levels to predict the risk of mortality in patients with acute coronary syndrome. N Engl J Med 1996;335(18):1342-9.

[12] Antman EM, Hand M, Armstrong PW, et al: 2007 focused update of the ACC/AHA 2004 guidelines for the management of patients with ST-elevation myocardial infarction: A report of the American College of Cardiology/American Heart Association Task Force on Practice Guidelines: Developed in collaboration With the Canadian Cardiovascular Society: Endorsed by the American Academy of Family Physicians: 2007 Writing Group to Review New Evidence and Update the ACC/AHA 2004 Guidelines for the Management of Patients With ST-Elevation Myocardial Infarction, Writing on Behalf of the 2004 Writing Committee. Circulation 2008; 117:296.

[13] Bradley EH, Herrin J, Wang Y, et al: Strategies for reducing the door-to-balloon time in acute myocardial infarction. N Engl J Med 2006; 355:2308.

[14] Wang OJ, Wang Y, Lichtman JH, et al: "America's Best Hospitals" in the treatment of acute myocardial infarction. Arch Intern Med 2007; 167:1345.

[15] Bruins Slot MHE, van der Heijden GJMG, Rutten FH, van der Spoel OP, Gijs Mast E, BrederoAdC, Doevendans PA, Glatz JFC, Hoes AW. Heart-type fatty acid-binding protein in acute myocardial infarction evaluation (FAME): background and design of a diagnostic study in primary care. BMC CardiovascDisord 2008;8:8.

[16] Azzazy HM, Christenson RH. Cardiac markers of acute coronary syndromes: is there a case for point-of-care testing? ClinBiochem 2002;35:13–27.

[17] Newby LK. Markers of cardiac ischemia, injury, and inflammation.ProgCardiovasc Dis 2004;46:404–16.

[18] Balk EM, Ioannidis JP, Salem D, et al. Accuracy of biomarkers to diagnose acute cardiac ischemia in the emergency department: a meta-analysis. Ann Emerg Med 2001;37:478–94.

[19] Alpert JS, Thygesen K, Antman E, et al. Myocardial infarction redefined: a consensus document of The Joint European Society of Cardiology/American College of Cardiology Committee for the redefinition of myocardial infarction. J Am CollCardiol 2000;36:959–69.

[20] Panteghini M. Acute coronary syndrome: biochemical strategies in the troponin era. Chest 2002;122:1428–35

[21] Roongsritong C, Warraich I, Bradley C. Common causes of troponin elevations in the absence of acute myocardial infarction: incidence and clinical significance. Chest 2004;125:1877–84

[22] Cantwell RV, Aviles RJ, Bjornsson J, et al. Cardiac amyloidosis presenting with elevations of cardiac troponin I and angina pectoris. ClinCardiol 2002;25:33–7.

[23] Aviles RJ, Wright RS, Aviles JM, et al. Long-term prognosis of patients with clinical unstable angina pectoris without elevation of creatine kinase but with elevation of cardiac troponin i levels. Am J Cardiol 2002;90:875–8.

[24] Antman EM, Tanasijevic MJ, Thompson B, et al. Cardiac-specific troponin I levels to predict the risk of mortality in patients with acute coronary syndromes. N Engl J Med 1996;335:1342–9

[25] Hamm CW, Giannitsis E, Katus HA. Cardiac troponin elevations in patients without acute coronary syndrome. Circulation 2002;106:2871–2

[26] Apple FS, Murakami MM, Pearce LA, et al. Predictive value of cardiac troponin I and T for subsequent death in end-stage renal disease. Circulation 2002;106:2941–5

[27] Donnino MW, Karriem-Norwood V, Rivers EP, et al. Prevalence of elevated troponin I in end-stage renal disease patients receiving hemodialysis. AcadEmerg Med 2004;11:979–81.

[28] Aviles RJ, Askari AT, Lindahl B, et al. Troponin T levels in patients with acute coronary syndromes, with or without renal dysfunction. N Engl J Med 2002;346:2047–52

[29] Polanczyk CA, Lee TH, Cook EF, et al. Cardiac troponin I as a predictor of major cardiac events in emergency department patients with acute chest pain. J Am CollCardiol 1998;32:8–14.

[30] Kleine AH, Glatz JF, Van Nieuwenhoven FA, Van der Vusse GJ. Release of heart fatty acid-binding protein into plasma after acute myocardial infarction in man.Mol Cell Biochem 1992;116(1-2):155-62.

[31] Chan CP, Sum KW, Cheung KY, Glatz JF, Sanderson JE, Hempel A, et al. Development of a quantitative lateral-flow assay for rapid detection of fatty acidbinding protein. J Immunol Methods 2003;279(1-2):91-100.

[32] Nakata T, Hashimoto A, Hase M, Tsuchihashi K, Shimamoto K. Human heart-type fatty acid-binding protein as an early diagnostic and prognostic marker in acute coronary syndrome. Cardiology 2003;99(2):96-104.

[33] Pelsers MM, Hermens WT, Glatz JF. Fatty acid-binding proteins as plasma markers of tissue injury.ClinChimActa 2005;352(1-2):15-35.

[34] Ishii J, Wang JH, Naruse H, Taga S, Kinoshita M, Kurokawa H, et al. Serum concentrations of myoglobin vs human heart-type cytoplasmic fatty acid-binding protein in early detection of acute myocardial infarction. ClinChem 1997;43(8 Pt 1):1372-8.

[35] Naroo GY, Ali SM, Butros V et al. Elevated heart-type fatty acid-binding protein predicts early myocardial injury and aids in the diagnosis of non-ST elevation myocardial infarction. Hong Kong Journal of Emergency Medicine 2009;16(3):141-147.

[36] Azzazy HME, Pelsers MMAL, Christenson RH. Unbound free fatty acids and heart type binding protein: diagnostic assays and clinical applications. ClinChem 2006;52(1):19–29.

[37] Ecollan P, Collet JP, Boon G,Tanguy ML, Fievet ML, Haas R, Bertho N, Siami S, Hubert JC, Coriat P, Montalescot G. Pre-hospital detection of acute myocardial infarction with ultra-rapid human fatty acid-binding protein (H-FABP) immunoassay. Int J Cardiol. 2007 Jul 31;119(3):349-54. Epub 2006 Nov 13.

12

Coronary Bypass Grafting in Acute Coronary Syndrome: Operative Approaches and Secondary Prevention

Stephen J. Huddleston[1] and Gregory Trachiotis[2]
[1]*The Johns Hopkins Hospital,*
[2]*George Washington University and Veterans Affairs Medical Center*
United States of America

1. Introduction

Many patients who present with acute coronary syndrome (ACS) are candidates for coronary artery bypass grafting (CABG). Approximately 500,000 CABG operations are performed each year in the United States, and many of these patients present with acute coronary syndrome. In the Bypass Angioplasty Revascularization Investigation (BARI) trial comparing CABG and percutaneous coronary intervention for coronary artery disease, 64% of the patients presented with unstable angina (Rosamond, Flegal et al. 2008). According to 2007 ACC/AHA guidelines (Anderson, Adams et al. 2007), left main stenosis greater than 50% and three-vessel coronary artery disease represent a class I indication for coronary artery bypass grafting in patients with unstable angina or non-ST elevation myocardial infarction. In addition, patients with 2-vessel coronary artery disease and either diabetes or left ventricular dysfunction may benefit from coronary artery bypass grafting (Class II recommendation). Regardless of the modality of revascularization, patients with acute coronary syndrome benefit from antagonists of platelet activity such as aspirin and clopidogrel since these agents reduce the risk of major adverse events. However, antiplatelet agents also increase the risk of bleeding in patients who will ultimately proceed to coronary artery bypass graft surgery. Usually the benefits of early initiation of antiplatelet therapy outweigh the risks. The purpose of this review is to summarize current antiplatelet therapy in acute coronary syndrome, with particular emphasis on patients who will undergo coronary artery bypass, and the appropriate operative strategies will be discussed. We will also review the current recommendations for secondary prevention after coronary artery bypass grafting.

2. Antiplatelet therapy

Platelet activation and aggregation play a critical role in the pathogenesis of coronary thrombosis, and antiplatelet therapy has become a central tenet of the treatment strategy in acute coronary syndrome. Platelet aggregation and activation can be inhibited pharmacologically at several points in the cascade leading up to platelet aggregation, and several of these antiplatelet agents are commonly used perioperatively in the setting of acute coronary syndrome. Aspirin inhibits the formation of thromboxane A2 thereby preventing glycoprotein (Gp) IIb/IIIa-mediated activation of platelets. Ticlodipine and clopidogrel inhibit ADP release from platelets and thereby prevent Gp IIb/IIIa activation, and eptifibatide blocks GpII B/IIIa-mediated platelet aggregation. The pharmacokinetics of platelet inhibition and inactivation by each type of agent is of particular importance regarding the timing of CABG because of the bleeding risk associated with antiplatelet therapy. However, the timing of CABG in the setting of ACS is often flexible, with perhaps less than 1% of patients with ACS requiring emergent CABG (Serebruany, Malinin et al. 2004), so much of the bleeding risk associated with antiplatelet therapy can often be mitigated by waiting several days before CABG is performed.

Regardless of whether patients with ACS undergo percutaneous coronary intervention or CABG, the overwhelming body of evidence supports the use of antiplatelet therapy in ACS. In one large meta-analysis of studies of patients with ACS (Seshadri, Whitlow et al. 2002), the risk of serious vascular events including non-fatal myocardial infarction or stroke was reduced by 25%. Although aspirin was associated with a significantly reduced risk of major vascular events, the adenosine diphosphate (ADP)-receptor antagonists ticlodipine and clopidogrel were associated with an additional 10-12% risk reduction. In a direct comparison of aspirin and clopidogrel in the randomized Clopidogrel versus Aspirin in Patients at Risk for Ischemic Events (CAPRIE) trial, clopidogrel was associated with an 8.7% relative reduction of risk of ischemic stroke, myocardial infarction, or vascular death compared with aspirin, with no signicant difference in the safety profiles of the two drugs (1996). Furthermore, the beneficial effects of aspirin and clopidogrel in ACS are additive. In the Clopidogrel in Unstable angina to prevent Recurrent Events (CURE) trial, unstable angina and non-ST elevation myocardial infarction (NSTEMI), patients taking both clopidogrel and aspirin had less chance of cardiac death, non-fatal MI, or stroke at 30 days and 1 year compared to those only taking aspirin (Yusuf, Zhao et al. 2001). Taken together, these studies all confirm that antiplatelet therapy with both aspirin and clopidogrel should be intitiated early in ACS.

In patients with ST-elevation myocardial infarction (STEMI), clopidogrel in addition to aspirin improves outcomes. In the Clopidogrel and Metoprolol in Myocardial Infarction (COMMIT) trial, clopidogrel in addition to aspirin was associated with a significant decrease in the composite endpoint of death, reinfarction, or stroke compared to aspirin alone (Sabatine, Cannon et al. 2005). The Clopidogrel as Adjunctive Reperfusion Therapy-Thrombolysis In Myocardial Infarction (CLARITY-TIMI) compared aspirin alone to clopidogrel in addition to aspirin in patients with STEMI and demonstrated a 36% reduction in relative risk of the early composite endpoint of occlusion of the infarct-related artery, recurrent MI, or death, and there was a 20% relative risk reduction of the late composite endpoint of death from cardiovascular cause, recurrent MI, or recurrent ischemia leading to urgent revascularization (Sabatine, Cannon et al. 2005). Importantly, there was no increase in bleeding complications in either the COMMIT or the CLARITY-TIMI trial. Based on such compelling findings, the current AHA/ACC guidelines for patients with ACS recommend that aspirin and clopidogrel be given as soon as possible (Anderson, Adams et al. 2007). The typical loading dose for clopidogrel is 300mg or 600mg. Usually for patients undergoing stent placement, 600mg of clopidogrel is given, while patients who are found to be candidates for CABG are given 300mg of clopidogrel.

New ADP-receptor antagonist antiplatelet agents include prasugrel and ticagrelor. Both decrease the relative risk of ischemic events when used with aspirin (Ebrahimi, Dyke et al.

2009; Wallentin, Becker et al. 2009). However, prasugrel is associated with increased risk of bleeding complications, especially related to CABG. In contrast, ticagrelor was not associated with increased risk of bleeding related to CABG.
Several clinical trials have examined the outcomes of patients with ACS who were treated with antiplatelet therapy before undergoing CABG. In the CURE trial, patients who proceeded to CABG after receiving clopidogrel as opposed to placebo had a decreased relative risk of the composite endpoint of death, MI or stroke prior to CABG (RR 0.56 95% CI 0.29-1.08, absolute risk reduction 1.8%). As long as clopidogrel was stopped 5 days prior to CABG there was no increase in risk of life-threatening bleeding. The CLARITY-TIMI trial and the ACUITY (Acute Catheterization and Urgent Intervention Triage strategy) trials demonstrated similar improved outcomes without increased risk of bleeding in patients who underwent CABG after being treated with clopidogrel (Ferraris, Ferraris et al. 2005).

3. Coronary artery bypass grafting and acute coronary syndrome

Using antiplatelet agents in patients with ACS raises the risk of bleeding in those patients that undergo CABG, however several factors including the pharmacokinetic profile, individual patient sensitivity to the agent, and timing of the surgery determine the exact risk posed. Clinical trials are often difficult to compare because of varying classification of bleeding complications leading to differing conclusions. The Aspirin Guideline Taskforce of the Society of Thoracic Surgeons reviewed 21 studies examining the effect of preoperative aspirin on bleeding after CABG (Ebrahimi, Dyke et al. 2009). The dose of aspirin varied significantly between studies, so comparison of the findings is difficult. However, there appears to be a small increase in chest tube drainage and blood loss and a small increase in need for blood transfusion associated with preoperative aspirin, all of which may be dose related. Nonetheless, the mortality benefit of aspirin preoperatively in ACS outweighs the small risk of bleeding, leading to a class IIa recommendation to continue aspirin for urgent/emergent CABG patients. Some studies have shown an increased risk of perioperative bleeding in patients treated with both aspirin and ADP receptor antagonists such as clopidogrel who proceed to CABG (Yende and Wunderink 2001; Hongo, Ley et al. 2002; Genoni, Tavakoli et al. 2003). Therefore, clopidogrel should be stopped for 5-7 days before CABG when possible (ACC/AHA class I recommendation).
Because of the increased risk of bleeding after CABG in patients on dual antiplatelet therapy, one strategy would be to wait until coronary anatomy is defined on coronary angiography. However, this would delay antiplatelet therapy for all patients with a decrement in the benefit for all patients, most of whom do not end up undergoing CABG. The number of patients with ACS who proceed to CABG is probably between 7-14% (Bhatt, Roe et al. 2004; Fox, Anderson et al. 2007), and salvage CABG after failed percutaneous coronary intervention is relatively uncommon. The risk of bleeding after CABG, as well as the risk of reoperation for bleeding, overall is fairly low. Thus, the vast majority of patients will benefit from starting dual antiplatelet therapy early in ACS, and many patients would be harmed by delaying therapy.

4. Operative strategies

Usually CABG can be delayed in ACS to allow ADP-receptor blockers to be metabolized and excreted allowing platelet function to recover. If anticoagulation is critical, as is usually the case in ACS, short acting anticoagulants such as unfractionated heparin and Gp IIb/IIIa inhibitors can be used up until shortly before going to the operative room. Patients with ACS who have ongoing ischemia or are hemodynamically unstable and have received ADP-receptor antagonists may benefit from bridge percutaneous coronary intervention or intra-aortic balloon pump insertion. An algorithm for the management of patients with ACS that undergo CABG is presented in Figure 1.

Figure 1

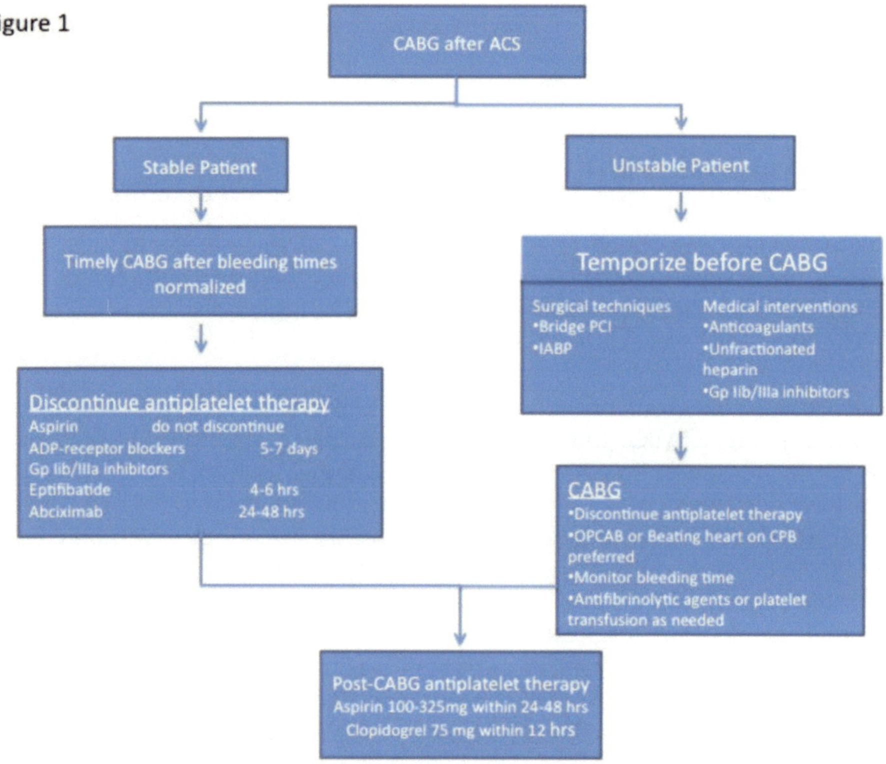

Fig. 1. Algorithm or the management of patients with ACS and indications for CABG.

Patients with ACS who are stable are observed while ADP receptor blockers are held for 5 days prior to surgery to eliminate the increased risk of bleeding and mortality (Ferraris, Ferraris et al. 2005; Ebrahimi, Dyke et al. 2009). Aspirin is continued up to the time of surgery. If there is particular concern about the grade of coronary stenosis or evidence of ongoing ischemia, the patient may be continued on unfractionated heparin and/or Gp IIb/IIIa inhibitors up until the time of surgery. The bleeding time or platelet function time can be used to assess platelet function and the bleeding risk preoperatively. This may be useful in assessing bleeding risk and planning for CABG. The dose of clopidogrel may be proportional to the risk of bleeding after CABG. In patients who receive the 600 mg loading dose of clopidogrel, CABG should be delayed 5-7 days for the platelet function to recover. However, in patients who received the lower 300 mg loading dose and are maintained on 75 mg per day of clopidogrel, CABG may be safely performed after holding clopidogrel for 1-3 days. A logical strategy is to administer 300mg of clopidogrel in addition to aspirin at the time of presentation in patients with ACS. When coronary angiography is performed, an additional 300mg of clopidogrel may be given if percutaneous coronary intervention is performed, while in those that will undergo CABG, no additional clopidogrel is given and low dose aspirin is continued.

In patients with ACS and high grade left main coronary artery stenosis or left main equivalent who have received high dose clopidogrel or thrombolytics, insertion of an intra-aortic balloon pump (IABP) will improve coronary perfusion and decrease cardiac demand by afterload reduction. Preoperative IABP insertion in these situations provides hemodynamic stability and reduces hospital mortality (Wiviott, Braunwald et al. 2007).

CABG may be performed on cardiopulmonary bypass with cardioplegic arrest or off-pump (OPCAB). The advantages and disadvantages of OPCAB have been studied and reviewed extensively, yet remain controversial (Moore, Pfister et al. 2005). OPCAB avoids full heparinization and the systemic inflammatory response syndrome associated with cardiopulmonary bypass. Early studies suggested that off-pump CABG is associated with fewer adverse cardiovascular events and reduced early postoperative morbidity and mortality (Rastan, Eckenstein et al. 2006; Magee, Alexander et al. 2008). However, more recent data demonstrate a slightly higher rate of incomplete revascularization and a greater need for subsequent revascularization, as well as slightly reduced long-term mortality (Puskas, Kilgo et al. 2008). However, much of the outcome after OPCAB may be surgeon and center dependent, and this should be taken into account when formulating operative plans for patients with ACS undergoing CABG.

5. Secondary prevention

CABG for patients with ACS reduces angina, reduces the risk of myocardial infarction, and improves long-term survival, particularly when the internal thoracic artery is grafted to the left anterior descending artery (Anderson, Adams et al. 2007). However, secondary prevention strategies are critical for the long-term benefit of revascularization to be realized. Lifestyle modification such as diet modification, an exercise regimen, and smoking cessation are necessary. Pharmacologic secondary prevention consisting of lipid-lowering agents, antihypertensives (primarily with beta blockers), and antiplatelet medications is also required to decrease the risk of progression of coronary artery disease and graft occlusion. A strategy for antiplatelet therapy after CABG in patients with ACS is presented in Figure 2. All patients should be continued on aspirin postoperatively to reduce the risk of vein graft occlusion (ACC/AHA class I recommendation). This also protects against the risk of future cardiovascular, cerebrovascular, and peripheral vascular ischemic events. In patients with ACS who have undergone coronary artery stent placement, clopidogrel is required in addition to aspirin to reduce major cardiac events (Muller, Buttner et al. 2000). In the CURE trial, patients with ACS treated with clopidogrel in addition to aspirin had decreased cardiac events, stroke and hospitalizations at 1 year regardless of whether they underwent PCI or CABG (Yusuf, Zhao et al. 2001). Therefore, in our practice, patients with ACS who undergo on-pump CABG or OPCAB are treated with 600mg aspirin suppository upon postoperative admission to the intensive care unit. When they are extubated, clopidogrel 75mg daily is administered, in addition to aspirin 81mg daily. Dual antiplatelet therapy is continued in all patients with ACS for 9-12 months.

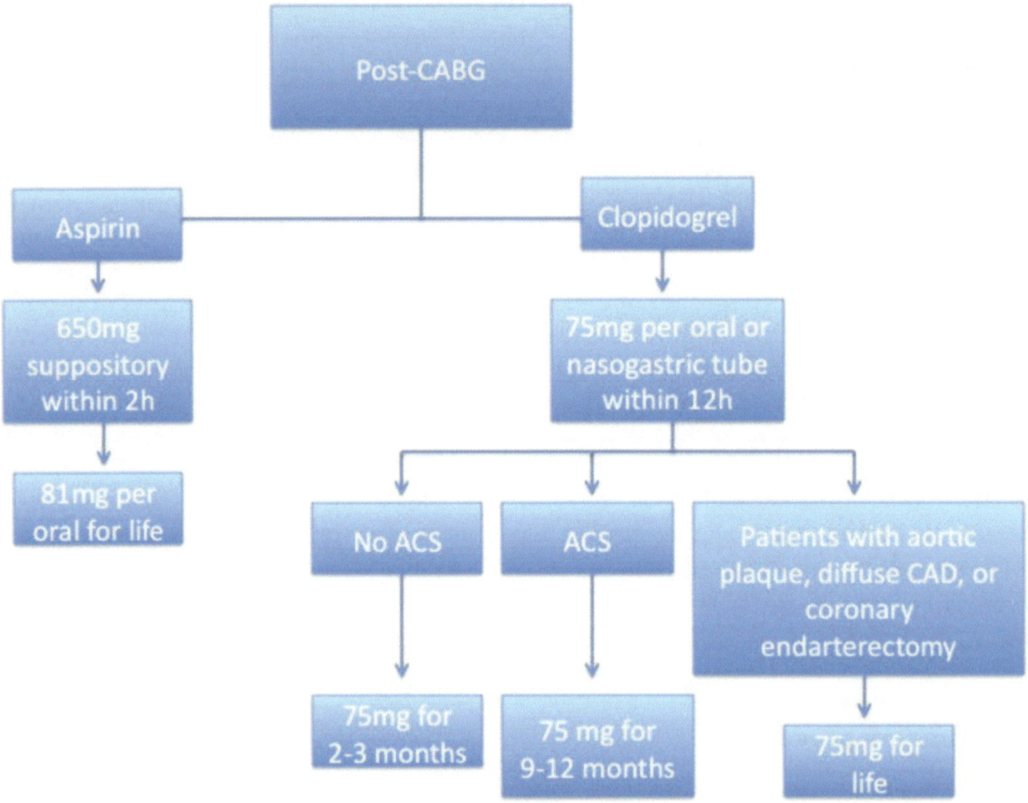

Fig. 2. Strategy for antiplatelet therapy for secondary prevention of CAD after CABG.

All patients with a history of a cardiovascular event should be started on a beta blocker and 3-hydroxy-3-methylglutaryl coenzyme A (MHG -CoA) reductase inhibitors (statins) for secondary prevention of cardiovascular events unless otherwise contraindicated (1994; Sacks, Pfeffer et al. 1996; 1998). Angiotensin converting enzyme inhibitors should be initiated in all patients with CAD and a left ventrticular ejection fraction less than 40%, diabetes, hypertension, or chronic kidney disease (Smith, Allen et al. 2006). ACE inhibitors may be considered in lower risk patients with well-controlled risk factors. If ACE inhibitors are not tolerated or are contraindicated, angiotensin receptor blockers (ARBs) may be considered. Patients with heart failure may also benefit from ARBs. Medication compliance is required for successful secondary prevention and must be ensured to reap the benefits of revascularization.

6. Conclusions

Antiplatelet therapy with aspirin and clopidogrel imparts a clear benefit in major adverse cardiovascular events and mortality after acute coronary syndrome. Although these agents may pose additional bleeding risk in the small percentage of patients with ACS that proceed to CABG, the risk is far outweighed by the benefits, and much of the bleeding can be diminished by delaying CABG when possible. Short acting anticoagulants and IABP insertion may temporize while allowing platelet function to recover after discontinuing clopidogrel. Following bleeding times postoperatively can clarify the need for platelet transfusion in the event of bleeding. OPCAB may have offer some benefits by avoiding full heparinization and avoiding the inflammatory response associated with cardiopulmonary bypass. Secondary prevention with antiplatelet therapy, beta blockade, lipid lowering therapy, and ACE inhibitors or ARBs is critical to the long term success of revascularization.

7. References

(1994). "Randomised trial of cholesterol lowering in 4444 patients with coronary heart disease: the Scandinavian Simvastatin Survival Study (4S)." *Lancet* 344(8934): 1383-9.

(1996). "A randomised, blinded, trial of clopidogrel versus aspirin in patients at risk of ischaemic events (CAPRIE). CAPRIE Steering Committee." *Lancet* 348(9038): 1329-39.

(1998). "Prevention of cardiovascular events and death with pravastatin in patients with coronary heart disease and a broad range of initial cholesterol levels. The Long-Term Intervention with Pravastatin in Ischaemic Disease (LIPID) Study Group." *N Engl J Med* 339(19): 1349-57.

Anderson, J. L., C. D. Adams, et al. (2007). "ACC/AHA 2007 guidelines for the management of patients with unstable angina/non-ST-Elevation myocardial infarction: a report of the American College of Cardiology/American Heart Association Task Force on Practice Guidelines (Writing Committee to Revise the 2002 Guidelines for the Management of Patients With Unstable Angina/Non-ST-Elevation Myocardial Infarction) developed in collaboration with the American College of Emergency Physicians, the Society for Cardiovascular Angiography and Interventions, and the Society of Thoracic Surgeons endorsed by the American Association of Cardiovascular and Pulmonary Rehabilitation and the Society for Academic Emergency Medicine." *J Am Coll Cardiol* 50(7): e1-e157.

Bhatt, D. L., M. T. Roe, et al. (2004). "Utilization of early invasive management strategies for high-risk patients with non-ST-segment elevation acute coronary syndromes: results from the CRUSADE Quality Improvement Initiative." *Jama* 292(17): 2096-104.

Ebrahimi, R., C. Dyke, et al. (2009). "Outcomes following pre-operative clopidogrel administration in patients with acute coronary syndromes undergoing coronary artery bypass surgery: the ACUITY (Acute Catheterization and Urgent Intervention Triage strategY) trial." *J Am Coll Cardiol* 53(21): 1965-72.

Ferraris, V. A., S. P. Ferraris, et al. (2005). "The Society of Thoracic Surgeons practice guideline series: aspirin and other antiplatelet agents during operative coronary revascularization (executive summary)." *Ann Thorac Surg* 79(4): 1454-61.

Fox, K. A., F. A. Anderson, Jr., et al. (2007). "Intervention in acute coronary syndromes: do patients undergo intervention on the basis of their risk characteristics? The Global Registry of Acute Coronary Events (GRACE)." *Heart* 93(2): 177-82.

Genoni, M., R. Tavakoli, et al. (2003). "Clopidogrel before urgent coronary artery bypass graft." *J Thorac Cardiovasc Surg* 126(1): 288-9.

Hongo, R. H., J. Ley, et al. (2002). "The effect of clopidogrel in combination with aspirin when given before coronary artery bypass grafting." *J Am Coll Cardiol* 40(2): 231-7.

Magee, M. J., J. H. Alexander, et al. (2008). "Coronary artery bypass graft failure after on-pump and off-pump coronary artery bypass: findings from PREVENT IV." *Ann Thorac Surg* 85(2): 494-9; discussion 499-500.

Moore, G. J., A. Pfister, et al. (2005). "Outcomes for off-pump coronary artery bypass grafting in high-risk groups: a historical perspective." *Heart Surg Forum* 8(1): E19-22.

Muller, C., H. J. Buttner, et al. (2000). "A randomized comparison of clopidogrel and aspirin versus ticlopidine and aspirin after the placement of coronary-artery stents." *Circulation* 101(6): 590-3.

Puskas, J. D., P. D. Kilgo, et al. (2008). "Off-pump coronary bypass provides reduced mortality and morbidity and equivalent 10-year survival." *Ann Thorac Surg* 86(4): 1139-46; discussion 1146.

Rastan, A. J., J. I. Eckenstein, et al. (2006). "Emergency coronary artery bypass graft surgery for acute coronary syndrome: beating heart versus conventional cardioplegic cardiac arrest strategies." *Circulation* 114(1 Suppl): I477-85.

Rosamond, W., K. Flegal, et al. (2008). "Heart disease and stroke statistics--2008 update: a report from the American Heart Association Statistics Committee and Stroke Statistics Subcommittee." *Circulation* 117(4): e25-146.

Sabatine, M. S., C. P. Cannon, et al. (2005). "Addition of clopidogrel to aspirin and fibrinolytic therapy for myocardial infarction with ST-segment elevation." *N Engl J Med* 352(12): 1179-89.

Sacks, F. M., M. A. Pfeffer, et al. (1996). "The effect of pravastatin on coronary events after myocardial infarction in patients with average cholesterol levels. Cholesterol and Recurrent Events Trial investigators." *N Engl J Med* 335(14): 1001-9.

Serebruany, V. L., A. I. Malinin, et al. (2004). "Risk of bleeding complications with antiplatelet agents: meta-analysis of 338,191 patients enrolled in 50 randomized controlled trials." *Am J Hematol* 75(1): 40-7.

Seshadri, N., P. L. Whitlow, et al. (2002). "Emergency coronary artery bypass surgery in the contemporary percutaneous coronary intervention era." *Circulation* 106(18): 2346-50.

Smith, S. C., Jr., J. Allen, et al. (2006). "AHA/ACC guidelines for secondary prevention for patients with coronary and other atherosclerotic vascular disease: 2006 update: endorsed by the National Heart, Lung, and Blood Institute." *Circulation* 113(19): 2363-72.

Wallentin, L., R. C. Becker, et al. (2009). "Ticagrelor versus clopidogrel in patients with acute coronary syndromes." *N Engl J Med* 361(11): 1045-57.

Wiviott, S. D., E. Braunwald, et al. (2007). "Prasugrel versus clopidogrel in patients with acute coronary syndromes." *N Engl J Med* 357(20): 2001-15.

Yende, S. and R. G. Wunderink (2001). "Effect of clopidogrel on bleeding after coronary artery bypass surgery." *Crit Care Med* 29(12): 2271-5.

Yusuf, S., F. Zhao, et al. (2001). "Effects of clopidogrel in addition to aspirin in patients with acute coronary syndromes without ST-segment elevation." *N Engl J Med* 345(7): 494-502.

13

Markers of Endothelial Activation and Impaired Autonomic Function in Patients with Acute Coronary Syndromes – Potential Prognostic and Therapeutic Implication

Arman Postadzhiyan, Anna Tzontcheva and Bojidar Finkov
Medical University, Clinic of Cardiology, St. Anne University Hospital, Sofia, Bulgaria

1. Introduction

Atherosclerosis is increasingly considered as a low grade inflammatory response of the arterial wall to a variety of stimuli [Fuster&Lewis, 1994; Libby, 2001]. It is accepted that the adhesion of circulating leukocytes and monocytes to endothelial cells (EC) and subsequent transendothelial migration are an important step in the initiation and the development of atherosclerotic lesions [Hillis&Flapan, 1998; Jang, 1994]. This process is mediated by receptors expressed on the surface of vascular EC - cell adhesion molecules (CAM) under the action of an enhanced oxidative stress, lipopolysaccharide and proinflammatory cytokines. Vascular cell adhesion molecule (VCAM-1) and intercellular adhesion molecule (ICAM-1) are two members of the immunoglobulin gene superfamily that play important but different roles in the adhesion of blood cells to the vascular endothelium. The significance of these molecules in the course of atherogenesis is confirmed by their immunohistochemically established elevated expression in the atherosclerotic plaques [Cybulsky&Gimbronejr, 1991; O'Brien et al., 1993] and by experimental models proving a delayed lesion development in case of their absence [Cybulsky et al., 2001].

Circulating forms of adhesion molecules that have been described are probably generated by cleavage to a site close to membrane insertion. The amount of ICAM-1 released has been demonstrated to be directly correlated with the surface expression of ICAM-1 in EC in culture and a correlation between plasma VCAM-1 and VCAM-1 mRNA has been reported in human atherosclerotic aorta [Leuwenberg et al., 1992; Pigott et al., 1992].

Levels of soluble cell adhesion molecules have been postulated to be useful risk predictor of cardiovascular events in healthy populations and various settings of ischemic heart disease [de Lemos et al., 2000; Hwang et al., 1997; Mulvihill et al., 2000, 2001; O'Malley et al., 2001; Ridker et al., 1998]. Nonetheless, the pathologic role of different soluble adhesion molecules in various stages of coronary artery disease is not fully defined.

Two electrocardiographic markers - ventricular arrhythmias (VA), [Bigger et al., 1981; Farrell et al., 1991; Kostis et al., 1987] and impaired cardiac autonomic function, as indicated by depressed heart rate variability (HRV), [Bigger at al., 1992; Farrell et all, 1991;

Hartikainen et al., 1996; Kleiger et al., 1987; Lanza et al., 1998, 2006; La Rovere et al., 1998] have been shown to predict mortality among patients recovering from acute myocardial infarction (MI). However there are only limited data about the prognostic value of depressed HRV in the whole spectrum of patients with ACS and few attempts to quantify the exact value of soluble adhesion molecules and HRV in the cumulative risk assessment of patients with ACS [Kennon et al., 2008; Lanza et al., 2006].
Previous studies have shown that statin treatment improve the prognosis in patients with acute coronary syndromes [Kinlay et al., 2003; Ridker at al., 2005]. The reduction of clinical events secondary to lipid lowering has traditionally been attributed to reduction of cholesterol deposition and facilitation of cholesterol efflux from coronary plaques. However, several studies have recently suggested that the beneficial effects of statins in atherosclerotic disease may not be limited to the lipid-lowering effects of these drugs. Possible explanations for the observed reduction of morbidity and mortality with statin use include improvement of endothelial function, plaque stabilisation, and inhibition of the inflammatory response associated with atherosclerosis [Liao 2003; Ray&Cannon, 2005]. In the last years an antiarrhythmic effect of statins has been suggested and reported as a possible contributing mechanism.
The aim of this study was:

1. To assess heart rate variability and soluble adhesion molecules ICAM-1 (intercellular adhesion molecule-1) and VCAM-1 (vascular cells adhesion molecule-1) in patients with coronary artery disease and healthy control and to evaluate the usefulness of the markers of impaired autonomic function and endothelial activation as predictors of adverse prognosis in patients with acute coronary syndromes.
2. The impact of early initiation of low and moderate-dose rosuvastatin treatment on autonomic function and concentrations of soluble adhesion molecules during the first 12 weeks post ACS without ST segment elevation.

2. Methods

2.1 Study protocol

The study consisted of two phases. In the first phase two groups of patients with coronary artery disease (acute coronary syndromes without ST segment elevation and stable angina pectoris) and one control group of subjects were included for comparisons of soluble levels of adhesion molecules and heart rate variability. Between December 2001 and July 2002, a total number of 136 patients were involved in the study. Patients were divided into three groups according to the clinical diagnosis. The first group consisted of 75 patients with non-ST segment elevation ACS (unstable angina and non ST elevation myocardial infarction). Unstable angina (UA) patients (n=57) had ischemic chest pain at rest within the preceding 48 hours that had developed in the absence of an extracardiac precipitating cause with either ST segment depression of >0.1 mV or T wave inversion in two or more contiguous leads on the presenting 12 lead ECG. Patients with non ST elevation myocardial infarction (n=18) had similar diagnostic criteria along with elevation of serum creatine kinase, without the evolution of pathological q waves. The second group consisted of 36 patients with stable angina pectoris (SAP) who had typical exertional angina pectoris and positive stress test. Patients with angina at rest were excluded from this group. The control group comprised of 25 healthy volunteers in the same age of distribution, without angina symptoms and with normal physical examination and stress test. Subjects with acute or chronic inflammatory diseases, malignancies, renal insufficiency, and severe liver disease, on immunosuppressive and antibiotic treatment were excluded from the study. Also excluded were patients with acute ST elevation myocardial infarction, diabetes mellitus, and history of myocardial infarction, surgical intervention or major trauma within the preceding month.

A six months follow-up of patients with ACS was assessed by regular clinical examination for every month. Primary outcome was defined as cardiac death, non-fatal myocardial infarction or recurrent hospital admission for severe unstable angina. After the 6-month period of observation the study population was divided into two groups - with favorable course of the disease and with occurrence of adverse coronary events.

In the second phase other 30 patients with ACS were allocated into two groups, and received rosuvastatin 10 mg/day (n =16, mean age 57.25±2.2 years) or rosuvastatin 20 mg/day (n =14, mean age 57.64±3.1 years). The randomization was carried out by the adaptive dynamic random allocation method irrespective of serum lipids levels. A follow-up assessment of both HRV on ambulatory ECG monitoring and adhesion molecules levels was performed during study period of 12 weeks. All patients were under treatment with the same medications during the acute phase of the episode (aspirin, nitrates, beta blockers, ACE inhibitors), according to the guidelines.

2.2 Biochemical analysis

Blood samples from ACS patients were collected after admission in the ICU prior to the onset of the antiischemic and anticoagulant therapy with a closed Vacutainer system (Beckton Dickinson, NJ, USA) and after 12 weeks for patients included into the second phase of the study. In SAP group and in controls, blood samples were collected at the time of clinical admission. The serum was separated after centrifugation at 3000 g for 10 min until 1 hour after taking the samples and sent in Department of Clinical Laboratory, Saint Anne University hospital for analyses of creatine kinase, cholesterol and triglycerides levels as a part of routine patient management. Two aliquots of the serum were centrally stored at -80°C and sent in batches to the Department of Clinical Laboratory and Clinical Immunology, Medical university, Sofia (for analyses of cTnT and hsCRP) and to the Section of Molecular Immunology, Bulgarian Academy of Sciences, Sofia (for analyses of VCAM-1 and ICAM-1). Determination of cTnT, hsCRP and soluble adhesion molecules levels was performed at the end of the study period, blinded to patients' histories and allocated treatment.

Quantitative detection of serum concentrations of sVCAM-1 and sICAM-1 was performed using an enzyme linked immunosorbent assay (ELISA) technique employing a commercially available assay kit (BenderMed Sysytems, Vienna, Austria). The intra- and interassay coefficients of variation were 3.1%, 5.2% for VCAM-1 and 4.1%, 7.6% for ICAM-1 respectively. The levels of cardiac troponin T (cTnT) were determined by a third generation troponin STAT electrochemiluminescent immunoassay on the ELECSYS 1010 (Roche Diagnostics, Basel, Switzerland) with the detection limit at 0.01 ng/ml and a total coefficient of variation (CV) of 6% at 5.07 ng/ml and 9.3% CV at 0.10 ng/ml. High-sensitivity C-reactive protein was measured with a CardioPhase hsCRP immunonephelometric assay (Dade Behring Inc) on BN systems. The detection limit was 0.175 mg/l with a total CV of 7.6% at 0.41 mg/l.

2.3 Holter monitoring

Patients underwent 24 h ECG Holter monitoring within 24 h of admission with two-channel tape recorders and monitoring two bipolar chest leads. Cardiac autonomic function was assessed by frequency-domain HRV analyses for the entire 24 hours. Frequency domain HRV was assessed in the frequency range of 0 to 0.5 Hz by fast-Fourier transform spectral analysis, with a spectral resolution of 0.0005 Hz. The amplitude of the following frequency-domain HRV variables was obtained: very low frequency (0.0033 to 0.04 Hz), low frequency (0.04 to 0.15 Hz), and high frequency (0.15 to 0.40 Hz). Further, the ratio of low to high frequency was calculated.

2.4 Statistical analysis

Any quantitative parameters under investigation were presented as a mean value and standart deviation. Any qualitative parameters under investigation were presented as a number and percentage. Student's t test or paired sample t-test was used to compare the quantitative parameters in the groups with a normal distribution. Mann-Whitney's or Wilcoxon signed rank non-parametric analysis is applied to compare the quantitative parameters of non-Gaussian distribution such as cTnT, hsCRP, sICAM-1, sVCAM-1 and parameters of HRV. Comparison of the categorical variables was performed by Pearson's x2test and Fisher's test. Receiver-operating characteristics (ROC) analysis was performed to estimate the potential of the variable tested to discriminate between patients with and without cardiovascular events during follow-up. To identify variables as independent predictors of CV events we calculated various multivariate Cox regression models with stepwise adjustment for univariate predictors possibly confounding the examined variable. Probability values of $p<0,05$ were considered statistically significant. All analyses were performed with SPSS, 9.0 version for Windows.

3. Results

3.1 Markers of endothelial activation and impaired autonomic function in patients with acute coronary syndromes – Potential prognostic implication

3.1.1 Characteristics of the study population

Table 1 demonstrates clinical characteristics and biochemical data of all study groups. There were no significant differences among study groups regarding age, gender, family history and smoking status. The patients with coronary artery disease (acute coronary syndromes and stable angina) had significantly higher rates of hypertension and dyslipidaemia compared with healthy control group. The presence of coronary risk factors was equal among groups with acute coronary syndromes and stable angina pectoris. Eight of the patients in the control group (32%) were on antihypertensive medications. The corresponding number of patients on antihypertensive medications in ACS group was 48 (64%) and 21 (61%) in stable angina pectoris group. All soluble ICAM-1, VCAM-1 and hsCRP significantly discriminated between patients with ACS and SAP ($p=0.014$, 0.05 and 0.025 respectively) and control subjects ($p<0.001$, 0.05 and 0.048). Soluble ICAM-1 and hsCRP were also elevated in patients with SAP compared with control group whereas no difference in sVCAM-1 was found ($p<0.001$, 0.05 and 0.4). In opposite, all the parameters of the frequency domain HRV tented to be lower in patients with ACS compared with stable angina and control group. In healthy subjects VLF, LF and HF were elevated, but LF/HF ratio was lower in comparison with stable angina patients ($p=0.006$).

Variable	ACS Group 1	Stable AP Group 2	P1	Control Group 3	P2	P3
Number	75	36		25		
Age	57.8±8.8	57.8±8.7	1	55.6±9.2	0.3	0.4
Male gender	41 (54.7%)	15(41.7%)	0.2	12 (48%)	0.7	0.8
Family history	36 (48%)	15(41.7%)	0.5	11 (44%)	0.8	1
Hypertension	51 (68%)	27 (75%)	0.5	11 (44%)	0.05	0.01
Smoking	38 (50.7%)	14(38.9%)	0.31	11 (44%)	0.65	0.8
Cholesterol mmol/l	6.24±1.25	6.21±1.41	0.92	5.41±0.79	0.002	0.01
Tryglycerides mmol/l	1.94±1.06	1.82±1.21	0.62	1.27±0.42	0.003	0.03
BMI>25	43 (57.3%)	26(72.2%)	0.15	12 (48%)	0.49	0.06
Preivious MI	19 (25.3%)	4 (11.1%)	0.13	0 (0%)	0.003	0.14
sVCAM-1 ng/ml	1447.3±52.9	1362.4±114.9	0.05	1318.6±78.4	0.05	0.419
sICAM-1 ng/ml	465.5±15.9	387.2 ±29.2	0.014	108.6 ±14.7	<0.001	<0.001
hsCRP mg/l	15.5 ±3.95	2.33 ±0.39	0.025	1.45±0.24	0.048	0.05
VLF ms	101.4±9.3	195.2±45.3	0.003	213.9±45.1	<0.001	0,78
LF ms	71.1±8.05	187.6±46.7	<0.001	199.7±43.5	<0.001	0.85
HF ms	42.1±8.6	87±27.6	0.04	128.4±37.1	0.001	0.37
LF/HF ms	2.67±0.3	4.09±0.7	0.03	2.12±0.39	0.43	0.06

P1 group 1 vs group 2
P2 group 1 vs group 3
P3 group 2 vs group 3

Table 1. Baseline characteristics of study population

3.1.2 Baseline characteristics of patients with ACS according to clinical outcome

During the six month follow-up of the patients with acute coronary syndromes three patients (4%) died suddenly, seventeen (22.7%) suffered a non-fatal myocardial infarction and eight (10.7%) had recurrent UA, for a major adverse cardiovascular event rate of 37.3%. The majority of ischemic events occurred within 30 days of the initial episode of non ST elevation acute coronary syndrome - 16 (57.14%). Simultaneously, the risk of development of non-fatal AMI and rehospitalization for recurrent UA remained significant even during a longer period of observation as 12 (42,8%) of the subsequent complications occurred during the period between the 30th day and the 6th month.

On Table 2 the demographic, clinical and laboratory data of the patients with major cardiovascular events were compared with those of the patients with favorable outcome. Both groups do not differ concerning the classical risk factors for the development of ischemic heart disease such as age, gender, history of arterial hypertension, tobacco smoking, obesity, familial history and indices of lipid profile. The patients have received identical drug therapy including heparin (97,3%), acetysal (90,7%), β-blocker (73,3%), nitrate (100%), ACE-inhibitor (48%) and diuretics (17,3%). The patients with subsequent complications presented more often with Killip class over 1 (28,6% versus 8,5%, p=0,047) and with a significantly lower left ventricular ejection fraction on the echocardiographic examination performed between day 3 and day 7 of the hospitalization (54,6% versus 60,4%, p=0,003). Concentrations of sVCAM-1 (1488,75 ng/ml versus 1071,45 ng/ml, p<0,001), sICAM-1 (516,7 vs 433,3 ng/ml, p=0,010), hsCRP (32.6 vs 5.31 mg/l, p=0.001) and cTnT (0,72 vs 0,115 ng/ml, p<0,001) at presentation were significantly raised in patients who went on to have ischemic events during the six months of follow-up. None of the parameters of HRV was significantly associated with the occurrence of the composite endpoint. Although the prognostic information of frequency domain HRV indices was low, we found out that 2 variables - reduced LF (27±1.7 vs 65.1±10 ms, p=0.05) and LF/HF ratio (0.5±0.2 vs 2.94±0.4, p=0.004) were significantly predictive of death, but no for other endpoints (Fig 1)

	No event n (%)	Event n (%)	p
Number	47	28	
Males	26 (55.3)	15 (53.6)	1
Age, y	57.36 ±8.2	58.6 ±10.1	0.559
Hypertension	34 (72.3)	17 (60.7)	0.318
Smoking	23 (48.9)	15 (53.6)	0.812
Previous MI	12 (25.5)	7 (25)	1
Family history	20 (42.6)	16 (57.1)	0.242
BMI>25	25 (53.2)	18 (64.3)	0.470
Kilip>1	4 (8.5)	8 (28.6)	0.047
Cholesterol mmol/l	6.30 ±1.22	6.13 ±1.31	0.581
Triglycerides mmol/l	2.07 ±1.19	1.70 ±0.75	0.145
Ejection fraction %	60.4 ±7.65	54.6 ±8.45	0.003
Troponin T ng/ml	0.115 ±0.01	0.72 ±0.16	<0.001
hsCRP mg/l	5.31 ±1.66	32.59 ±9.45	0.001
sVCAM-1 ng/ml	1071.5 ±54.08	1488.8 ±90.3	<0.001
sICAM-1 ng/ml	433.3 ±20.01	516.7 ±23.8	0.010
VLF ms	114.5±13.4	89.2±11.6	0.16
LF ms	73.7±12.2	65.2±10.1	0.62
HF ms	56.6±16.4	32.5±6.5	0.143
LF/HF ms	1.98±0.3	2.98±0.4	0.07

Table 2. Baseline characteristics of patients with and without cardiovascular events during follow-up

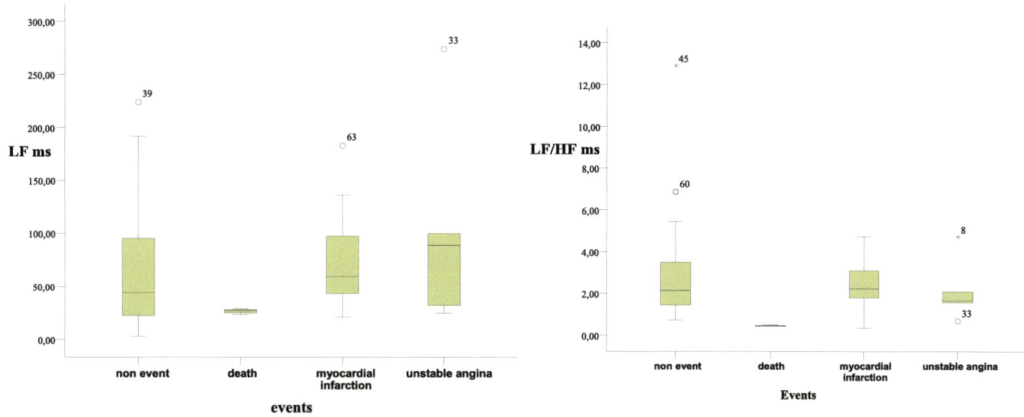

Fig. 1. LF and LF/HF in patients according to the prognosis during the study period

Table 3 presents the associations between soluble adhesion molecules, high sensitivity C-reactive protein and troponin T in patients with ACS. There is a moderately strong positive correlation between the levels of sICAM-1 and sVCAM-1 (Spearman's r=0,205, p=0,028). Levels of sICAM-1 showed a strong correlation with hsCRP. The correlation between sVCAM-1 and hsCRP was r=0.144, p=0.11. In acute coronary syndromes levels of the myocardial necrosis marker troponin T correlated highly significant with hsCRP (r=0.451, p=0.001), but showed no interdependence with sVCAM-1 (r=0.106, p=0.383) and sICAM-1 (r=0.129, p=0.286).

		sVCAM-1	sICAM-1	hsCRP
sVCAM-1	r	1	0,205	0,144
	p	-	0,028	0,11
sICAM-1	r	0,205	1	0,438
	p	0,028	-	<0,001
hsCRP	r	0,144	0,438	1
	p	0,11	<0,001	-
cTnT	r	0,106	0,129	0,451
	p	0,383	0,286	<0,001

Table 3. Associations between soluble adhesion molecules, high sensitivity C-reactive protein and troponin T

A nonsignificant inverse correlation was found between sVCAM-1 levels and all HRV variables studied with the strongest association with low frequency amplitude. The correlation coefficients of hsCRP and cTnT with HRV parameters were low and without clinical significance. (table 4)

		VLF	LF	HF	LF/HF
hsCRP	r	0,128	-0,02	0,16	-0,19
	p	0,35	0,87	0,24	0,16
sVCAM-1	r	-0,10	-0,24	-0,12	-0,06
	p	0,46	0,08	0,41	0,67
sICAM-1	r	-0,08	0,014	0,03	0,009
	p	0,55	0,92	0,82	0,95
cTnT	r	0,125	0,017	0,15	-0,07
	p	0,36	0,9	0,27	0,57

Table 4. Associations between HRV and soluble adhesion molecules, high sensitivity C-reactive protein and troponin T

3.1.3 Soluble adhesion molecules and cardiovascular events

The ROC analysis was performed to provide an index for assessment of the accuracy of the variable investigated to discriminate between subjects with cardiovascular complications and those without it. The data obtained from it demonstrate threshold concentrations of 0,01 ng/ml for cTnT (area under the curve 0,803, p=0,001), 4 mg/l for hsCRP (AUC 0,859, p=0,001), 1153,4 ng/mL for sVCAM-1 (AUC 0,786, p=0,001) and 438 ng/mL for sICAM-1 (AUC 0,671, p=0,017) Fig 2.

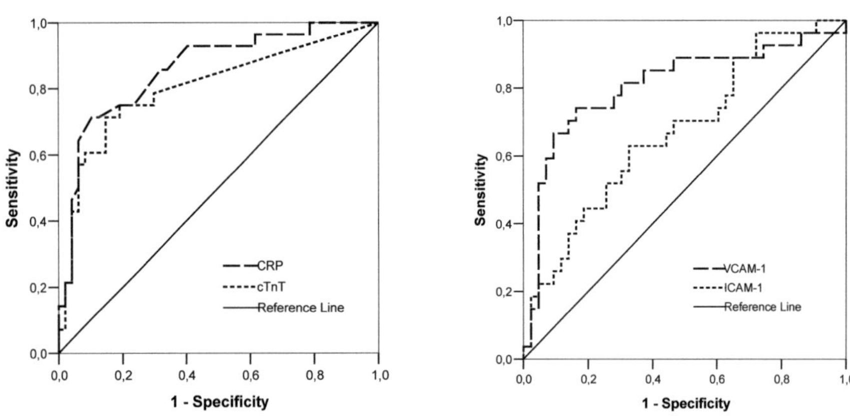

Variable	AUC	SE	95% Confidence Interval	
CRP	0,859	0,045	0,770	0,948
cTnT	0,803	0,057	0,692	0,914
VCAM-1	0,786	0,059	0,669	0,902
ICAM-1	0,671	0,066	0,542	0,800

AUC – area under the curve, SE – standard error

Fig. 2. Receiver-operator characteristic curves of the investigated biomarkers as a test for predicting major adverse coronary events in patients with acute coronary syndromes

A total of 37 patients (49.3%) had a concentration of sVCAM-1>1153.4 ng/ml and the ischemic event rate for these patients was 78.6%. The remaining 38 patients had sVCAM-1 concentrations <1153.4 ng/ml and the ischemic event rate in this group was 21.4% (Pearson x2= 15,28, p<0,001). As Figure 3 A shows the difference was mainly driven by an increased rate of non-fatal myocardial infarction and rehospitalsation for unstable angina in the group of patients with high sVCAM-1 levels. Although the incidence rate of the ischemic complications in the patients with sICAM-1>438 ng/ ml was 66,7% while in the patients with subthreshold concentration of this parameter it was only 33,3%, a statistically reliable difference was lacking (Pearson x2=2,71,p<0,140, Figure 3 B). The sensitivity of a concentration of sVCAM-1>1153.4 ng/ml for predicting future ischemic events was 79%, with a specificity of 68%. The negative predictive value was 84%. The sensitivity of sICAM-1>438 ng/ml for predicting a future ischemic events was 66%, with a specificity of 53% and negative predicting value of 72%.

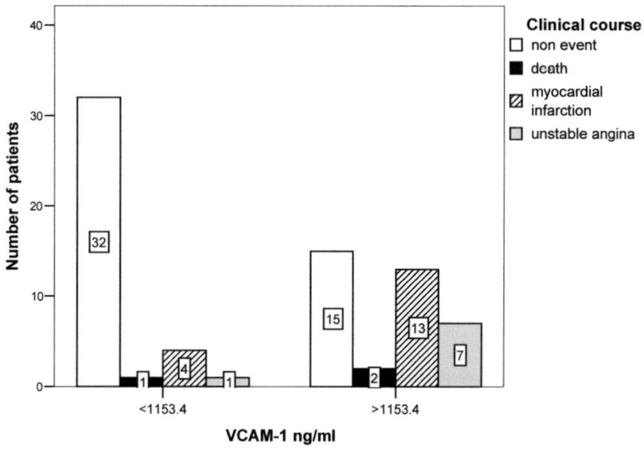

a

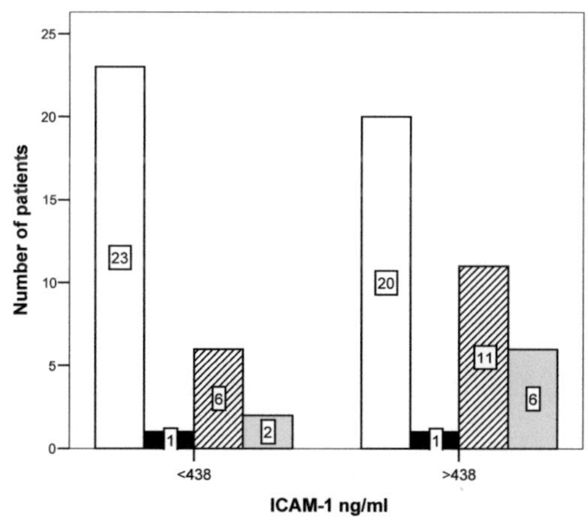

b

Fig. 3. Cardiovascular events in patients according to concentration of sVCAM-1 (A) and sICAM-1 (B)

3.1.4 Multivariate risk stratification

In a multivariate analysis that included baseline characteristics and biochemical markers (Table 5) sVCAM-1 remained an independent and powerful predictor of increased cardiac risk at 6 months follow-up. The odds ratio associated with the highest value of sVCAM-1 was 4.62 (95% CI 1.8-11.4, p=0.0009) without adjustment and remained significantly elevated after adjustment for Killip class and left ventricular ejection fraction in model 2 (RR 4.63, 1.8-11.7, p=0.0012), troponin T in model 3 (RR 3.93, 1,5-10, p=0.04) and C-reactive protein in model 4 (RR 2.22, 0.8-5.7, p=0.05) Figure 4.

	Odds ratio	95% CI	P
Sex - Males	0.93	0.44 - 1.97	0.86
Age > 65 y	1.48	0.68 - 3.21	0.31
Hypertension	1.38	0.64 - 2.96	0.39
Smoking	1.11	0.52 - 2.34	0.77
BMI > 25	1.38	0.6 - 2.9	0.41
Hypercholesterolemia	1.11	0.45 - 2.76	0.80
Family history	1.58	0.7 - 3.34	0.23
Previous MI	1.00	0.42 - 2.37	0.98
ST depression > 0.5 mm	2.11	0.85 - 5.2	0.10
Killip > 1	2.73	1.19 - 6.22	0.016
EF < 50%	2.75	1.24 - 6.11	0.0125
ICAM-1 > 438 ng/ml	1.81	1.82 - 4.04	0.15
VCAM-1 > 1153.4 ng/ml	4.62	1.86 - 11.4	0.0009
hsCRP > 4 mg/l	9.85	3.39 - 28.5	<0.0001
cTnT > 0.01 ng/ml	5.29	2.13 - 13.1	0.0003

Table 5. Univariate Cox proportional regression analyses

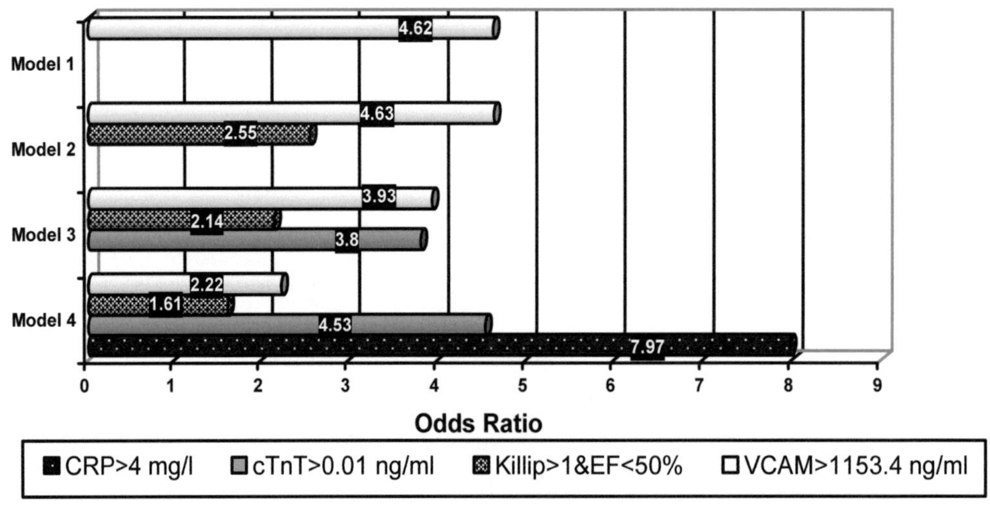

Fig. 4. Multivarate Cox regression models on VCAM-1 as predictor of major adverse coronary events during 6 month follow-up

In order to assess the exact role of the increased soluble adhesion molecules levels we analyzed the combined predictive value of these two molecules with that of the already established prognostic indicators among ACS patients - troponin T and hs C-reactive protein. Division of the patients into 4 groups based on their sCAM and cTnT levels revealed that sVCAM-1 is an independent prognostic indicator of major adverse coronary events during the six months follow-up. In the patients admitted to the ICU without any detectable levels of the marker of cardiomyocyte necrosis (n=39) the incidence rate of the ischemic events was 1,3% when combined with low levels of sVCAM-1 and 6,7% when combined with sVCAM-1> 1153,4 ng/ml (Pearson $\chi 2=6{,}03$, $p<0{,}024$, Figure 5 A). Simultaneously, the high sICAM-1 levels do not improve the prognostic value of troponin T as there was no statistically significant difference in the incidence rate of the complications in the patients with a negative cTnT test in dependence on the low or high sICAM-1 levels (the incidence of the complications was 2,9% and 5,7%, respectively) (Figure 5 B).

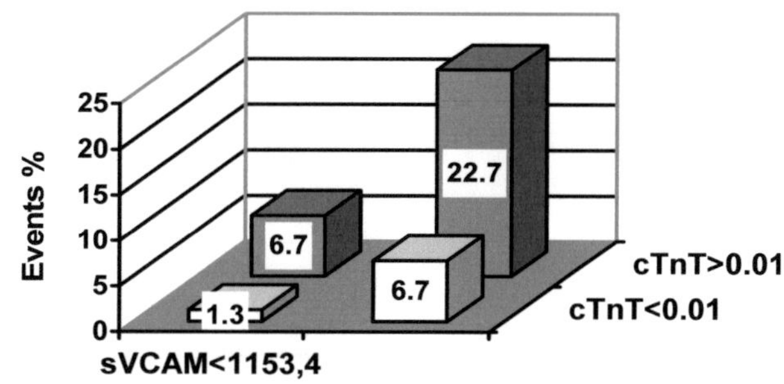

a

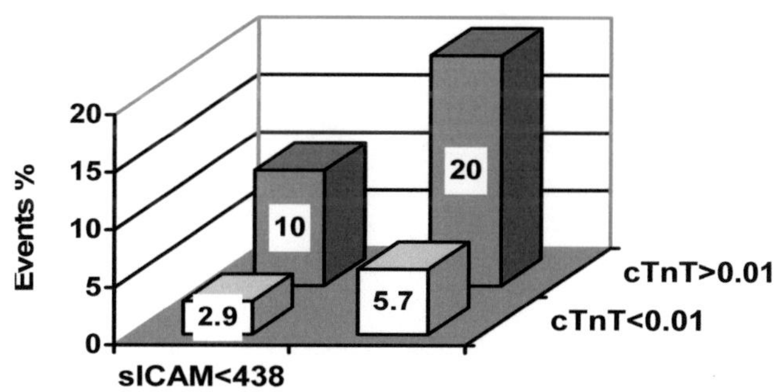

b

Fig. 5. Incidence of cardiovascular events according to soluble VCAM-1 and cTnT levels (A) and soluble ICAM-1 and cTnT levels (B)

Furthermore, the predictive value of VCAM-1 was independent of systemic inflammation as evidenced by C-reactive protein. High VCAM-1 serum levels indicated increased cardiac risk both in patients with high CRP serum levels (25.3%% vs 6.7%, p=0.024) and in those with low CRP serum levels (4% vs 1.3%, p=0.05), Figure 6.

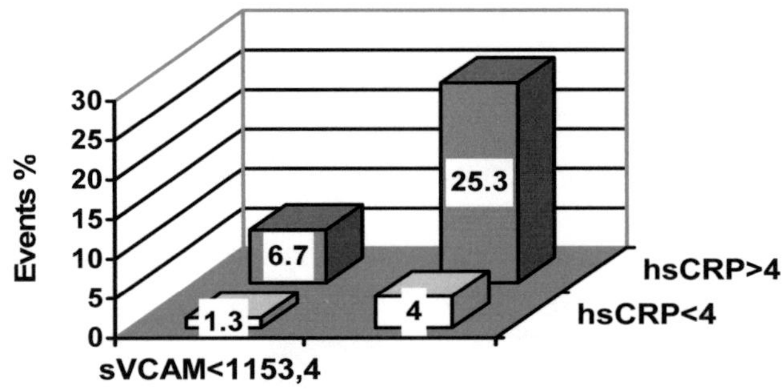

a

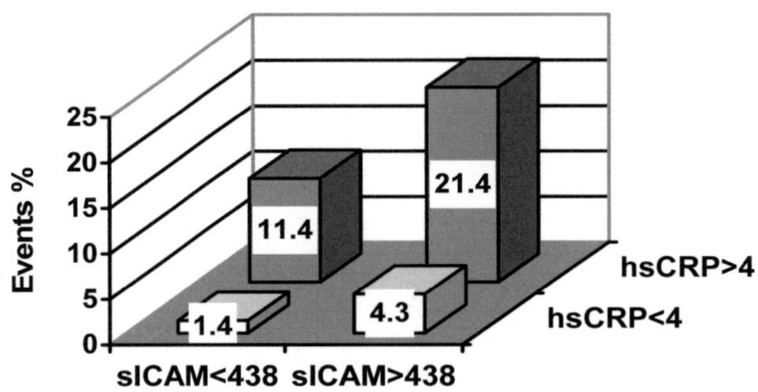

b

Fig. 6. Incidence of cardiovascular events according to soluble VCAM-1 and hsCRP levels (A) and soluble ICAM-1 and hsCRP levels (B)

3.2 Markers of endothelial activation and impaired autonomic function in patients with acute coronary syndromes – Potential therapeutic implication

3.2.1 Characteristics of the study population

During the second phase of the study 30 patients with ACS were allocated into two groups, and received rosuvastatin 10 mg/day (n =16, mean age 57.25±2.2 years) or rosuvastatin 20 mg/day (n =14, mean age 57.64±3.1 years) for 12 weeks. Baseline characteristics for each group are presented in Table 6, showing no significant differences between the two treatment groups. Furthermore, no significant differences in lipids, HRV and markers of endothelial activation were observed at baseline.

Variable	Rosuvastatin 10 mg n=16	Rosuvastatin 20 mg n=14	p
Age	57,25±2,22	57,64±3,1	0.34
Male gender	7 (23%)	9 (30%)	0.22
Hypertension	9 (30%)	9 (30%)	0.72
Smoking	7 (23.3%)	6 (20%)	0.62
Family history	5 (16.7%)	7 (23.3%)	0.46
cTnT	0,29±0.13	0,46±0,18	0.91
EF %	58,5±2,1	58,8±2,6	0.46
BMI	26,8±1	26,9±1	0.34
Cholesterol mmol/l	5,66±0,28	6,07±0,32	0.4
Tryglycerides mmol/l	1,76±0,17	1,93±0,25	0.6
HDL-C mmol/l	0,99±0,03	0,91±0,03	0.14
LDL-C mmol/l	3,86±0,29	4,27±0,28	0.3
sVCAM-1 ng/ml	1235(831.3-1476.3)	1327,4(1039.5-1989.7)	0.21
sICAM-1 ng/ml	476,8(424,3-516,8)	439,4(362,1-607,3)	0.92
VLF ms	97±18,7	90,7±16,7	0.80
LF ms	43,3±8,2	44,5±7,1	0.91
HF ms	19,8±5,8	20,9±6,7	0.89
LF/HF ms	3,34±0,5	3,58±0,5	0.77

Table 6. Baseline characteristics

3.2.2 Effects of rosuvastatin on lipid profile and markers of endothelial and autonomic activation

The changes in lipid values from baseline to 12 weeks in the two treatment groups are shown in Table 7.

	Rosuvastatin 10 mg			Rosuvastatin 20 mg		
	Baseline	3 months	p	Baseline	3 months	p
Cholesterol mmol/l	5,66±0,28	4,49±0,18	<0.001	6,07±0,32	4,24±0,16	<0.001
Tryglycerides mmol/l	1,76±0,17	1,3±0,13	<0.001	1,93±0,25	1,37±0,18	<0.001
HDL-C mmol/l	0,99±0,03	1,05±0,04	<0.001	0,91±0,03	1,06±0,03	<0.001
LDL-C mmol/l	3,86±0,29	2,67±0,2	<0.001	4,27±0,28	2,27±0,11	<0.001

Table 7. Effects of rosuvastatin on lipid profile

Serum levels of total cholesterol, triglycerides and LDL-cholesterol in patients decreased after 3 months of treatment with rosuvastatin. The decrease in total cholesterol and LDL cholesterol was significantly larger in the more aggressively treated group ($p<0.05$ for all comparisons).

	Rosuvastatin 10 mg			Rosuvastatin 20 mg		
	Baseline	3 months	p	Baseline	3 months	p
sVCAM-1 median ng/ml 25- and 75-percentile	1235 (831.3-1476.3)	1120,2 (839,7-1341,2)	0.43	1327,4 (1039.5-1989.7)	962,4 (603,4-1570,3)	0,01
sICAM-1 median ng/ml 25- and 75-percentile	476,8 (424,3-516,8)	385,5 (348,5-453,9)	0,004	439,4 (362,1-607,3)	324,7 (188,5-447,5)	0.01
VLF ms	97±18,7	99,5±16,5	0,8	90,7±16,7	113,3±20,5	0,35
LF ms	43,3±8,2	63,8±14,9	0,2	44,5±7,1	56,7±13,4	0,23
HF ms	19,8±5,8	37±11,6	0,23	20,9±6,7	42,2±7,2	0,009
LF/HF ms	3,34±0,5	2,87±0,5	0,31	3,58±0,5	1,73±0,2	0,003

Table 8. Effects of Rosuvastatin on Adhesion Molecules and HRV levels

After 3 months, patients in the 20 mg rosuvastatin group demonstrated a significant decrease in serum levels of sICAM-1 and sVCAM-1 (Table 8, Figure 7 and 8). Also in the 10 mg-rosuvastin group, there was a significant decrease of sICAM-1 (Figure 9). However, no changes in sVCAM-1 levels were observed in this group of patients (Table 8, Figure 10). There were no significant differences in changes between the two treatment groups for either soluble adhesion molecules levels, but for sICAM-1 we found out a trend towards lower concentrations in the moderately treated group ($p=0.07$).

No correlations were found between changes in LDL-cholesterol over 12 weeks and changes in s-ICAM-1 ($r=0.198$, $p=0.29$), sVCAM-1 ($r=0.193$, $p=0.31$) and HRV during the same period. The Spearman's correlation coefficients between hsCRP and sICAM-1 ($r=0.059$, $p=0,7$) and sVCAM-1 ($r=0.15$, $p=0,4$) are low and not statistically significant.

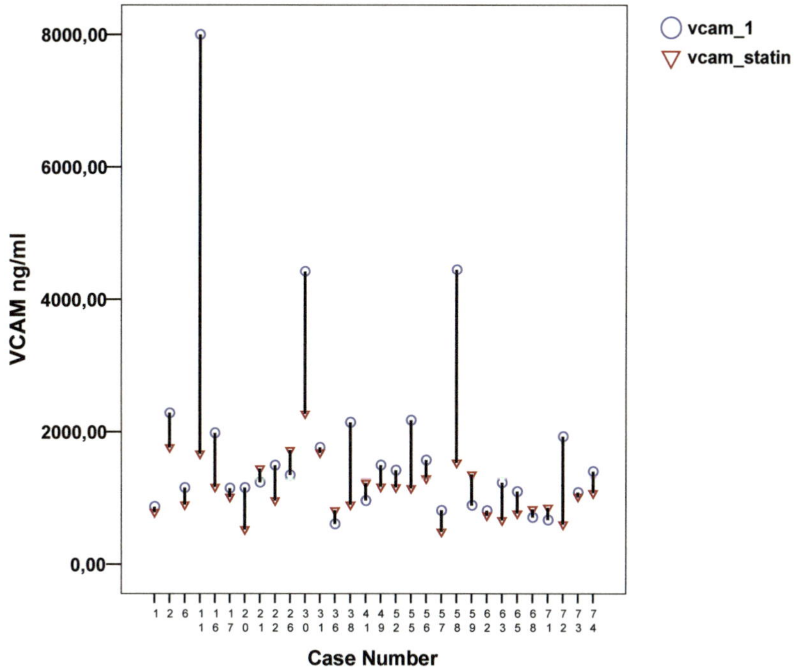

Fig. 7. Intra-individual changes in levels of s-VCAM-1 in patients during the study.

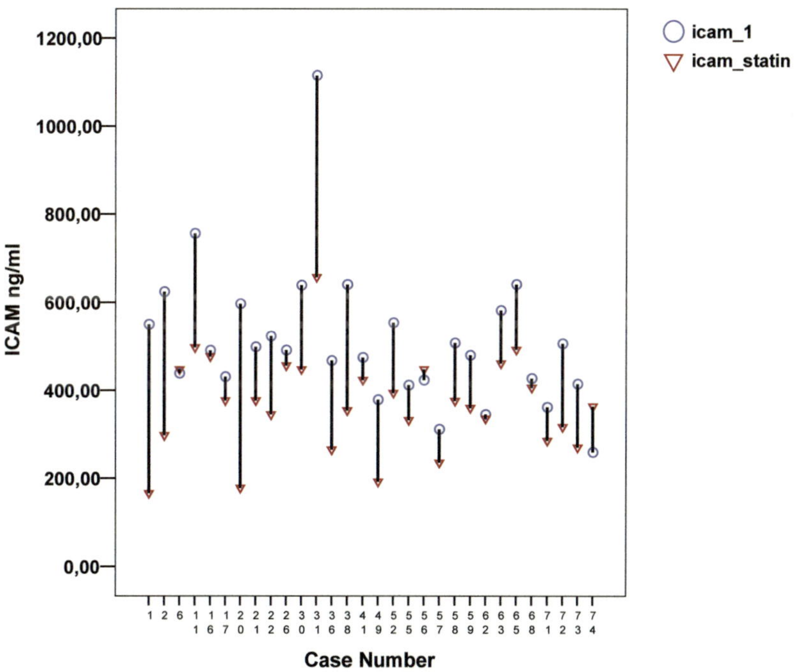

Fig. 8. Intra-individual changes in levels of s-ICAM-1 in patients during the study.

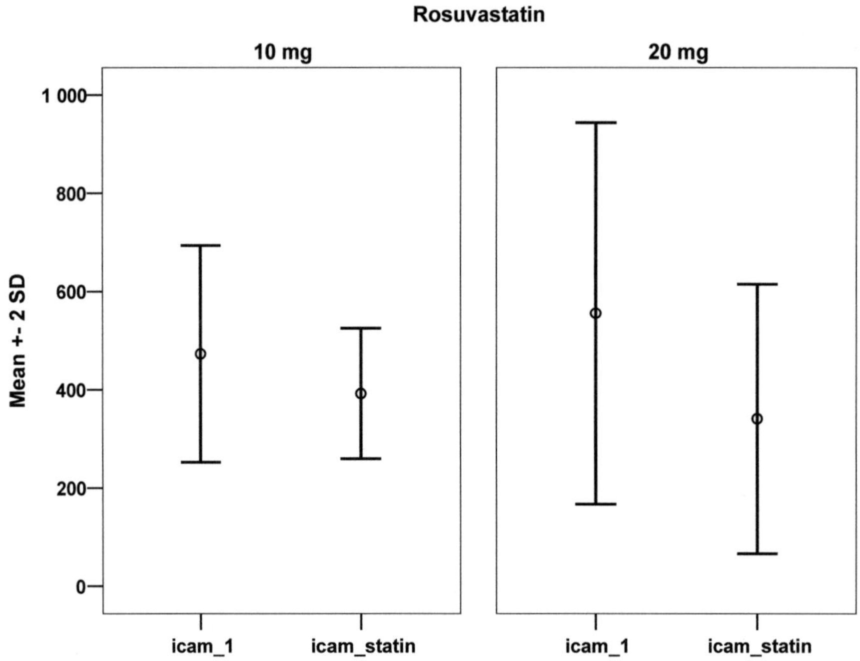

Fig. 9. Mean changes ± 2 SD of sICAM-1 in the two rosuvastatin treated groups

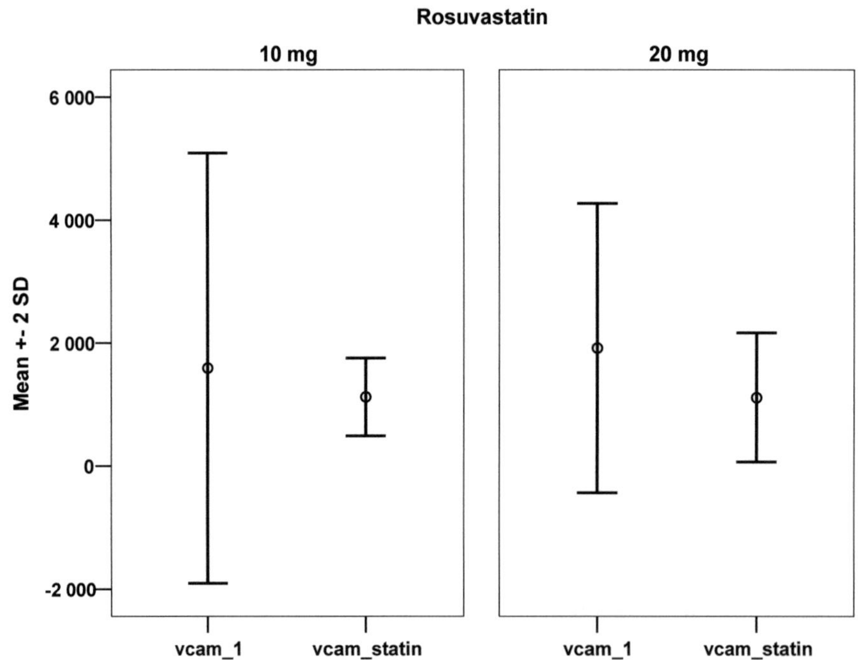

Fig. 10. Mean changes ± 2 SD of sVCAM-1 in the two rosuvastatin treated groups

In ACS group, a significant inverse correlation was observed between markers of endothelial activation and HRV variables, with the strongest association being found for sVCAM-1 and HF amplitude (r =−0.506, p= 0.004) and LF amplitude (r=-0,4, p=0.02). In addition, sympathovagal balance was shifted to greater vagal predominance with 20 mg rosuvastatin (increase of HF and decrease of low frequency/ high frequency ratio) when compared to lower dose of 10 mg, p=0.05, Table 9.

			LDL	vcam 1	icam 1	VLF	LF	HF	LF/HF
Spearman's rho	LDL	Correlation Coefficient	1,000	,193	,198	,049	,029	,130	-,098
		Sig. (2-tailed)	.	,308	,294	,804	,882	,509	,620
	vcam 1	Correlation Coefficient	,193	1,000	,384(*)	-,158	-,423(*)	-,506	,207
		Sig. (2-tailed)	,308	.	,036	,405	,020	,004	,273
	icam 1	Correlation Coefficient	,198	,384(*)	1,000	,089	-,144	-,234	,210
		Sig. (2-tailed)	,294	,036	.	,654	,465	,231	,284
	VLF	Correlation Coefficient	,049	-,158	,089	1,000	,694	,431(*)	,125
		Sig. (2-tailed)	,804	,405	,654	.	,000	,017	,511
	LF	Correlation Coefficient	,029	-,423(*)	-,144	,694	1,000	,656	,091
		Sig. (2-tailed)	,882	,020	,465	,000	.	,000	,634
	HF	Correlation Coefficient	,130	-,506	-,234	,431(*)	,656	1,000	-,649
		Sig. (2-tailed)	,509	,004	,231	,017	,000	.	,000
	LF/HF	Correlation Coefficient	-,098	,207	,210	,125	,091	-,649	1,000
		Sig. (2-tailed)	,620	,273	,284	,511	,634	,000	.

* Correlation is significant at the 0.05 level (2-tailed).

Table 9. Associations between HRV and soluble adhesion molecules and LDL cholesterol

4. Discussion

The measurement of ICAM-1 and VCAM-1 in prospective studies is based on the presence of an inflammatory process in the artery wall which increases the expression of adhesion molecules and on the hypothesis that the serum levels of these molecules reflect their expression by the endothelial cells. In this study we had measured the two main representatives of the immunoglobulin gene superfamily of CAM and found significantly higher levels of both sVCAM-1 and sICAM-1 in patients with ACS as compared with those with SAP and healthy controls. Our finding that soluble adhesion molecules and especially sVCAM-1 are strongly and independently predictive for future CV events in patient with ACS extends previous observations describing the predictive value of inflammatory markers on future cardiac events. However, whereas the causative role of C-reactive protein in promoting the inflammatory component in development of plaque rupture remains controversial, our data implicate a direct mediator of an inflammatory vessel wall process. Several arguments support the hypothesis that sCAM may be more useful than other markers of inflammation in predicting clinical outcome:

First, all sICAM-1 and sVCAM-1 measured in our study are elevated in patients at risk for future cardiovascular events. Second, sCAM levels did not correlate with cTnT, a specific marker of cardiomyocyte necrosis and the most established prognostic marker in patients with ACS. The risk related to the high sVCAM-1 concentrations is independent of the cTnT that is evident from the increasing rate of complications in the groups with negative and positive cTnT in dependence on sVCAM-1 levels. These data suggest that VCAM-1 release actually precedes myocardial injury and that VCAM-1 elevation identifies patients with unstable atherosclerotic plaque formation even before complete microvascular obstruction. In contrast, we do not find any relationship between sICAM-1 and the risk of subsequent events in the course of the follow-up and we do not read any enhanced incidence rate of vascular events in the patients without laboratory evidence of a cardiomyocyte necrosis in dependence on the levels of this parameter. Third, sVCAM-1 levels did not correlate with C-reactive protein, a systemic marker of inflammation. Because hsCRP correlated with cTnT levels elevated CRP serum levels most likely reflect both a robust vascular inflammatory response and myocardial injury. The measurement of sVCAM-1 added to the predictive value of hsCRP in determining the risk of future cardiovascular events. Even patients with low hsCRP levels were found to be at significantly higher risk with elevated sVCAM-1 levels which suggest that endothelial activation and proteolytic cleavage of sCAM is a primary event and is followed by release of other systemic mediators and acute phase proteins such as C-reactive protein.

Prospective data of soluble adhesion molecules are sparse. The results of our study correspond to the data published in the literature about the relationship between sCAM and the risk of cardiovascular events and they find their explanation in some differences between the two adhesion molecules studied. In the large prospective trials ARIC and PHS of healthy individuals, sICAM-1, but not sVCAM-1 appears consistently related to incident CAD [de Lemos et al., 2000; Hwang et al., 1997; Ridker et al., 1998]. ICAM-1 expression is not only endothelial and ICAM-1 is constitutively expressed by a variety of cell types including cells of the hematopoietic lineage and fibroblasts. sICAM-1 correlates with acute phase reactants like CRP and provides similar predictive information to CRP in settings of primary prevention [Blankenberg et al., 2003; Mulvihill et al., 2002; Ridker et al., 1998; 2000]. sICAM-1 therefore appears as a general marker of a proinflammatory status with little prognostic information in patients with ACS after controlling the data for troponin T and C-reactive protein (Figure 5 and 6). By contrast, VCAM-1 is not expressed in baseline condition, but is rapidly induced by pro-atherosclerotic conditions in animal models and humans [Cybulsky&Gimbronejr, 1991; O'Brien et al., 1993]. It seems that sVCAM-1 represents an appropriate marker of plaque burden or activity of a potential clinical importance as a prognostic indicator under the conditions of secondary prevention rather than in healthy individuals without endothelial dysfunction [Blankenberg et al., 2003; Mulvihill et al., 2002]. A similar hypothesis is supported by the data proving the independent predictive value of sVCAM-1 in the patients with angiographically proven coronary artery disease [Blankenberg et al., 2001], with diabetes mellitus [Jager et al., 2000] and with ACS [Mulvihill et al., 2001, 2002] as well as its absence in healthy individuals [de Lemos et al., 2000].

The relationship between depressed HRV and mortality is difficult to ascertain as the exact physiological mechanisms responsible for the various HRV components are still incompletely known [Task Force of the European Society of Cardiology and the North American Society of Pacing and Electrophysiology, 1996; Tsuji et al., 1996]. Decreased values of HRV variables, including LF, may reflect reduced vagal tone or predominant sympathetic influence to the heart. The presence of frequent or complex non-sustained VA in the context of sympathovagal imbalance can increase the susceptibility to fatal VA, in particular during myocardial ischaemia [Kent et al., 1973; Lanza et al., 1998, 2006; Schwartz et al.,1988]. On the other hand, VA and depressed HRV are unlikely to be associated with the triggers of acute MI, as they were not predictive of non-fatal MI in hospital or at six-month follow up.

Recent experimental findings have suggested that the nervous autonomic system can significantly modulate inflammatory reactions [Wang et al., 2003]. In particular, vagal stimulation has been shown to decrease inflammatory reactions in animals by inhibiting tissue macrophage activation, an effect mediated by stimulation of the alpha-7 subunit of the macrophage nicotine receptor by the vagal neurotransmitter acetylcholine, whereas adrenergic activity has been reported to favor sympathectomy and towards inflammatory reactions. Conversely, several products of inflammation have been shown to have potential influence on nervous autonomic activity by central and/or peripheral mechanisms [Lanza et al.,2006; Tracey,2002]. The low and no significant correlations between markers of endothelial activation and HRV in the present study emphasize that neural influence unlikely explained the observed predictive value of soluble adhesion molecules in patients with ACS.

ACS is a diffuse process involving the entire coronary vasculature [Buffon et al., 2002]. Although mechanical revascularization by percutaneous coronary intervention may address the culprit lesion, recurrent events may reflect disease progression or instability elsewhere in the vascular tree. Stabilization of vulnerable plaques or modulation of the so-called vulnerable patient is becoming recognized as an important target for systemic therapy [Libby&Aikawa 2003; Naghavi et al., 2003a, 2003b]. The rapid pleiotropic effects of statins on inflammation, endothelial function, and coagulation are likely to be particularly beneficial in patients with ACS in whom these systems are deranged.

Inhibition of HMG CoA reductase by statins inhibits cholesterol synthesis and isoprenoid production. This results in reduced prenylation of small G-proteins such as Rho and, in turn, NF-κB activation. By inhibiting HMG CoA reductase, statins can prevent the biosynthesis of isoprenoids such as farnesyl pyrophosphate and geranylgeranyl pyrophosphate. Inhibition of Rho geranylgeranylation by statins can reduce leukocyte adhesion and fibronolytic activity [Rasmussen et al., 2003; Yoshida et al.,2001]. A recent report suggests additional mechanism which is independent of mevalonate production - statins bind to a novel allosteric site within the ß2-integrin leukocyte function–associated antigen–1 (LFA- 1), preventing binding to the counterreceptor on the endothelial surface (ICAM-1) [Weitz-Schmidt et al., 2001].

In addition, statins can induce endothelial nitric oxide synthase (eNOS) accumulation in endothelial cells, an effect dependent on the inhibition of Rho geranylgeranylation, reduce the activation of monocyte/macrophage system, the cytotoxicity of T-lymphocytes and the balance between Th-1/Th-2 subclass. Hence, statins modify the immune response in ACS via reductions in inflammatory cell number, adhesion, and activation at potentially vulnerable sites along the wall [Liao, 2002; Libby&Aikawa 2003].

In animal models HMG-CoA reductase inhibitors have been shown to reduce renal sympathetic nerve traffic [Pliquett et al., 2003]. To date, the underlying mechanism by which statins reduce sympathetic outflow has not been elucidated. An effect on central nitric oxide (NO) and reactive oxygen species (ROS) formation, as well as regulation of the AT1-receptor expression, have been proposed as possible explanations [Gao et al., 2005; Gomes et al., 2010; Hirooka et al., 2010; Patel et al., 2001].

Contradictory results have been published about the effect of statins on sICAM-1 and sVCAM-1 plasma/serum concentrations in patients with various clinical manifestation of ischemic heart disease. In a number of small population studies, different authors have noted that treatment with statins diminished sICAM-1 concentrations in subjects with hypercholesterolemia or CHD [Ascer et al., 2004; Patti et al., 2006]. However, Wiklund et al., 2002 observed a small and inconsistent effect of simvastatin and atorvastatin treatment in hypercholesterolemic patients. Furthermore, Jilma et al., 2003, demonstrated that atorvastatin, simvastatin, or pravastatin did not modify sICAM-1 concentrations after 3 months of treatment in subjects with moderate hypercholesterolemia. Blanco-Colio et al. 2007, investigate the effect of 10-, 20-, 40- and 80 mg Atorvastatin on sICAM-1 and MCP-1 levels in 2117 patients with CHD in Achieve Cholesterol Targets Fast with Atorvastatin Stratified Titration Trial and didn't found statistically significant differences between the various doses used. Although atorvastatin had a weak effect on sICAM-1 concentrations in the whole population [-2.2 % change (95% confidence interval -3.8 to -0.6%); P =.006], in the highest quartile all doses of atorvastatin diminished sICAM-1 plasma levels by more than 10% in subjects at high cardiovascular risk, indicating that atorvastatin has a greater effect in subjects with higher systemic inflammation. In the large PROVE-IT TIMI 22 study Ray et al. 2006 didn't found significant difference between intensive (80 mg Atorvastatin) and standart (40 mg Pravastatin) regiment on sICAM-1 levels at 30 days. However, when considered the relation among statin therapy, sICAM-1 levels, and clinical outcomes, the authors found that the risk of adverse events for patients with a sICAM-1 level >231 ng/ml appeared more marked among those allocated to standard dose statin therapy (each odds ratio >2.1). The observed pattern raises the hypothesis that the risk associated with sICAM-1 may be attenuated by treatment with intensive statin therapy (each odds ratio <1.5).

In this study we have analyzed the effect of two rosuvastatin regimens on sICAM-1 and sVCAM-1 concentration in patients with high risk ACS defined by the levels of soluble adhesion molecules. We observed that the treatment with rosuvastatin diminish both markers of endothelial activation during 12 week follow-up. We found out a trend towards lower concentrations of sICAM-1 in patients randomized to 20 mg Rosuvastatin, in addition to the previously observed significant lowering of low-density lipoprotein and C-reactive protein. There was no correlation between sCAMs and low-density lipoprotein and hsCRP at month 3 and the effect of rosuvastatin on soluble CAMs did not appear to be explained by changes in lipids or inflammatory markers.

However, standart statin therapy did not significantly alter sVCAM-1 levels at 3 months. The present observations with sVCAM-1 are analogous to the observations with aspirin and clopidogrel in which each drug decreases the risk of adverse clinical events in subjects with high CRP levels but do not decrease CRP significantly [Chew et al., 2001; Kennon et al., 2001; Ridker et al., 1997]. A potential mechanistic explanation for our clinical observations is, that among subjects with increased endothelial activation, a more potent statin regimen could bind to lymphocyte function-associated antigen-1 on inflammatory cells to a greater extent, thus interfering with downstream effects of increased endothelial activation rather than decreasing endothelial activation itself. This hypothesis raises the possibility that novel therapeutic strategies that target inhibition of adhesion molecules may be of benefit in ACS, as has been demonstrated in animal models and in patients with inflammatory bowel disease [Gill et al., 2005; Van Assche et al., 2005].

An interesting finding was the observed beneficial effect of more intense statin regiment on some parameters of autonomic function. During the study period we found out a significant increase of high frequency component with represents the parasympathetic contribution to the spectrum, whereas low frequency remained unchanged. As a result, the LF/HF ratio, measure of autonomic balance was reduced significantly in patients received 20 mg Rosuvastatin. The results of the correlation analysis clearly suggest that some of the beneficial effects of more potent statin dose may be driven by the effect on endothelial and autonomic function [Lanza et al., 2006; Patti et al., 2006]. Supports for this hypothesis are the results of the meta-analysis of Patti et al, who found that high-dose statin pretreatment before percutaneous coronary intervention leads to a significant reduction in periprocedural myocardial infarction and 30-day adverse events. It is noteworthy that the effect is most pronounced, but is not limited in patients with elevated markers of inflammatory activity [Patti et al., 2011]. Our findings must be confirmed by larger studies. It may contribute to the achievement of specific treatment goals for each patient with proper drug selection and dose titration in high risk patients such as those with elevated markers of endothelial activation and depressed HRV.

5. Conclusions

In patients with ACS, soluble adhesion molecules are independent predictors of subsequent MACE and reduced HRV of medium-term mortality, suggesting that markers of endothelial activation and impaired autonomic function should be taken into account in the risk stratification of these patients.

Our findings support the hypothesis that statins decrease endothelial injury and activation in patients with acute coronary syndromes. In addition we found that more aggressive regiment with early initiation of 20 mg Rosuvastatin significantly decreases sICAM-1 levels and better preserve parasympathetically mediated variable of HRV. Future studies are required to elucidate the optimal dose of statin treatment in patients with ACS and high levels of markers of inflammatory and endothelial activation or impaired autonomic function.

6. References

Ascer E, Bertolami MC, Venturinelli ML, et al (2004). Atorvastatin reduces proinflammatory markers in hypercholesterolemic patients. *Atherosclerosis*, Vol. 177, pp. 161 -6.

Bigger JT, Weld FM, Rolnitzki LM (1981). Prevalence, characteristics and significance of ventricular tachycardia (three or more complexes) detected with ambulatory electrocardiographic recording in the late hospital phase of acute myocardial infarction. *Am J Cardiol*, Vol. 48, pp.815–23.

Bigger JT, Fleiss JL, Steinman RC, et al (1992). Frequency-domain measures of heart period variability and mortality after myocardial infarction. *Circulation*, Vol. 85, pp. 164–71.

Blankenberg S, Rupprecht HJ, Bickel C, Peetz D, Hafner G, Tiret L, et al. (2001) Circulating cell adhesion molecules and death in patients with coronary artery disease. *Circulation* , Vol. 104: pp. 1336–42.

Blankenberg S, Barbaux S, Tiret L (2003). Adhesion molecules and atherosclerosis. *Atherosclerosis*, Vol. 170, pp. 191-203

Blanco-Colio LM, Martın-Ventura JL, de Teresa E, Farsang C, Gaw A, et all of the ACTFAST investigators (2007). Elevated ICAM-1 and MCP-1 plasma levels in subjects at high cardiovascular risk are diminished by atorvastatin treatment. Atorvastatin on Inflammatory Markers study: A substudy of Achieve Cholesterol Targets Fast with Atorvastatin Stratified Titration. *Am Heart J*, Vol. 153, pp. 881-8.

Buffon A, Biasucci LM, Liuzzo G, D'Onofrio G, Crea F, Maseri A (2002). Widespread coronary inflammation in unstable angina. *N Engl J Med*, Vol. 347, pp. 5–12.

Chew DP, Bhatt DL, Robbins MA, Mukherjee D, Roffi M, Schneider JP, Topol EJ, Ellis SG (2001). Effect of clopidogrel added to aspirin before percutaneous coronary intervention on the risk associated with C-reactive protein. *Am J Cardiol*, Vol.88, pp.672- 674.

Cybulsky MI&Gimbronejr MA (1991). Endothelial expression of a mononuclear leukocyte adhesion molecule during atherogenesis. *Science*, Vol. 251, pp. 788–91.

Cybulsky MI, Iiyama K, Li H et al (2001). A major role for VCAM-1, but not ICAM-1, in early atherosclerosis. *J Clin Invest*, Vol. 107, pp. 1255-1262

de Lemos JA, Hennekens CH, Ridker PM (2000). Plasma concentration of soluble vascular cell adhesion molecule-1 and subsequent cardiovascular risk. *J Am Coll Cardiol*, Vol. 36, pp. 423–6.

Farrell TG, Bashir Y, Cripps T, et al.(1991). Risk stratification for arrhythmic events in postinfarction patients based on heart rate variability, ambulatory electrocardiographic variables and the signal-averaged electrocardiogram. *J Am Coll Cardiol*, Vol. 18, pp. 687–97.

Fuster V.&Lewis A. (1994). Conner Memorial Lecture. Mechanisms leading to myocardial infarction: insights from studies of vascular biology. *Circulation*, Vol. 90, pp. 2126-2146.

Gao L, Wang W, Li YL, Schultz HD, Liu D, Cornish KG, et al (2005). Simvastatin therapy normalizes sympathetic neural control in experimental heart failure: Roles of angiotensin II type 1 receptors and NAD(P)H oxidase. *Circulation*, Vol. 112, pp.1763 - 1770.

Gill V, Doig C, Knight D, Love E, Kubes P (2005). Targeting adhesion molecules as a potential mechanism of action for intravenous immunoglobulin. *Circulation*, Vol. 112, pp. 2031–2039.

Gomes, ME; Tack, CT; Verheugt, FW at al (2010). Sympathoinhibition by Atorvastatin in Hypertensive Patients. *Circ J*, Vol. 74, pp. 2622 - 2626

Hartikainen JEK, Malik M, Staunton A, et al (1996). Distinction between arrhythmic and nonarrhythmic death after acute myocardial infarction based on heart rate variability, signal-averaged electrocardiogram, ventricular arrhythmias and left ventricular ejection fraction. *J Am Coll Cardiol*, Vol. 28, pp. 296–304.

Hillis GS&Flapan AD (1998). Cell adhesion molecules in cardiovascular disease: a clinical perspective. *Heart* , Vol. 79, pp. 429- 431.

Hirooka Y, Sagara Y, Kishi T, Sunagawa K (2010). Oxidative stress and central cardiovascular regulation: Pathogenesis of hypertension and therapeutic aspects. *Circ J*, Vol. 74, pp. 827 - 835.

Hwang SJ, Ballantyne CM, Sharrett AR, Smith LC, Davis CE, Gottojr AM, et al. (1997). Circulating adhesion molecules VCAM-1, ICAM-1 and E-selectin in carotid atherosclerosis and incident coronary heart disease cases: the Atherosclerosis Risk In Communities (ARIC) study. *Circulation*, Vol. 96, pp. 4219–25.

Jager A, van Hinsbergh VW, Kostense PJ, Emeis JJ, Nijpels G, Dekker JM, et al. (2000) Increased levels of soluble vascular cell adhesion molecule 1 are associated with risk of cardiovascular mortality in type 2 diabetes: the Hoorn study. *Diabetes*, Vol. 49, pp. 485–91.

Jang Y, Lincoff AM, Plow EF, Topol EJ (1994). Cell adhesion molecules in coronary artery disease. *J Am Coll Cardiol* , Vol. 24, pp. 1591- 601.

Jilma B, Joukhadar C, Derhasching U, et al (2003). Levels of adhesion molecules do not decrease after 3 months of statin therapy in moderate hypercholesterolemia. *Clin Sci (Lond)*, Vol. 104, pp. 189 - 93.

Kennon S, Price CP, Mills PG, Ranjadayalan K, Cooper J, Clarke H, Timmis AD (2001). The effect of aspirin on C-reactive protein as a marker of risk in unstable angina. *J Am Coll Cardiol*, Vol. 37, pp. 1266 –1270.

Kennon S, Price CP, Mills PG et al (2003). Cumulative risk assessment in unstable angina: clinical, electrocardiographic, autonomic, and biochemical markers. *Heart*, Vol. 89, pp36-41

Kent KM, Smith ER, Redwood DR, et al (1973). Electrical stability of acutely ischemic myocardium: influences of heart rate and vagal stimulation. *Circulation*, Vol. 47, pp. 291–8.

Kinlay S, Schwartz GG, Olsson AG, et al. (2003). Myocardial Ischemia Reduction with Aggressive Cholesterol Lowering Study Investigators. High-dose atorvastatin enhances the decline in inflammatory markers in patients with acute coronary syndromes in the MIRACL study. *Circulation*, Vol. 108, pp. 1560–1566.

Kleiger RE, Miller JP, Bigger JT et al., The Multicenter Postinfarction Research Group, (1987). Decreased heart rate variability and its association with increased mortality after acute myocardial infarction. *Am J Cardiol*, Vol. 59, pp. 256–62.

Kostis JB, Friedman LM, Goldstein S et al., for the BHATB Study Group, (1987). Prognostic significance of ventricular ectopic activity in survivors of acute myocardial infarction. *J Am Coll Cardiol*, Vol. 10, pp. 231–42.

Lanza GA, Guido V, Galeazzi MM, et al (1998). Prognostic role of heart rate variability in patients with a recent acute myocardial infarction. *Am J Cardiol*, Vol. 82, pp. 1323–8.

Lanza GA, Cianflone D, Rebuzzi AG, et al. for the Stratificazione Prognostica dell'Angina Instabile Study Investigators (2006). Prognostic value of ventricular arrhythmias and heart rate variability in patients with unstable angina. *Heart*, Vol. 92, pp.1055-1063;

Lanza, GA, Sguegliaa GA, Cianflone D et al. for the SPAI (Stratificazione Prognostica dell'Angina Instabile) Investigators (2006). Relation of Heart Rate Variability to Serum Levels of C-Reactive Protein in Patients With Unstable Angina Pectoris. *Am J Cardiol*, Vol. 97, pp. 1702–1706

La Rovere MT, Bigger JT Jr, Marcus FI, et al (1998). Baroreflex sensitivity and heart rate variability in prediction of total cardiac mortality after myocardial infarction. ATRAMI (autonomic tone and reflexes after myocardial infarction) investigators. *Lancet*, Vol. 351, pp.478–84.

Leuwenberg JF, Smeets EF, Neefjes JJ et al (1992). E-selectin and intercellular adhesion molecule-1 are relased by activated human endothelial cells in vitro. *Immunology*, Vol. 77, pp. 543-9.

Liao JK (2002). Beyond lipid lowering: the role of statins in vascular protection. *Int J Cardiol*, Vol. 86, pp. 5–18.

Libby P. (2001). Current concepts of the pathogenesis of the acute coronary syndromes. *Circulation*, Vol. 104, pp. 365-372

Libby P&Aikawa M (2003). Mechanisms of plaque stabilization with statins. *Am J Cardiol*, Vol. 91(suppl 4A), pp. 4B–8B.

Mulvihill N, Foley JB, Murphy R et al (2000). Evidence of prolonged inflammation in unstable angina and non Q wave myocardial infarction. *J Am Coll Cardiol*, Vol. 36, pp 1210-6.

Mulvihill N, Foley JB, Murphy R et al (2001). Risk stratification in unstable angina and non-Q-wave myocardial infarction using soluble cell adhesion molecules. *Heart*, Vol. 85, pp. 623-627

Mulvihill N, Foley JB, Crean P, Walsh M (2002). Prediction of cardiovascular risk using soluble cell adhesion molecules. *Eur Heart J*, Vol. 23, pp. 1569-1574

Naghavi M, Libby P, Falk E, Casscells SW, Litovsky S, Rumberger J, Badimon JJ, Stefanadis C, Moreno P, Pasterkamp G, et al (2003). From vulnerable plaque to vulnerable patient: a call for new definitions and risk assessment strategies, part I. *Circulation*, Vol. 108, pp. 1664 -1672.

Naghavi M, Libby P, Falk E, Casscells SW, Litovsky S, Rumberger J, Badimon JJ, Stefanadis C, Moreno P, Pasterkamp G, et al (2003). From vulnerable plaque to vulnerable patient: a call for new definitions and risk assessment strategies, part II. *Circulation*, Vol. 108, pp. 1772–1778.

O'Brien KD, Allen MD, McDonald TO, Chait A, Harlan JM,Fishbein D, et al. (1993). Vascular cell adhesion molecule-1 is expressed inhuman coronary atherosclerotic plaques.

Implications for the mode of progression of advanced coronary atherosclerosis. *J Clin Invest,* Vol. 92, pp. 945–51.

O'Malley T, Ludlam CA, Riemermsa RA, Fox K (2001). Early increase in levels of soluble intercellular adhesion molecule-1 (sICAM-1). Potential risk factor for the acute coronary syndromes. *Eur Heart J,* Vol. 22, pp. 1226-34

Patel KP, Li YF, Hirooka Y (2001). Role of nitric oxide in central sympathetic outflow. *Exp Biol Med,* Vol. 226, pp. 814 - 824.

Patti G, Chello M, Pasceri V, et al (2006). Protection from procedural myocardial injury by atorvastatin is associated with lower levels of adhesion molecules after percutaneous coronary intervention. *J Am Coll Cardiol,* Vol. 48, pp. 1560 -6.

Patti G, Cannon C, Murphy SA et al (2011). Clinical benefit of statin pretreatment in patients undergoing percutaneous coronary intervention. A collaborative patient-level meta-analysis of 13 randomized studies. *Circulation,* Vol 123, pp 1622-1632.

Pigott R, Dillon LP, Hemingway IH et al. (1992). Soluble forms of ICAM-1 and VCAM-1 are present in the supernatants of cytokine activated cultured endothelial cells. *Biochem Biophys Res Comm,* Vol. 187, pp. 584-9.

Pliquett RU, Cornish KG, Peuler JD, Zucker IH (2003). Simvastatin normalizes Autonomic neural control in experimental heart failure. *Circulation,* Vol. 107, pp.2493 - 2498.

Rasmussen LM, Hansen PR, Nabipour MT, et al. (2001). Diverse effects of inhibition of 3-hydroxy-3-methylglutaryl-CoA reductase on the expression of VCAM-1 and E-selectin in endothelial cells. *Biochem J,* Vol. 360, pp. 363–370.

Ray KK &Cannon CP (2005). Early Time to Benefit with Intensive Statin Treatment: Could It Be the Pleiotropic Effects? *Am J Cardiol,* Vol. 96 [suppl F], pp. 54F–60F

Ray KK, Morrow DA, Shui A, et al (2006). Relation between soluble intercellular adhesion molecule-1, statin therapy, and long-term risk of clinical cardiovascular events in patients with previous acute coronary syndrome (from PROVE IT-TIMI 22). *Am J Cardiol,* Vol. 98, pp.861 -5.

Ridker PM, Cushman M, Stampfer MJ, Tracy RP, Hennekens CH (1997). Inflammation, aspirin, and the risk of cardiovascular disease in apparently healthy men. *N Engl J Med,* Vol. 336, pp. 973–979.

Ridker PM, Hennekens CH, Roitman-Johnson B, et al. (1998). Plasma concentration of soluble intercellular adhesion molecule 1 and risks of future myocardial infarction in apparently healthy men. *Lancet,* Vol. 351, pp. 88–92.

Ridker PM, Hennekens CH, Buring JE, Rifai N (2000). C-reactive protein and other markers of inflammation in the prediction of cardiovascular disease in women. *New Engl J Med* , Vol. 342, pp. 836–43.

Ridker PM, Cannon CP, Morrow D, et al. (2005). Pravastatin or Atorvastatin Evaluation and Infection Therapy-Thrombolysis in Myocardial Infarction 22 (PROVE IT-TIMI 22) Investigators. C-reactive protein levels and outcomes after statin therapy. N *Engl J Med,* Vol. 352, pp. 20–28

Schwartz PJ, Vanoli E, Stramba-Badiale M, et al (1988). Autonomic mechanisms and sudden death: new insights from analysis of baroreceptor reflexes in conscious dogs with and without a myocardial infarction. *Circulation,* Vol. 78, pp. 969–79.

Seljeflot I, Tonstad S, Hjermann I, et al (2002). Reduced expression of endothelial cell markers after 1 year treatment with simvastatin and atorvastatin in patients with coronary heart disease. *Atherosclerosis,* Vol. 162, pp. 179 - 85.

Task Force of the European Society of Cardiology and the North American Society of Pacing and Electrophysiology (1996). Heart rate variability: standards of measurement, physiological interpretation and clinical use. *Circulation*, Vol. 93, pp.1043–65.

Tracey KJ (2002). The inflammatory reflex. *Nature*, Vol. 420, pp. 853– 859.

Tsuji H, Venditti FJ Jr, Manders ES, et al (1996). Determinants of heart rate variability. *J Am Coll Cardiol*, Vol. 28, pp. 1539–46.

Van Assche G& Rutgeerts P. (2005). Physiological basis for novel drug therapies used to treat the inflammatory bowel diseases. I. Immunology and therapeutic potential of antiadhesion molecule therapy in inflammatory bowel disease. *Am J Physiol Gastrointest Liver Physiol*, Vol. 288(suppl), pp. G169–G174.

Wang H, Yu M, Ochani M, et al (2003). Nicotinic acetylcholine receptor alpha7 subunit is an essential regulator of inflammation. *Nature*, Vol. 421, pp. 384 –388.

Weitz-Schmidt G, Welzenbach K, Brinkmann V, et al (2001). Statins selectively inhibit leukocyte function antigen-1 by binding to a novel regulatory integrin site. *Nat Med*, Vol. 7, pp. 687–92.

Wiklund O, Mattson-Hulten L, Hurt-Camejo E, et al (2002). Effects of simvastatin and atorvastatin on inflammatory markers in plasma. *J Intern Med*, Vol. 251, pp. 338 - 47.

Yoshida M, Sawada T, Ishii H, et al. (2001). HMG-CoA reductase inhibitor modulates monocyte-endothelial cell interaction under physiological flow conditions in vitro: involvement of Rho GTPase-dependent mechanism. *Arterioscler Thromb Vasc Biol*, Vol. 21, pp. 1165–1171.

14

Acute Coronary Syndrome from Angioscopic Viewpoint

Yasunori Ueda
Osaka Police Hospital, Osaka, Japan

1. Introduction

Acute coronary syndrome (ACS), i.e. acute myocardial infarction (MI) and unstable angina, is a life threatening disease, and its treatment after onset has greatly improved; however, we are not satisfied with the long-term outcome of the patients with ACS. Furthermore, we cannot adequately prevent the onset of ACS, although we know many risk factors of ACS, e.g. diabetes mellitus, dyslipidemia, hypertension, obesity, and smoking.

As plaque disruption and thrombosis is known as the major cause of ACS, many investigations to identify vulnerable plaques that are prone to disrupt have been performed but failed to identify high-risk lesions of future ACS event. Major reason for this failure may be that disruption of plaques does not always cause ACS and probably very few percentages of disrupted plaques may actually cause ACS. In order to know adequately about the mechanisms for the onset of ACS and to prevent it effectively, we have to clarify those missing factors that are essential for the disrupted plaques to cause ACS.

In this chapter, we would like to elucidate and discuss on the known and unknown mechanisms for the onset of ACS from the angioscopic point of view.

2. Culprit lesions of acute coronary syndrome

The culprit lesions of ACS[1, 2] have disrupted yellow plaque and thrombus in >90% of cases. The surface of the yellow plaques is irregular and has the adhesion of white or mixed thrombus. The plaque is defined as ruptured[3, 4] if the protrusion of yellow necrotic core is observed; otherwise, it is defined as eroded (or non-ruptured). Thrombus[2] directly adhering to the plaque surface is usually white, and it becomes reddish when blood flow is disturbed by massive white thrombus and the fibrin network captures many red blood cells in it, i.e. mixed or red thrombus. In the same way, thrombus becomes yellow when the fibrin network of white thrombus contains protruded necrotic core, i.e. yellow thrombus.

After reperfusion therapy[1] or coronary intervention with balloon or stent, the culprit lesion of ACS gradually loses its thrombogenicity. In the patients with acute MI, 64% of patients still have thrombus at their culprit lesion at one month after reperfusion, while it becomes as low as 5% at 6 months. The prevalence of thrombus at one month is higher in the patients with diabetic patients than in the non-diabetic patients (78% vs. 45%), suggesting that the healing process of disrupted plaque is deteriorated in the diabetic patients.

As >90% of ACS patients have disrupted yellow plaque in their culprit lesions, both ruptured and eroded plaques, which are detected in about 70% and 30% of cases, respectively, by pathologic studies, should be detected as yellow plaques[5]. We have recently revealed[4] that both ruptured and non-ruptured yellow plaques detected by angioscopy have similar atherosclerotic characteristics including thin-cap fibroatheroma (TCFA) when examined by VH-IVUS (Figure 1).

3. Detection of vulnerable plaques by angioscopy

Because the majority of ACS culprit lesions have disrupted yellow plaques, yellow plaques should be the vulnerable plaques that are prone to disrupt. Yellow plaques are classified into 3 grades[6] according to its yellow color intensity: grade 1, slight yellow; grade 2, yellow; and grade 3, intensive yellow (Figure 2). We have revealed that yellow plaques of higher yellow color grade have the higher incidence of having thrombus on it, i.e. higher incidence of disruption, suggesting that those plaques are more vulnerable. Furthermore, the yellow plaques of higher yellow color grade have the higher incidence of positive remodeling and the thinner fibrous cap[7], which supports the idea that those yellow plaques are more vulnerable.

Although we have experienced >5,000 cases of angioscopic examinations and found huge number of yellow plaques, it was quite rare that the plaque caused ACS shortly after the examination. However, the prospective follow-up of the angioscopically examined patients have revealed[8] that patients with more than 2 yellow plaques per vessel have the higher incidence of ACS event than the patients with 1 or no yellow plaque per vessel during the mean follow-up interval of 4.8 years. Formation of yellow plaques occurs equally in the culprit and non-culprit vessels of MI as it is regarded pan-coronary process of atherosclerosis progression[9] (Figure 3). Therefore, the patients who have many yellow plaques in their coronary arteries are regarded as vulnerable patients. Judging from the results of this and other angioscopic studies, the probability of each yellow plaque to disrupt and to cause ACS may be estimated[5] as 25%/year and 0.3-1%/year, respectively.

4. Silent plaque disruption and missing factors for the onset of acute coronary syndrome

Disrupted yellow plaques are sometimes found in the asymptomatic patients or in the non-culprit segments of ACS patients, which are called silent plaque disruptions[10, 11]. Factors required for the disrupted plaques to cause symptomatic ACS are unknown, which is an important but unsolved issue for clarifying the mechanism of ACS onset. However, thrombogenic potential of blood, thrombogenic potential of necrotic core that would be exposed to blood by plaque rupture, underlying stenosis or stenosis caused by the protrusion of necrotic core at the site of plaque rupture, and/or vasoconstriction may play a role for the onset of ACS after the disruption of vulnerable plaques[12]. Investigations to clarify the contributions of these or other factors have not been reported adequately. Although the thrombogenicity of blood, i.e. vulnerable blood, has been regarded one of important factors, reports on this issue are limited. We have recently reported[13] that originally defined parameter of blood thrombogenicity (blood vulnerability index) is significantly and extremely higher in the patients with acute MI than in the patients with stable coronary heart disease.

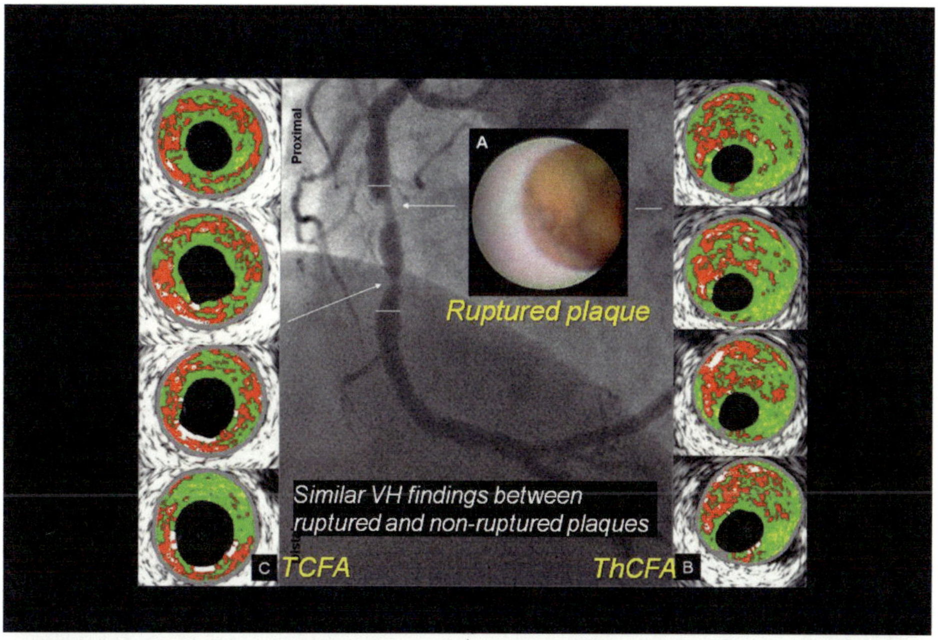

A

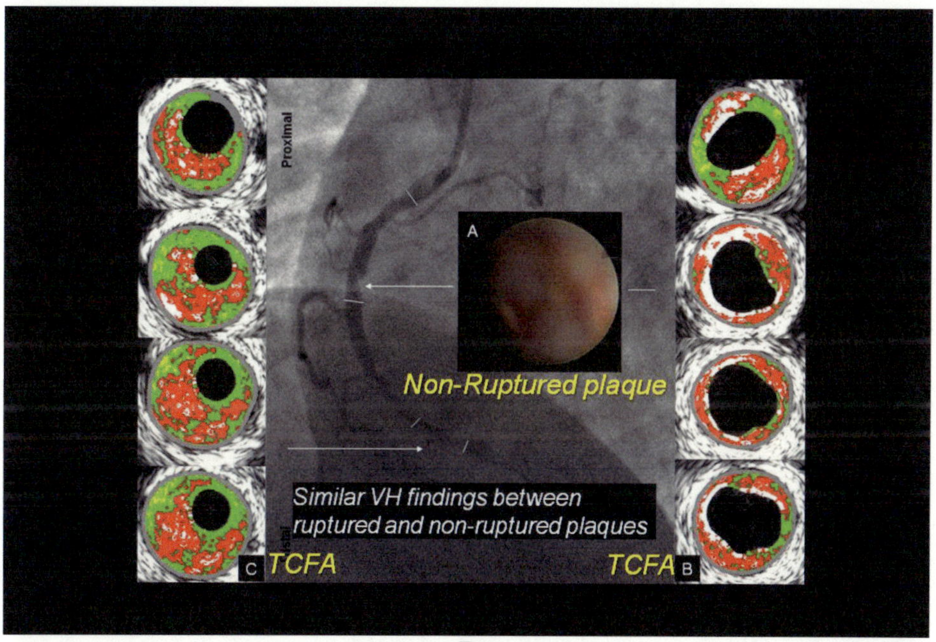

B

Most of ACS culprit lesions have disrupted yellow plaque, which is classified into ruptured or non-ruptured yellow plaque by angioscopy. Non-rupture would include small rupture and erosion of pathologic classifications. Both of ruptured and non-ruptured yellow plaques have similar atherosclerotic characteristics by VH-IVUS. (From reference #4)

Fig. 1. Culprit lesions of ACS

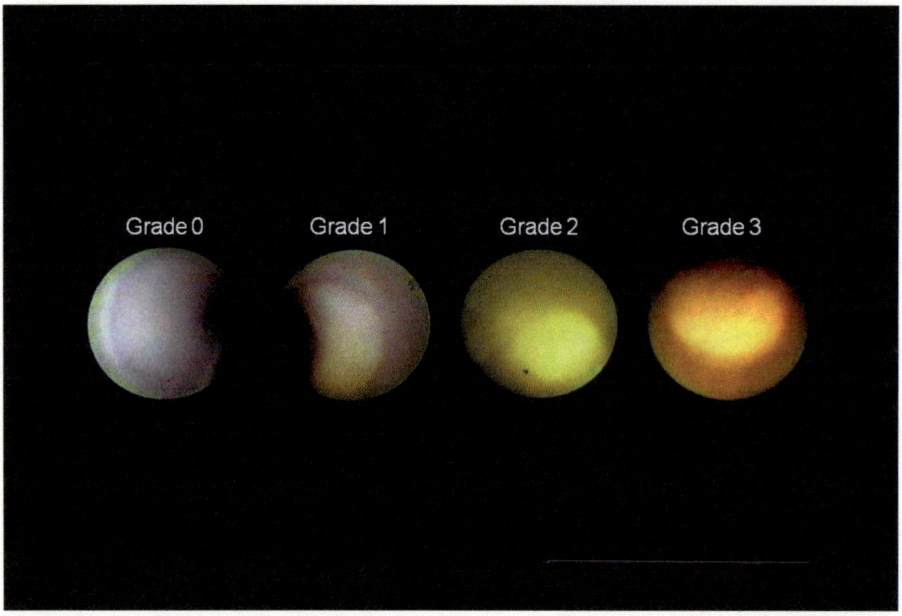

Yellow plaques are classified into 3 grades according to these standard colors: grade 1, slight yellow; grade 2, yellow; and grade 3, intensive yellow. Grade 0 indicates white color. Yellow plaques of the higher grade are regarded more vulnerable as they have higher frequency of plaque disruption. (From reference #6)

Fig. 2. Classification of yellow plaques according to their color

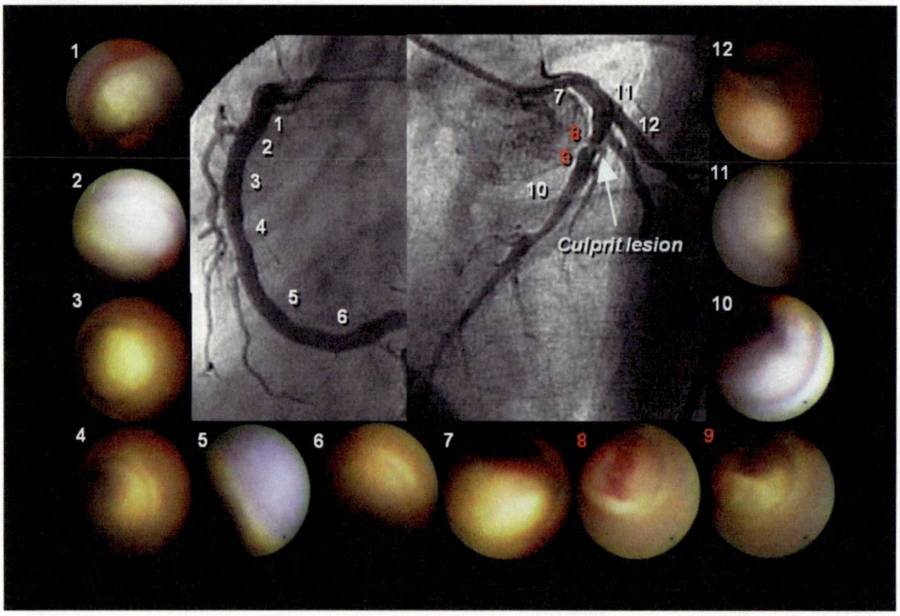

The yellow plaque at the culprit lesion is disrupted having thrombus on it. There are multiple yellow plaques in the non-culprit segments both in culprit and non-culprit vessels. The formation of yellow plaques is regarded pan-coronary process. (From reference #9)

Fig. 3. Coronary arteries in acute MI patients

5. Stent thrombosis and atherosclerosis

Bare metal stent (BMS) is gradually covered by neointima and the coverage is usually completed by 3-6 months after implantation[14]. Neointima at 3-6 months is generally white and its surface is smooth; and stent is not seen buried under neointima. Yellow plaques under stent are also covered and buried under the neointima. Neointima becomes thinner and rather transparent at about 3 years again[15], although its surface is smooth and thrombus is not detected on its surface. Therefore, the implantation of BMS stabilizes the vulnerable plaques by the formation of thick fibrous neointima over the plaques, which is called sealing effect of BMS. It takes about 10 years for the formation of vulnerable plaques in the fibrous healthy neointima over BMS leading to its disruption and onset of ACS. Very late stent thrombosis (VLST) in the BMS is indeed quite rare especially within a few years after implantation.

On the other hand, neointima formation over drug-eluting stent (DES) is generally very poor[16, 17]; and stent is usually seen through very thin neointima or partly uncovered in the majority of cases (Figure 4). The incidence of thrombus at the stented lesion is significantly higher in the 1st generation DES (Cypher and Taxus DES) than in BMS. Furthermore, the stented lesions become yellow after Cypher DES implantation[17, 18], suggesting that DES promotes progression of atherosclerosis (Figure 5). However, Endeavor DES is known to have larger late loss but have as good neointima formation as observed in BMS; and thrombus is rarely detected in this DES. Although the angioscopic findings on the newer DES has not been fully clarified, Xience V and Nobori DES appear to have as thin neointima as 1st generation DES but have lower incidence of thrombus than 1st generation DES.

The mechanisms for the onset of VLST have not been fully clarified; however, uncovered stent strut, uncovered disrupted plaque, new disruption of uncovered yellow plaque, and new disruption of newly formed yellow plaque may be the probable thrombogenic sources[19] that can cause VLST. After BMS and Endeavor DES implantation, thick and white fibrous neointima completely covers stent and plaques; and the incidence of VLST is known to be very low. However, as the neointima over Xience V and Nobori DES is thin and may not reduce the risk of new yellow plaque disruption, we should be careful about the incidence of VLST after the implantation of these stents. From the angioscopic point of view, Endeavor DES would be the safest DES among the DES examined by angioscopy. BMS that has not developed restenosis would be the best condition that should be achieved by newly developed DES in the future, i.e. complete coverage by rather thick white smooth neointima.

6. Regression of vulnerable plaques by statin treatment

Statin treatment is known to reduce both plaque volume evaluated by IVUS and yellow color evaluated by angioscopy[20, 21]. However, it has not been clarified which of plaque volume and plaque color is more directly associated with the risk of plaque disruption or the risk of ACS. According to the results of TWINS study[20], yellow color of plaques regressed significantly from baseline to 28 weeks but did not change thereafter until 80 weeks under atorvastatin treatment; on the other hand, plaque volume decreased gradually but significantly from baseline to 28 weeks and to 80 weeks. Early effect of statin treatment to reduce the risk of ACS might be reflected by the early regression of yellow color.

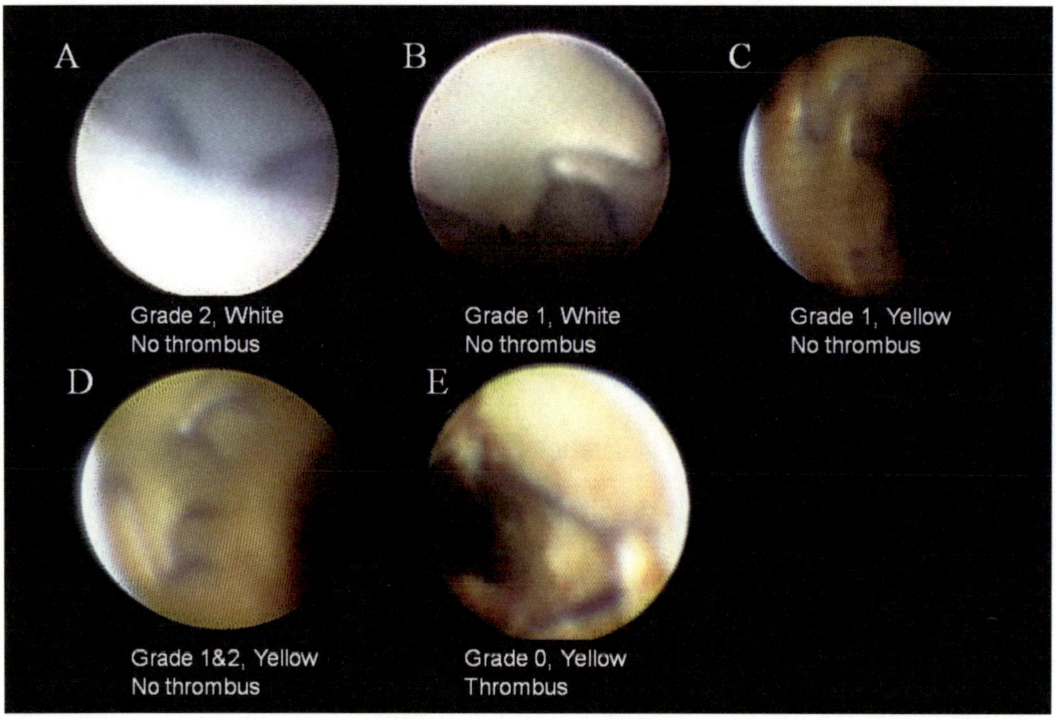

Various conditions of neointima coverage are observed at 1-year follow-up after DES implantation. A: White and good (grade 2) neointima coverage is observed without thrombus formation. B: Thin (grade 1) neointima coverage is observed without thrombus formation; and the vessel wall under stent is white. C: Thin (grade 1) neointima coverage is observed without thrombus formation; however, the vessel wall under stent is yellow. D: Neointima coverage grade is partly 1 and partly 2. Both of vessel wall under stent and neointima over stent are yellow. Yellow atherosclerotic neointima is often observed after Cypher stent implantation but never after BMS implantation. E: Uncovered stent strut is observed on the yellow disrupted plaque. Thrombus is detected on the yellow plaque and on the stent strut. (From reference #17)

Fig. 4. Angioscopic appearance of DES implanted lesions at follow-up

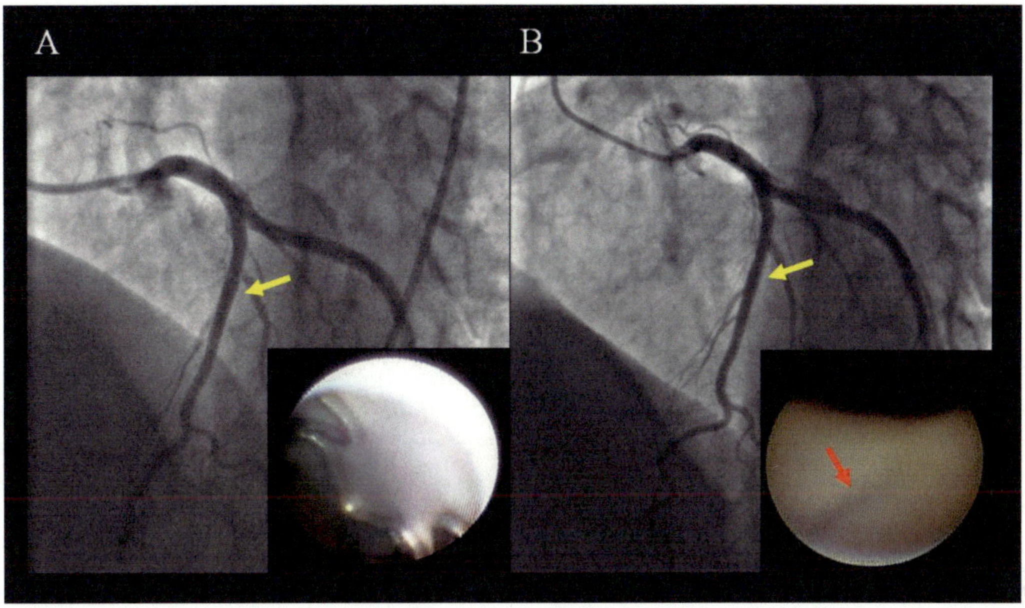

Cypher stent was implanted on a white vessel wall (A). However, at 1-year follow-up (B), neointima that covered the stent was yellow, suggesting the early formation of atherosclerosis in the neointima. Yellow arrow indicates where the stent was implanted. Red arrow indicates the stent strut. (From reference #17)

Fig. 5. Rapid progression of atherosclerosis in the neointima after DES implantation

7. Investigation of missing factors and hypothesis on the mechanisms of ACS onset

According to the results of PROSPECT trial[22], in addition to the presence of TCFA, large plaque burden and narrow minimum lumen area were the risk of future coronary event. Although ACS is known to occur from angiographically mild to moderate stenosis, findings in PROSPECT trial may be consistent with this. Underlying stenosis that can be detected only by IVUS and large plaque burden that may cause abrupt progression of stenosis on rupturing may be important for the onset of ACS. Presence of relatively severe stenosis might be essential for the formation of occlusive thrombus at the disrupted plaque. The larger necrotic core might possibly have the higher thrombogenicity; however, there are very few investigations on the difference of necrotic core thrombogenicity. Vasoconstriction has been speculated to play an important role, although no investigation has ever demonstrated its contribution to the onset of ACS. We have reported[13] that blood thrombogenicity (blood vulnerability index) is significantly and extremely higher in the patients with acute MI than in the patients with stable coronary heart disease. This high blood thrombogenicity might be either a cause or a result of ACS. However, none of stable coronary heart disease patients including those who had silent plaque disruption had that high blood vulnerability index. Therefore, silent plaque disruption will never result in the extreme increase of blood vulnerability index. Furthermore, ACS patients who were taking dual antiplatelet therapy also had high blood vulnerability index, suggesting that dual antiplatelet therapy was not adequately effective to prevent this increase of blood vulnerability index and thus failed to prevent the onset of ACS.

Process of positive feedback and cyclic flow variation might play an important role for the onset of ACS: i.e. a plaque disruption causes thrombus formation that increases thrombogenicity of blood and more thrombus would be formed; if the occlusive thrombus is formed, it may cause cyclic flow variation depending on the severity of stenosis and the amount of thrombus formed, which may further increase the thrombogenicity of blood; and the thrombus may finally occlude the artery. In this process, the amount of thrombus must be influenced by the thrombogenicity of both blood and exposed necrotic core; and the severity of stenosis would be determined by the underlying stenosis, the stenosis increased by the protrusion of necrotic core on plaque rupturing, and the stenosis caused by vasoconstriction that may be induced by thrombus formation.

It is well known that silent plaque disruption is frequently detected in the patients with ACS[23], suggesting that plaque disruption and/or thrombogenesis is generally promoted in ACS patients (Figure 6). Blood thrombogenicity would be increased in ACS patients as mentioned above. Another idea is that coronary vessels generally have inflammation in ACS patients, i.e. coronary flu syndrome, which might possibly be the initiation mechanism of ACS.

These mechanisms should be examined more intensively by clinical and basic investigations; and blocking some of these steps may be able to prevent the onset of ACS.

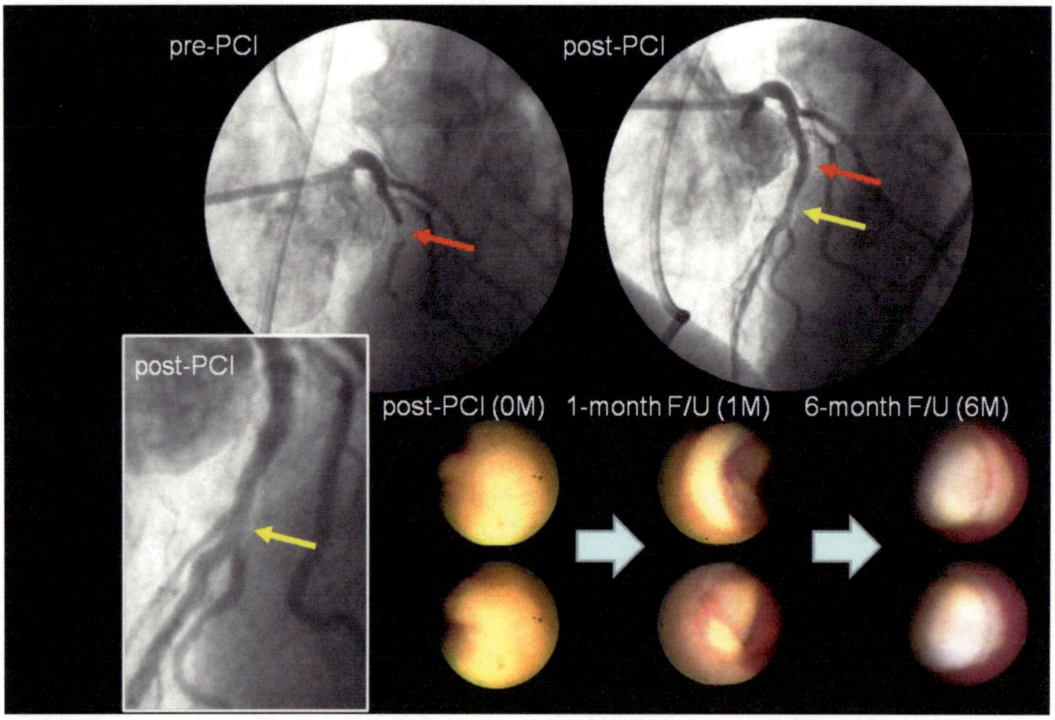

In a patient with acute MI (culprit lesion at red arrow), a silent plaque disruption (at yellow arrow) was detected. The healing process of silently disrupted yellow plaque was observed as the regression of yellow color intensity and the disappearance of thrombus by 6 months. (From reference #23)

Fig. 6. Silent plaque disruption and its healing in the non-culprit segments in acute MI patients

8. References

[1] Ueda Y, Asakura M, Yamaguchi O, Hirayama A, Hori M, Kodama K. The healing process of infarct-related plaques. Insights from 18 months of serial angioscopic follow-up. J Am Coll Cardiol. 2001;38:1916-1922.

[2] Ueda Y, Asakura M, Hirayama A, Komamura K, Hori M, Kodama K. Intracoronary morphology of culprit lesions after reperfusion in acute myocardial infarction: serial angioscopic observations. J Am Coll Cardiol. 1996;27:606-610.

[3] Mizote I, Ueda Y, Ohtani T, Shimizu M, Takeda Y, Oka T, Tsujimoto M, Hirayama A, Hori M, Kodama K.. Distal protection improved reperfusion and reduced left ventricular dysfunction in patients with acute myocardial infarction who had angioscopically defined ruptured plaque. Circulation. 2005;112:1001-1007.

[4] Sanidas EA, Maehara A, Mintz GS, Kashiyama T, Guo J, Pu J, Shang Y, Claessen B, Dangas GD, Leon MB, Moses JW, Stone GW, Ueda Y. Angioscopic and virtual histology intravascular ultrasound characteristics of culprit lesion morphology underlying coronary artery thrombosis. Am J Cardiol. 2011;107:1285-1290.

[5] Ueda Y, Ogasawara N, Matsuo K, Hirotani S, Kashiwase K, Hirata A, Nishio M, Nemoto T, Wada M, Masumura Y, Kashiyama T, Konishi S, Nakanishi H, Kobayashi Y, Akazawa Y, Kodama K. Acute coronary syndrome: insight from angioscopy. Circ J. 2010;74:411-417.

[6] Ueda Y, Ohtani T, Shimizu M, Hirayama A, Kodama K. Assessment of plaque vulnerability by angioscopic classification of plaque color. Am Heart J. 2004;148:333-335.

[7] Kubo T, Imanishi T, Takarada S, Kuroi A, Ueno S, Yamano T, Tanimoto T, Matsuo Y, Masho T, Kitabata H, Tanaka A, Nakamura N, Mizukoshi M, Tomobuchi Y, Akasaka T. Implication of plaque color classification for assessing plaque vulnerability: a coronary angioscopy and optical coherence tomography investigation. JACC Cardiovasc Interv. 2008;1:74-80.

[8] Ohtani T, Ueda Y, Mizote I, Oyabu J, Okada K, Hirayama A, Kodama K. Number of yellow plaques detected in a coronary artery is associated with future risk of acute coronary syndrome: detection of vulnerable patients by angioscopy. J Am Coll Cardiol. 2006;47:2194-2200.

[9] Asakura M, Ueda Y, Yamaguchi O, Adachi T, Hirayama A, Hori M, Kodama K. Extensive development of vulnerable plaques as a pan-coronary process in patients with myocardial infarction: an angioscopic study. J Am Coll Cardiol. 2001;37:1284-1288.

[10] Ueda Y, Hirayama A, Kodama K. Plaque characterization and atherosclerosis evaluation by coronary angioscopy. Herz. 2003;28:501-504.

[11] Masumura Y, Ueda Y, Matsuo K, Akazawa Y, Nishio M, Hirata A, Kashiwase K, Nemoto T, Kashiyama T, Wada M, Muller JE, Kodama K. Frequency and location of yellow and disrupted coronary plaques in patients as detected by angioscopy. Circ J. 2011;75:603-612.

[12] Muller JE, Tofler GH, Stone PH. Circadian variation and triggers of onset of acute cardiovascular disease. Circulation 1989;79;733-743.

[13] Matsuo K, Ueda Y, Nishio M, Hirata A, Asai M, Nemoto T, Kashiwase K, Kodama K. Thrombogenic potential of whole blood is higher in patients with acute coronary

syndrome than in patients with stable coronary diseases. Thromb Res. 2011, in press.
[14] Ueda Y, Nanto S, Komamura K, Kodama K. Neointimal coverage of stents in human coronary arteries observed by angioscopy. J Am Coll Cardiol. 1994;23:341-346.
[15] Asakura M, Ueda Y, Nanto S, Hirayama A, Adachi T, Kitakaze M, Hori M, Kodama K. Remodeling of in-stent neointima, which became thinner and transparent over 3 years: serial angiographic and angioscopic follow-up. Circulation. 1998;97:2003-206.
[16] Oyabu J, Ueda Y, Ogasawara N, Okada K, Hirayama A, Kodama K. Angioscopic evaluation of neointima coverage: sirolimus drug-eluting stent versus bare metal stent. Am Heart J 2006;152:1168-1174.
[17] Higo T, Ueda Y, Oyabu J, Okada K, Nishio M, Hirata A, Kashiwase K, Ogasawara N, Hirotani S, Kodama K. Atherosclerotic and thrombogenic neointima formed over sirolimus drug-eluting stent: an angioscopic study. JACC Cardiovasc Imaging. 2009;2:616-624.
[18] Nakazawa G, Otsuka F, Nakano M, Vorpahl M, Yazdani SK, Ladich E, Kolodgie FD, Finn AV, Virmani R. The pathology of neoatherosclerosis in human coronary implants bare-metal and drug-eluting stents. J Am Coll Cardiol. 2011;57:1314-1322.
[19] Higo T, Ueda Y, Matsuo K, Nishio M, Hirata A, Asai M, Nemoto T, Murakami A, Kashiwase K, Kodama K. Risk of in-stent thrombus formation at one year after drug-eluting stent implantation. Thromb Res. 2011, in press.
[20] Hirayama A, Saito S, Ueda Y, Takayama T, Honye J, Komatsu S, Yamaguchi O, Li Y, Yajima J, Nanto S, Takazawa K, Kodama K. Qualitative and quantitative changes in coronary plaque associated with atorvastatin therapy. Circ J. 2009;73:718-725.
[21] Kodama K, Komatsu S, Ueda Y, Takayama T, Yajima J, Nanto S, Matsuoka H, Saito S, Hirayama A. Stabilization and regression of coronary plaques treated with pitavastatin proven by angioscopy and intravascular ultrasound--the TOGETHAR trial. Circ J. 2010;74:1922-1928.
[22] Stone GW, Maehara A, Lansky AJ, de Bruyne B, Cristea E, Mintz GS, Mehran R, McPherson J, Farhat N, Marso SP, Parise H, Templin B, White R, Zhang Z, Serruys PW; PROSPECT Investigators. A prospective natural-history study of coronary atherosclerosis. N Engl J Med. 2011;364:226-35.
[23] Okada K, Ueda Y, Matsuo K, Nishio M, Hirata A, Kashiwase K, Asai M, Nemoto T, Kodama K. Frequency and Healing of Nonculprit Coronary Artery Plaque Disruptions in Patients With Acute Myocardial Infarction. Am J Cardiol. 2011;107:1426-1429.